DATE DUE

Examination of the Shoulder

The Complete Guide

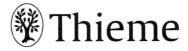

Examination of the Shoulder
The Complete Guide

Edward G. McFarland, M.D.
Vice Chairman
Department of Orthopaedic Surgery
Professor
Division of Sports Medicine and Shoulder Surgery
The Johns Hopkins University School of Medicine
Baltimore, Maryland

Editors

Tae Kyun Kim, M.D., Ph.D.
Assistant Professor
Department of Orthopaedic Surgery
Seoul National University
Bundang Hospital
Seoul, Korea

Hyung Bin Park M.D., Ph.D.
Assistant Professor
Department of Orthopaedic Surgery
College of Medicine
Gyeong Sang National University
Chinju, South Korea

George El Rassi M.D., Ph.D.
Consultant
Department of Orthopaedic Surgery
Saint George University Medical Center
Beirut, Lebanon

Harpreet Gill M.D., Ph.D.
Consultant
Department of Orthopaedics
Government Medical College
Rajindra Hospital
Patiala, India

Ekavit Keyurapan, M.D.
Clinical Instructor
Department of Orthopaedic Surgery
Mahidol University
Siriraj Hospital
Bangkok, Thailand

The author and publisher would like to thank the following company for their kind support of this book:

DePuy Mitek
Raynham, Massachusetts

Thieme Medical Publishers, Inc.
333 Seventh Ave.
New York, NY 10001

Editor: Esther Gumpert
Vice President, Production and Electronic Publishing: Anne T. Vinnicombe
Production Editor: Print Matters, Inc.
Sales Manager: Ross Lumpkin
Chief Financial Officer: Peter van Woerden
President: Brian D. Scanlan
Compositor: Compset
Printer: Maple-Vail

Library of Congress Cataloging-in-Publication Data

McFarland, Edward G.
Examination of the shoulder: the complete guide/Edward G. McFarland; editors, Tae Kyun Kim . . . [et al.].
    p.; cm.
    Includes bibliographical references and index.
    ISBN 1-58890-371-0 (US)—ISBN 3-13-141091-4 (GTV)
      1. Shoulder joint—Diseases—Diagnosis.   2. Shoulder joint—Wounds and injuries—Diagnosis.   3. Physical diagnosis.   4. Musculoskeletal system—Diseases—Diagnosis.
      [DNLM: 1. Shoulder.   2. Orthopedics—methods.   3. Physical Examination—methods.   WE 810 M478e 2005]   I. Kim, Tae Kyun.   II. Title.
    RD557.M33 2005
    617.5'72'075—dc22   2005050646

Important note: Medical knowledge is ever-changing. As new research and clinical experience broaden our knowledge, changes in treatment and drug therapy may be required. The authors and editors of the material herein have consulted sources believed to be reliable in their efforts to provide information that is complete and in accord with the standards accepted at the time of publication. However, in view of the possibility of human error by the authors, editors, or publisher of the work herein or changes in medical knowledge, neither the authors, editors, or publisher, nor any other party who has been involved in the preparation of this work, warrants that the information contained herein is in every respect accurate or complete, and they are not responsible for any errors or omissions or for the results obtained from use of such information. Readers are encouraged to confirm the information contained herein with other sources. For example, readers are advised to check the product information sheet included in the package of each drug they plan to administer to be certain that the information contained in this publication is accurate and that changes have not been made in the recommended dose or in the contraindications for administration. This recommendation is of particular importance in connection with new or infrequently used drugs.

Some of the product names, patents, and registered designs referred to in this book are in fact registered trademarks or proprietary names even though specific reference to this fact is not always made in the text. Therefore, the appearance of a name without designation as proprietary is not to be construed as a representation by the publisher that it is in the public domain.

Printed in the United States of America

5 4 3 2 1

TMP ISBN 1-58890-371-0
GTV ISBN 3-13-141091-4

To my wife, Michele, and my daughters, Julianne, Lily, and Isabel

Contents

Preface ix

Acknowledgments xiii

Foreword by Dr. Frank Jobe xv

Contributors xvii

Chapter 1   General Principles of Shoulder Examination 1

Chapter 2   Shoulder Range of Motion 15

Chapter 3   Strength Testing 88

Chapter 4   Rotator Cuff Disease and Impingement 126

Chapter 5   Instability and Laxity 162

Chapter 6   Examination of the Biceps Tendon and Superior
             Labrum Anteriorand Posterior (SLAP) Lesions 213

Chapter 7   The Acromioclavicular and Sternoclavicular Joints 244

Appendix: Statistical Terms and Analysis 258

Index 262

Preface

This book aims to do two things. First, it is meant to be a complete handbook of examination of the shoulder that can be used by any person who will be examining shoulders. Any person of any level of medical training should be able to look at any of these examination methods and be able to use them clinically. A DVD is provided demonstrating how to perform the examinations and it includes examples of abnormal examinations. Although many of the tests are readily available in other available texts, many physical examination signs have historical significance or may have been described in other countries. It is hoped that this book will be an exhaustive review of these signs, but it is possible that some may have slipped through the cracks of our literature review. Signs that have not been described in the mainstream literature may have been omitted, but we feel that the list here is fairly complete.

The second goal of this book is to evaluate critically how we examine shoulders so that we can improve our examination of this joint. The goal is for the person examining the shoulder to understand that some tests used and reported in the literature are useful and some are not. It is our belief that one reason the examination of the shoulder is difficult is that other texts have not provided any evidence on whether the tests are good or not. This book will attempt to evaluate the examination tests and will discuss their usefulness for the clinician. This goal will be accomplished by reviewing the literature available on each test to determine the exact clinical usefulness and accuracy of the test.

This book will also introduce a few new concepts of shoulder examination based on this review of the literature, discussions with colleagues, and our personal observations. Some of these concepts are new and will be noted as such. Although we believe these signs should stand the test of scientific analysis, we do think that they should be evaluated with respect to their use in the clinical situation.

For example, the use of laxity testing has a role in determining the degree of translation of the shoulder with certain motions. The use of laxity testing does have an influence on how we classify shoulder instability, and a schema using this new knowledge will be presented in this book. However, the goal is to make the shoulder examination clearer and more accessible to both the novice and the experienced clinician who evaluate shoulders.

This book has as its hypothesis that the physical examination of the shoulder is difficult for several reasons (**Table P-1**). First, the shoulder glenohumeral joint is covered by muscle, and it is difficult to put one's fingers on specific structures. Because many physicians learned the knee examination first, many seem to think that the shoulder is like the knee.

TABLE P–1 Factors That Make the Shoulder Examination Difficult

Structures are difficult to palpate and covered by muscle.
A click is nonspecific for any one diagnosis.
Pain patterns are not specific.
Pain from one condition can present in variable ways.
More than one condition can exist at the same time.
Some pathologies in the shoulder are normal, age-related changes.
Not all pathologies in the shoulder may be symptomatic.
Two conditions may coexist but not be causally related.
Knowledge of the normal shoulder structure and function is incomplete and continues to evolve.
Knowledge of pathological processes affecting the shoulder are incomplete and continue to evolve.
The best treatments for some conditions are unknown and continue to evolve.

Consequently, physicians have mistakenly believed that a click in the shoulder means there is a labrum tear, just like a click in the knee often means there is a meniscal tear. It is now known that the labrum does not behave much like a meniscus clinically, and that bucket handle or flap tears of the labrum that can get caught in the joint are quite rare. This misconception has spawned a series of physical examination signs for torn labrums incorrectly based on the presence of a click in the shoulder. This book will critically examine that idea and show that although a click may make one suspicious of a labrum tear, it does not reliably make the diagnosis.

Second, the shoulder has a variety of pain distributions that are not specific. In the knee, pain along the anteromedial joint line typically is due to a meniscal tear or degenerative changes of the medial joint. There are several other entities that can cause medial knee pain, including arthritis of the hip, but these can be ruled out with a careful history and examination. Pain in the shoulder complex seems to defy easy definition, so that pain in the anterior shoulder, for example, can be due to a long list of pathologies.

Part of the difficulty in diagnosing pain in the shoulder is that the pain distributions of these different pathological processes often overlap and are often variable in their presentation. Patients with shoulder problems often will have pain in one place one day and pain in another place on another day. Although the deficiency may be our lack of knowledge about which pathological entities cause pain to be referred to certain spots, the reality seems to be that shoulder problems can be variable in their presentation and symptoms. This vague nature of the shoulder examination was best summed up by one of our residents when he commented, "The shoulder is not like the knee—it's more like the back." When examining the shoulder, we sometimes expect things to be more definitive than nature can deliver.

The third difficulty with the shoulder examination is that the shoulder can often have more than one clinical syndrome present at the same time. This leads to overlapping and variable symptoms, which can make an accurate diagnosis difficult. Sometimes this obscurity is compounded by the physician's desire to make it easy and to come up with just one diagnosis.

A good example of the challenge presented by more than one concurrent condition is the patient who presented with insidious onset of shoulder pain after doing some yard work for the first time in the springtime. The patient had proceeded to protect the shoulder and presented with a painful, stiff shoulder. The first physician assumed it was rotator cuff tendinitis by history and noticed that the patient had positive impingement signs. The patient was instructed in rotator cuff exercises but not stretching exercises. The patient did not get better and subsequently had a magnetic resonance imaging (MRI) evaluation, which demonstrated a partial rotator cuff tear. A cortisone shot into the subacromial space gave the patient no relief. The patient became worried, and surgery was considered based on his physical and MRI findings.

The patient next came to see us for another opinion, and upon closer examination he was found to have a very stiff shoulder with limited elevation and rotation. Also, as is usually the case with a stiff shoulder, the patient had positive signs for rotator cuff tendinitis due to his stiffness. The patient was treated for his stiff shoulder and got his motion back, and his pain went away. The first physician cannot be faulted in his assessment because the signs for impingement are frequently positive in patients with stiff shoulders. Unfortunately, the stiffness was the real problem, and the physical examination signs actually misled the physician into treating only one part of this particular patient's problem.

Likewise, the shoulder often has multiple pathologies present at the time of surgery, which makes an accurate assessment of the cause of the pain difficult. When a patient has two or more pathologic findings at the time of arthroscopic or open surgery, it becomes difficult to know which one is really causing the pain. A good example is the 45-year-old man with a supraspinatus tendon tear and a type II SLAP (superior labrum anterior to posterior) lesion. Which one was causing the pain down the arm? Which one was responsible for the anterior pain radiating into the biceps regions? Which one needs to be surgically corrected? If the patient does not get better with surgery, which pathology was not addressed adequately, and which has healed?

This problem with multiple pathologies present at the same time contributes in part to the lack of knowledge of how pathologic processes in the shoulder cause pain. For example, the pain of rotator cuff disease seems to many of us to be fairly straightforward. The pain is typically in the anterior shoulder and deltoid region. It is made worse with overhead activity. There may be a click or catch with motion or activity. Most people these days would say that the cause of the pain is an impingement of the rotator cuff against the acromion and coracoacromial ligament, as described by Neer and others.[1–5]

Unfortunately, the pain considered typical of rotator cuff disorders also can radiate into the biceps tendon region; thus, is the pain due to the rotator cuff or to biceps pathology? It is equally possible that both entities are causing pain in this region at the same time. If both entities exist together, it is difficult to determine which is causing the problem and which needs to be treated.

Even with something as seemingly straightforward as rotator cuff disease, there is no uniform opinion on where the pain is coming from. Is it the bursa? Is it the cuff itself hitting the acromion? There is evidence that the rotator cuff is underneath the acromion with elevation above 80 degrees, so could the pain be due to the inflamed cuff hitting the superior glenoid and not due to hitting the acromion? Could it be the greater tuberosity that is actually hitting the acromion, which we often see in patients with massive rotator cuff tears? Until the pathologic processes of the shoulder are better understood, the difficulties with the shoulder examination may persist.

Another difficulty with the shoulder is that pathologic conditions can exist and not be symptomatic. It is well known that rotator cuff disease progresses with age.[5–10] It is well known that full-thickness rotator cuff tears can be present and not be painful, including large to massive rotator cuff tears.[7,11–13] It is well known that degenerative joint disease at the acromioclavicular joint increases with age, and in most people it is entirely asymptomatic. Type I SLAP lesions increase with age, but it is unknown if they cause symptoms or not.

Knowledge of normal shoulder anatomy, biomechanics, and function has continued to evolve. The past 20 years have seen a significant increase in our understanding of the shoulder and how it works. The shoulder has been a difficult joint to study, however, because there are so many moving parts. There are many conflicting claims about the normal structure and function of the shoulder, and this evolution of knowledge can help us understand why some tests upon physical examination work and some do not.

Likewise, the knowledge of pathologic processes that affect the shoulder have been increasingly studied, and it is important when examining a shoulder to have an understanding of what conditions can affect the shoulder and in which ways. An understanding of the pathophysiological processes affecting the shoulder is important when trying to decipher the physical examination; unfortunately, we do not have complete knowledge of many disease entities affecting the shoulder.

A good example of the continuing evolution of the concepts of shoulder pathophysiology is the etiology of pain in the shoulder of the overhead athlete. There are many competing theories about what causes shoulder pain in these athletes. This controversy is discussed in several different chapters in this text because the pathophysiology of pain in the overhead athlete challenges every aspect of how we examine a shoulder. Is the pain due to a rotator cuff problem? Is it an instability problem? Is it due to a labrum alone? Does altered range of motion of the shoulder cause these problems? Are all of these pathologies related, or are they coincidental?

Progress in examination and treatment of the shoulder can only be made with careful scientific evaluation. Many people want the shoulder evaluation to be easy, but the reality may be that, although the mechanics of the examination are within the grasp of most individuals, the results of the examination may be difficult to interpret. Dr. Ralph Hertel, a Swiss orthopedic shoulder specialist, once commented that everyone wants shoulder evaluation and treatment to be easy, but "perhaps it is not easy" (personal communication). Although we hope that he is not right, and that the evaluation and treatment of the shoulder should be within the grasp of every health professional, the shoulder is different. The shoulder does not appear to be a joint that one can understand without thought and experience.

Currently, clinical diagnosis and treatment of the shoulder are performed based on a complex mix of past information, examination findings, and operative findings. It may be the reality that the diagnosis of disease entities cannot be made based predictably on one finding alone. It is the goal of this book to evaluate critically the shoulder examination, and by doing so we hope to make it more accessible to every health care professional. Sometimes admitting that we do not know allows us to make progress and to further decipher the mysteries of the shoulder.

REFERENCES

1. Neer CS II. Anterior acromioplasty for the chronic impingement syndrome in the shoulder: a preliminary report. J Bone Joint Surg Am 1972;54(1):41–50
2. Bigliani LU, et al. The relationship of acromial architecture to rotator cuff disease. Clin Sports Med 1991;10(4):823–838
3. Hawkins RJ, Hobeika PE. Impingement syndrome in the athletic shoulder. Clin Sports Med 1983;2(2):391–405
4. Flatow EL, et al. Excursion of the rotator cuff under the acromion: patterns of subacromial contact. Am J Sports Med 1994;22(6):779–788
5. Ogata S, Uhthoff HK. Acromial enthesopathy and rotator cuff tear: a radiologic and histologic postmortem investigation of the coracoacromial arch. Clin Orthop 1990;254:39–48
6. Norwood LA, Barrack R, Jacobson KE. Clinical presentation of complete tears of the rotator cuff. J Bone Joint Surg Am 1989;71(4):499–505
7. Milgrom C, et al. Rotator-cuff changes in asymptomatic adults: the effect of age, hand dominance and gender. J Bone Joint Surg Br 1995;77(2):296–298
8. Gill TJ, et al. The relative importance of acromial morphology and age with respect to rotator cuff pathology. J Shoulder Elbow Surg 2002;11(4):327–330
9. Lehman C, et al. The incidence of full thickness rotator cuff tears in a large cadaveric population. Bull Hosp Jt Dis 1995;54(1):30–31
10. Cofield RH, et al. Surgical repair of chronic rotator cuff tears: a prospective long-term study. J Bone Joint Surg Am 2001;83-A(1):71–77
11. Tempelhof S, Rupp S, Seil R. Age-related prevalence of rotator cuff tears in asymptomatic shoulders. J Shoulder Elbow Surg 1999;8(4):296–299
12. Worland RL, et al. Correlation of age, acromial morphology, and rotator cuff tear pathology diagnosed by ultrasound in asymptomatic patients. J South Orthop Assoc 2003;12(1):23–26
13. Sher JS, et al. Abnormal findings on magnetic resonance images of asymptomatic shoulders. J Bone Joint Surg Am 1995;77(1):10–15

Acknowledgments

This book is dedicated to my wife, Michele, for her love and loyalty despite my schedule and habits, and for the sense of wonder, she brings to each day. To my daughters, Julianne, Lily, and Isabel, that the may grow to be good people and humble scientists who are proud of their father. To my parents, Patience and Julian McFarland, for their guidance and support, and to my brothers, Andy, Paul, Doug, and Stephen, who I love deeply and for whom I have the deepest respect. To my surrogate parents during college, Sam and Freda Finch, and their son Dan, for their love and support all these years.

To the people who mentored me along the way, who inspired me and guided me in a medical career—Dan Haley, Dr. Hal Houston, Dr. Lowell Katz, Dr. Bernie Morrey, Dr. Frank Jobe, and especially to the memory of Dr. Richard Stauffer, who gave me a chance for which I am forever grateful. This book is for all the students, residents, and fellows who keep me young and ask the questions that remind us how much we do not really know. There are untold numbers of students and residents who have worked with me and have contributed to the database or various projects that are now portions of this book, and they deserve credit for working hard on a daily basis and for conscientiously "loading the truck."

There are many clinical fellows who assisted with the preoperative assessments and generally worked hard for my patients and for me, and I never thanked them enough. These individuals include Barry Hyman, Andy Cosgarea, Mike Wang, Greg Holt, Phil Volk, Mark Perazous, Brian Torpey, Mike McGee, Owen O'Neil, Adrian Medina, Thomas Cervoni, John Yap, Christine Morganti, Paul Sherbondy, Richard Savino, Anita Rao, Alex Bertot, Dave Anderson, and Sam Hu.

I must also thank my research fellows over the years, who have been some of my closest friends and who cheerfully spent a year or two here, and to whom I am deeply indebted for being friends and for reminding me of how small the world has become. These research fellows include Carlos Niera, Cheng Yen Hsu, Jin Sub Kim, Pornthep Mamanee, Carlos Caicedo, Prachan Banchasuek, Tae Kyun Kim, Efstathios Chronopoulos, Hyung Bin Park, Yakota Atshushi, Sung-Kai Lin, Harpreet Gill, George El Rassi, Harpal Selhi, and Ekavit Keyurapan. Special recognition goes to Ekavit Keyurapan for his Herculean effort to answer all the author queries and to get this book to press.

Dr. T. K. Kim has been one of my best friends and an inspiration to me. Without his presence, the world would have been a different place for me, and when I think of him there is the peace of our day at BooSeokSa. Everyone should have a friend and mentor like him once in their lives.

My secretaries, Carie Johnson and Brandy Vinson, contributed in a million wonderful ways with only minimal griping and deserve extra credit for keeping the place together. I am grateful to my coeditors and contributing authors, who did most of the work finalizing these chapters and providing needed consultation.

Lastly, I extend my heartfelt gratitude to the patients who chose me to be their physician and allowed me to be involved in their care, and who trusted God to do the rest.

Foreword

A painful shoulder can have a bewildering array of potential diagnoses. The shoulder is a particularly difficult complex system, consisting as it does of four distinct joints and 21 separate muscles. The examiner must sort the presenting complaints into a coherent diagnostic whole before selecting a comprehensive treatment program. Dr. Edward McFarland's text is a clear and thorough explication of all the salient points necessary in a shoulder examination.

There are a number of clinical groups who will find this book essential to their education. First, there are those who are still in training and acquiring the skills necessary to perform a satisfactory examination. These students, whether they are medical, orthopaedic, rehabilitative or kinesiologic, will find the clear illustrations, succinct text and complete instructions an unparalleled help in their studies.

Next, for those recently out in practice, seeing patients in a variety of ailment categories, Dr. McFarland's is a compact *reference* in the examination room for a quick review or recollection of the difference between the diagnostic criteria for a SLAP lesion vs. a rotator cuff problem vs. a traction injury of one of the girdle muscles.

Finally, continuing education is one of the hallmarks of our strong and illustrious profession. Physicians who are well established in their practice can learn from this compendium how to do all of the more recent, more sophisticated clinical examination tests. Expanding our investigative armamentarium allows us to be that much more precise in our shoulder diagnoses. We have come a long way in recent years in understanding not only how the shoulder works but also how and what to do to return it to optimal function in the face of increasing demands.

I can think of no stronger foundation for the delivery of efficient and effective care than a good examination. The bedrock of our understanding is the information gleaned from listening to the patient's history and by performing a good clinical examination. Radiographical and laboratory tests are secondary. If you have a thorough clinical examination of the sort outlined by Dr. McFarland, these other test modalities can be used as a confirmation, not an explanation of the problem.

Frank W. Jobe, M.D.

Contributors

Edward G. McFarland, M.D.
Vice Chairman
Department of Orthopaedic Surgery
Professor
Division of Sports Medicine
  and Shoulder Surgery
The Johns Hopkins University School of
  Medicine
Baltimore, Maryland

EDITORS

Tae Kyun Kim, M.D., Ph.D.
Assistant Professor
Department of Orthopaedic
  Surgery
Seoul National University
Bundang Hospital
Seoul, South Korea

Hyung Bin Park, M.D., Ph.D.
Assistant Professor
Department of Orthopaedic Surgery
College of Medicine
Gyeong Sang National University
Chinju, South Korea

George El Rassi, M.D., Ph.D.
Consultant
Department of Orthopaedic
  Surgery
Saint George University Medical Center
Beirut, Lebanon

Harpreet S. Gill, M.D., Ph.D.
Consultant
Department of Orthopaedic Surgery,
SPS Apollo Hospitals
Ludhiana, India

Ekavit Keyurapan, M.D.
Clinical Instructor
Department of Orthopaedic Surgery
Siriraj Hospital
Mahidol University
Bangkok, Thailand

CONTRIBUTORS

Richard Blalock
Undergraduate Student
Murray State University
Murray, Kentucky

Renan C. Castillo, B.A.
Assistant Scientist
Center for Injury Research and Policy
Department of Health Policy
  and Management
Bloomberg School of Public Health
The Johns Hopkins University
Baltimore, Maryland

Efstathios Chronopoulos, M.D.
Lecturer, Department of Orthopaedic Surgery
Athens University Hospital Agia Olga
Athens, Greece

Constantine A. Demetracopoulos, B.S.
Medical Student
The Johns Hopkins University School of Medicine
Baltimore, Maryland

Adam Farber, M.D.
Resident
Department of Orthopaedic Surgery
The Johns Hopkins University School of Medicine
Baltimore, Maryland

Nirav S. Kapadia, B.A.
Medical Student
The Johns Hopkins University School of Medicine
Baltimore, Maryland

Brian Krabak, M.D.
Assistant Professor, Physical Medicine and
    Rehabilitation
Assistant Professor, Orthopaedic Surgery
The Johns Hopkins University School of Medicine
Baltimore, Maryland

George Murrell, M.B.B.S., D.Phil.
Director
Orthopaedic Research Institute
Conjoint Associate Professor
University of New South Wales

Chief
Sports Medicine and Shoulder Service
The St. George Hospital
Kogarah, Australia

William Romani, Ph.D., M.H.A., P.T.
Assistant Professor, Physical Therapy
University of Maryland School of Medicine
Baltimore, Maryland

Eric L. Sauers, Ph.D., A.T.C.
Chairman
Department of Sports Health Care
Arizona School of Health Sciences
A. T. Still University
Phoenix, Arizona

Harpal Singh Selhi, M.B.B.S., M.S.
Assistant Professor
Department of Orthopaedic Surgery,
Dayanand Medical College and Hospital
Ludhiana, Punjab, India

Atsushi Yokota, M.D., Ph.D.
Department of Orthopaedic Surgery
Osaka Medical College
Osaka, Japan

1

General Principles of Shoulder Examination

Making an accurate diagnosis of shoulder conditions requires a consideration of the patient's history, a physical examination, and sometimes imaging studies. This chapter will discuss what we consider important principles when examining the shoulder complex. In some cases it may not be necessary to fulfill all the components of the "ideal" examination, but a thorough history and physical examination are particularly helpful when evaluating a patient with shoulder and upper extremity complaints. This chapter will also delineate some of the findings that can be discovered simply by observation of the patient.

There are several important aspects of the history that should be established in each patient (**Table 1–1**). The dominance of the extremity can have significant implications for treatment. Many patients will live with a disability in the nondominant extremity that would be unacceptable in their dominant shoulder. A good example is the professional baseball player who has a traumatic shoulder instability in his nondominant arm that does not affect his performance; if the instability was in the player's dominant extremity, then surgery would more likely be necessary. It is often helpful to have patients fill out a standardized history form to obtain information about their symptoms (**Fig. 1–1**).

The etiology of the onset of the problem is particularly important, specifically whether it was insidious or if there was a history of trauma. If the patient had no trauma, it is important to find out if he or she had tried any new activities in the days preceding the onset of pain. New activities often will initiate a rotator cuff tendinitis but also can aggravate a preexisting arthritis of the shoulder. A history of a "pop" followed by ecchymosis suggests a tendon tear, such as the long head of the biceps tendon or the pectoralis major tendon.

The severity of the symptoms at onset is important. If the pain begins insidiously and is not very severe at the

TABLE 1–1 Examination History of the Shoulder*

| General Information | Medical Information | Shoulder Complaints | | | |
		Symptoms	Injury Pattern	Symptom Characteristics	Related Symptoms
Age	Chronic or acute problem	Pain	Sudden versus acute onset	Location	Cervical
Dominant arm	Review of systems	Weakness or fatigue	Gradual versus chronic onset	Character and severity	Peripheral nerve
Participation in sports	Preexisting or recurrent shoulder problem	Instability/subluxation	Traumatic onset	Provocation	Brachial plexus
Level of competition	Other musculoskeletal problems	Stiffness	Recurrent pattern	Duration	Entrapment
		Catching/locking		Paresthesias/ referral pattern	
				Effect on sport/other disability	

*Source: Adapted with permission from Ellenbecker T. Clinical Examination of the Shoulder, Vol. 1. New York: Elsevier Science; 2004.

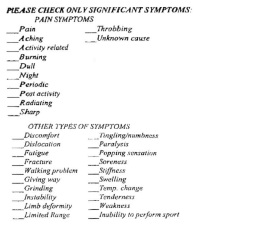

PLEASE CHECK ONLY SIGNIFICANT SYMPTOMS:

PAIN SYMPTOMS

___Pain	___Throbbing
___Aching	___Unknown cause
___Activity related	
___Burning	
___Dull	
___Night	
___Periodic	
___Post activity	
___Radiating	
___Sharp	

OTHER TYPES OF SYMPTOMS

___Discomfort	___Tingling/numbness
___Dislocation	___Paralysis
___Fatigue	___Popping sensation
___Fracture	___Soreness
___Walking problem	___Stiffness
___Giving way	___Swelling
___Grinding	___Temp. change
___Instability	___Tenderness
___Limb deformity	___Weakness
___Limited Range	___Inability to perform sport

FIGURE 1–1 Figure of standardized symptom checklist used in the office to help establish the nature and quality of the patient's complaints.

onset, then certain diagnoses may be considered over others. A sudden onset of severe pain without trauma could be brachial neuritis, a pinched cervical nerve, shingles, acute calcific tendinitis, a pathological fracture, or acute frozen shoulder. Slower onset of pain is typical of rotator cuff tendinitis, idiopathic frozen shoulder, cancer, and a multitude of other etiologies. If there is an acute event, the signs of a more serious injury include the inability to continue the activity or sport. Pain that makes a patient nauseous typically reflects a more severe problem.

Weakness of the shoulder or upper extremity is considered a neurologic complaint until proven otherwise. Weakness can be due to intrinsic shoulder problems, but it is imperative that the practitioner be considering other possible etiologies or combinations of etiologies causing the weakness. We have had several patients present to us who had seen physicians and given a diagnosis of rotator cuff dysfunction but who had weakness of the shoulder as a primary complaint. Both had no history of trauma, and both had a history of painless weakness. One example was a young woman in her 20s with arm weakness who had a cervical spine tumor. Another example was a more mature patient in his 60s who presented with similar insidious onset of weakness and who had Lou Gehrig's disease (amyotrophic lateral sclerosis). Weakness secondary to pain is common, but a complete upper extremity neurologic evaluation is recommended to make sure there is not a neurologic etiology.

Parasthesias have a neurologic etiology in most cases, and the patient should be asked about the distribution, duration, and severity of the sensory changes. Shoulder problems do not intrinsically cause parasthesias in most instances, and another source of the abnormal sensations should be pursued. Intrinsic shoulder problems that cause parasthesias include nerve entrapments in throwing athletes or workers.[1]

If the patient complains of pain, the distribution of the pain is important. Patients with acromioclavicular (AC) joint pain will typically (but not always) point right at the AC joint, whereas rotator cuff pain tends to be more global or into the deltoid. Gerber et al injected saline into the AC joint of volunteers, and the pain distribution was at the AC joint, with radiation into the trapezius.[2] Injection of saline into the subacromial space produced classic rotator cuff pain in the deltoid region. In some individuals with both AC arthritis and rotator cuff tendinitis, the pain may be present in both areas (**Fig. 1–2**). Inflammation and stiffness of the shoulder can both cause the pain to radiate down the arm; however, radiation down the arm to the hand should raise the suspicion of cervical disk disease.

Pain in the medial shoulder blade area is common, and the differential diagnosis includes thoracic outlet syndrome, a lung process, a rib problem, cervical disk disease, and, rarely, degenerative or pathological processes in the thoracic spine (**Fig. 1–3**). Medial shoulder blade pain may be due to incorrect use of the shoulder blade secondary to an intrinsic problem in the shoulder. In this case the patient is using the muscles of the shoulder blade to elevate the shoulder, and the increased or abnormal stress causes muscle fatigue and pain; however, the diagnosis of muscle pain in the medial scapular region should be a diagnosis of exclusion once other conditions have been ruled out.

Chest or rib pain not directly in the shoulder itself should prompt the examiner to inquire about shortness of breath or symptoms of angina. Anginal pain may radiate into the neck and down the arm, and the patient may place his or her hand over the region of the heart as the source of the pain; this is referred to as the "Levine sign" (**Fig. 1–4**).[3] Pain along the chest and medial to the midclavicle may be seen with sternoclavicular problems, but the differential diagnosis for anterior chest wall pain more typically includes thoracic outlet syndrome or cervical disk disease (**Fig. 1–5**). Pain in the axilla or ribs below the shoulder is uncommon, but the differential diagnosis includes a pathological rib process, a pulmonary problem, or thoracic outlet syndrome.

Referred pain to the shoulder from visceral causes has been reported (**Table 1–2**). Although the classic teaching is that gallbladder or liver disease can cause shoulder pain, the pain typically is located near the posterior shoulder blade and not in the shoulder (**Fig. 1–6**). Cardiac disease can cause shoulder and arm pain, and Horne et al have shown that angina pain radiated into the shoulder and arm in 66% of patients experiencing their first case of myocardial infarction.[4]

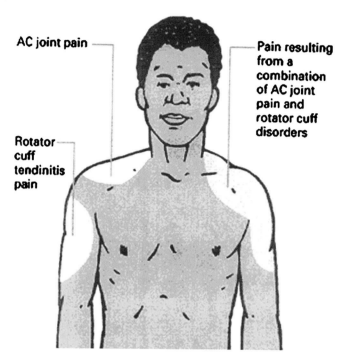

FIGURE 1–2 AC joint pain tends to be on the top of the shoulder and radiates into the trapezius region, whereas subacromial irritation tends to be present in the deltoid and lateral shoulder. (Adapted with permission from McFarland EG, Hobbs WR. The active shoulder: AC joint pain and injury. Your Patient Fitness 1998;12(4):23–27.)

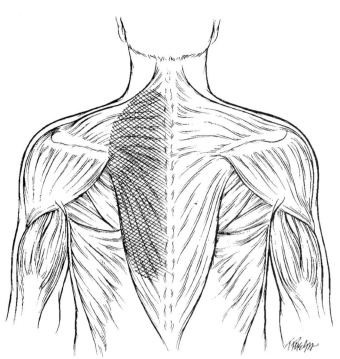

FIGURE 1–3 Drawing of typical location for posterior thorax pain as a result of cervical spine pathologies.

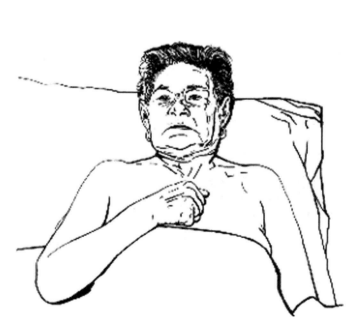

FIGURE 1–4 The Levine sign was described as a clenched fist over the chest and was felt to be indicative of angina. (Adapted with permission from Edmondstone WM. Cardiac chest pain: does body language help the diagnosis? BMJ 1995;311(7021):1660–1661.)

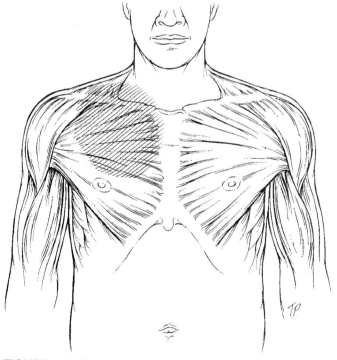

FIGURE 1–5 Pain along the anterior chest wall and medial to the clavicle is typically due to cervical spine (cervical level 4) pathology or due to thoracic outlet problems.

TABLE 1–2 Referred Shoulder Pain*

Right Shoulder		Left Shoulder	
Systemic Origin	**Location**	**Systemic Origin**	**Location**
Peptic ulcer	Lateral border, right scapula	Ruptured spleen	Left shoulder (Kehr's sign)
Myocardial ischemia	Right shoulder, down arm	Myocardial ischemia	Left pectoral/left shoulder
Hepatic/biliary acute cholecystitis	Right shoulder; between scapulae; right scapula area	Pancreas	Left shoulder
Liver abscess	Right shoulder	Ectopic pregnancy (rupture)	Left shoulder (Kehr's sign)
Gallbladder	Right upper trapezius		
Liver disease (hepatitis, cirrhosis, metastatic tumors)	Right shoulder, right subscapula		
Pulmonary: Pleurisy Pneumothorax Pancoast's tumor	Ipsilateral shoulder; upper trapezius	Pulmonary: Pleurisy Pneumothorax Pancoast's tumor	Ipsilateral shoulder; upper trapezius
Kidney	Ipsilateral shoulder	Kidney	Ipsilateral shoulder
		Postoperative laparoscopy	Left shoulder (Kehr's sign)

*Source: Adapted with permission from Ellenbecker T. Clinical Examination of the Shoulder, Vol. 1. New York: Elsevier Science; 2004.

Pain in multiple areas, particularly when not associated with any specific pattern, can be due to a severely inflamed shoulder. Included in the differential diagnosis of diffuse pain should be connective tissue disorders such as polymyositis, Lyme disease, medication myalgias, and fibromyalgia.

What makes the pain worse can be helpful in determining the diagnosis, but this is not diagnostic for any one entity (**Table 1–3**). Pain at night is a worrisome sign, especially if it occurs without the patient rolling over or lying on the shoulder. Progressive pain is also a red flag, especially if it continues to increase despite treatment. Pain that progresses to the need for narcotics suggests that there may be a more serious etiology of the pain.[5]

Which motions aggravate the pain can be of some assistance in making the diagnosis. Pain over shoulder level, especially into the deltoid or down the arm, can be indicative of rotator cuff disease, but it also can be seen with stiff shoulders. Patients with rotator cuff disease may have pain with motions behind the back, but patients with a frozen shoulder also may complain of this problem. In our analysis of patients by diagnostic group, we found that patients with rotator cuff had symptoms most often associated with using their back pocket, using their arm at shoulder level, and using their arm overhead. In contrast, patients with SLAP (superior labrum anterior to inferior) lesions showed difficulty performing most activities, regardless of degree of flexion at the shoulder (**Table 1–4**).

What makes the pain better may give some clues to the etiology of the pain, but this information will not typically make the diagnosis. Pain made better with anti-inflammatory agents usually indicates that the pain is not severe. Improvement with ice may indicate an inflammatory condition, but this finding is nonspecific. Improvement with massage may indicate a muscular condition, but this also is not diagnostic.

In patients who have an injury, the exact mechanism of injury can provide clues to the nature of the injury. Though not diagnostic, certain injury mechanisms are frequently associated with one injury type (**Table 1–5**). A fall onto the shoulder can cause fractures, rotator cuff tears, and SLAP lesions. A fall with the arm extended and externally rotated can result in dislocations or tears of the subscapularis tendon.

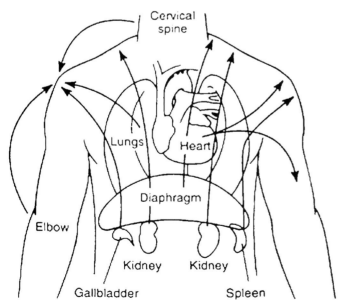

FIGURE 1–6 Visceral pain can be referred to the shoulder region in a variety of nonspecific patterns. (Adapted with permission from Ellenbecker T. Clinical Examination of the Shoulder, Vol. 1. New York: Elsevier Science; 2004.)

TABLE 1-3 Pattern of Shoulder Pain in Varying Shoulder Pathology*

Disease State[†]	N	At Rest[‡] (%)	During Activities[‡] (%)	Difficulty Sleeping at Night[§] (%)	Putting on/Removing Sweater[¶] (%)
Instability	167	14.6	44.5	44.3	10.5
Impingement	74	21.2	56.8	74.3	23.3
Osteoarthritis	80	53.2	82.3	82.5	57.9
AC joint	64	30.7	65.6	79.3	24.6
RCT	331	28.9	63.1	72.2	33.8
SLAP lesion	17	18.8	76.5	64.7	23.5

*Source: Data from The Johns Hopkins University shoulder database (unpublished data).

[†]Instability: anterior instability, anterior traumatic instability, multidirectional instability, occult instability, posterior instability. Impingement: external impingement. Osteoarthritis: glenohumeral osteoarthritis. AC joint: acromioclavicular joint arthritis, separation, osteolysis. RCT: rotator cuff tendinitis, partial tear, full tear. SLAP: superior labrum anterior to posterior.

[‡]Percentage of patients self-reporting severe or greater on a scale evaluating the quality of their pain.

[§]Percentage of patients self-reporting several days per week or more of difficulty sleeping at night due to pain.

[¶]Percentage of patients self-reporting severe pain or inability.

TABLE 1-4 Difficulty Performing Specific Activities with Varying Shoulder Pathology*

Disease State[†]	N	Activities (%)[‡]							
		Use Back Pocket	Wash Opposite Underarm	Eat with Utensil	Comb Hair	Use Arm at Shoulder Level	Dress	Use Hand Overhead	Carry Weight[§]
Instability	208	18.0	12.5	9.4	18.5	31.7	13.5	55.1	31.0
Impingement	103	42.6	28.2	17.8	39.4	59.2	35.3	78.4	66.0
Osteoarthritis	99	89.4	78.4	38.3	71.0	79.6	66.3	92.9	73.7
AC joint	78	39.7	33.3	17.3	32.5	47.4	36.4	69.3	62.2
RCT	376	39.7	34.0	20.1	39.0	61.2	35.8	77.4	58.1
SLAP lesion	19	47.4	47.4	33.3	44.4	52.6	47.4	73.7	38.9

*Source: Data from The Johns Hopkins University shoulder database (unpublished data).

[†]Instability: anterior instability, anterior traumatic instability, multidirectional instability, occult instability, posterior instability. Impingement: external impingement. Osteoarthritis: glenohumeral osteoarthritis. AC joint: acromioclavicular joint arthritis, separation, osteolysis. RCT: rotator cuff tendinitis, partial tear, full tear. SLAP: superior labrum anterior to posterior.

[‡]Variable for ability to perform activity from shoulder and elbow score; included here are only those who reported difficulty, with assistance, or not at all.

[§]10–15 lb with arm at side using a shoulder and elbow score.

TABLE 1-5 History and Possible Diagnosis

Trauma History	Injury Patterns
Fall on outstretched arm	proximal humerus fracture rotator cuff tear SLAP lesion
Fall onto the shoulder	AC separation rotator cuff tear fracture SLAP lesion
Arm abducted and externally rotated	anterior instability subscapularis tendon tear
Traction injury	SLAP lesion
Fall into hyperabducted arm	luxatio erecta (inferior dislocation)
Falling onto the point	AC lesion of the shoulder with the arm adducted greater tuberosity fracture
No trauma history	
Insidious onset of pain	degenerative joint disease tendinitis frozen shoulder
Insidious onset of severe pain	brachial neuritis shingles
Night pain	tumor
Weakness without pain	nerve injury muscle disease chronic rotator cuff tear

AC, acromioclavicular; SLAP, superior labrum anterior to posterior

TABLE 1-6 Specific Injuries Associated with Various Sports Activities

Football linemen	• posterior shoulder instability
Overhead athletes	• SLAP lesions • partial cuff tear • "occult" instability
Adolescent baseball pitchers	• proximal humeral apophysitis (Little League shoulder)
Bench press	• pectoralis major tendon tears
Bench presses, dips, push-ups	• osteolysis distal clavicle • AC arthritis
Kayaking	• supraspinatus partial tears
Archery	• anterior shoulder dislocations • posterior shoulder instability
Trapshooting	• coracoid stress fracture
Golf, rowing	• rib stress fractures

AC, acromioclavicular; SLAP, superior labrum anterior to posterior

Certain sports are associated with specific injuries, depending on the mechanism (**Table 1-6**). A tearing sensation that occurs when bench pressing or doing dips or pushups can indicate a tear of the pectoralis major tendon. An axial load on a slightly abducted arm can cause posterior instability. Some axial loads can cause fractures or chondral contusions. Statistical analysis of our patients

TABLE 1–7 Mechanism of Injury Associated with Varying Shoulder Pathology*

			Mechanism of Injury					
Disease State†	N	Insidious (%)	Sports Related (%)	Falling Down (%)	Traffic Accident (%)	Lifting Weights (%)	Work Related (%)	Home Related (%)
Instability	214	21.5	46.1	9.1	4.7	0.4	4.7	1.4
Impingement	108	45.4	12.0	9.3	9.3	4.6	12.0	1.9
Osteoarthritis	117	73.5	5.1	11.1	0.9	0.9	5.1	0.9
AC joint	88	35.2	18.2	9.1	13.6	3.4	15.9	1.1
RCT	392	41.6	10.2	24.0	5.1	3.8	7.4	4.3
SLAP lesion	20	30.0	10.0	20.0	15.0	0.0	15.0	10.0

**Source:* Data from The Johns Hopkins University shoulder database (unpublished data).

†Instability: anterior instability, anterior traumatic instability, multidirectional instability, occult instability, posterior instability. Impingement: external impingement. Osteoarthritis: glenohumeral osteoarthritis. AC joint: acromioclavicular joint arthritis, separation, osteolysis. RCT: rotator cuff tendinitis, partial tear, full tear. SLAP: superior labrum anterior to posterior.

TABLE 1–8 Five Principles of the Musculoskeletal Examination

Undress the patient
Compare both sides of the patient
Consider the joint above and below the patient's complaint
Perform a neurovascular examination
Radiograph the joint in at least two planes

revealed that shoulder instability is most often associated with sports-related injury, whereas rotator cuff tears present more frequently with insidious onset or resulting from a fall (**Table 1–7**).

The physical examination of any musculoskeletal body part should be methodical and thorough. The amount of detail required will be dictated by the clinical situation, and the recommendations that follow are meant to be guidelines, not absolute requirements in every case. In our estimation there are five principles when performing musculoskeletal examination that are particularly important in the shoulder (**Table 1–8**).

The first principle is to undress the patient. The topical anatomy is known to most examiners, and the examiner should evaluate the patient from the front and from the back (**Figs. 1–7** and **1–8**). Ecchymosis, atrophy, and deformity provide important clues to the diagnosis. For males, we recommend removing the shirt. For females, special gowns may be purchased or constructed (**Figs. 1–9** and **1–10**), or conventional gowns may be tied around the back (**Fig. 1–11**). When possible we recommend that women consider wearing athletic bras for their examination, but gowns are useful to help make the patient comfortable and relaxed (**Fig. 1–12**).

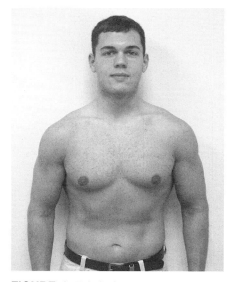

FIGURE 1–7 It is important to undress the patient to be able to evaluate the anterior musculature and symmetry of the patient.

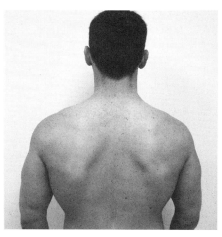

FIGURE 1–8 For males, the posterior thorax and shoulders can be observed with the shirt removed.

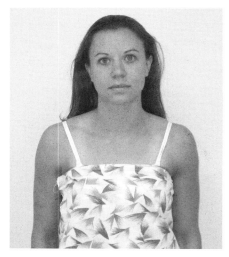

FIGURE 1–9 For females, it is helpful to use some sort of gown that will allow visualization of the entire shoulder.

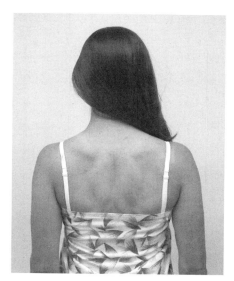

FIGURE 1–10 A gown with secure straps will make the patient more comfortable during the examination.

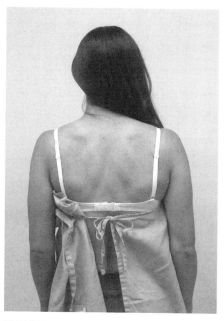

FIGURE 1–11 A conventional gown can be used in patients when there are no other alternatives.

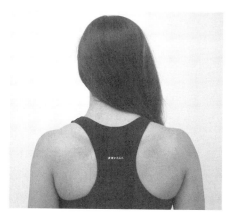

FIGURE 1–12 If possible, female patients can wear a sports bra during the examination.

A history of medical conditions should be acquired in every patient, and we recommend a generalized history sheet for screening new patients. Patients should be queried about a history of cancer. Medical questions that may have more relevance for the shoulder include a history of oral steroid use (which can cause avascular necrosis), systemic arthritis (rheumatoid, lupus erythematosus, etc.), Crohn's disease, ulcerative colitis, and psoriasis.

When observing patients from the front, it is important to look for asymmetry, atrophy, or deformity. Congenital absence of the pectoralis muscle is rare but can be detected if the patient is undressed (**Fig. 1–13**).

When observing the back of patients, it is important to look for deformity or atrophy. Congenital abnormalities such as a Sprengel's deformity or a web neck syndrome may be seen incidentally (**Fig. 1–14**).

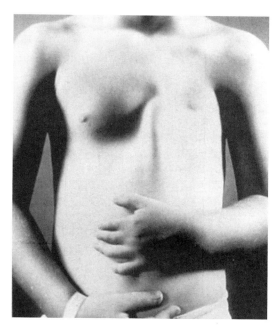

FIGURE 1–13 Congenital absence of the pectoralis muscle is uncommon but results in few functional deficits. (Adapted with permission from Rockwood C, ed. The Shoulder, Vol. 1, 3rd ed. Philadelphia: Saunders; 2004:136.)

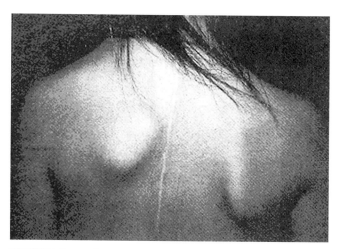

FIGURE 1–14 Sprengel's syndrome or web neck syndrome is a very uncommon abnormality best detected by physical examination.

TABLE 1–9 Muscle Atrophy Associated with Varying Shoulder Pathologies*

| Disease State[†] | N | Muscle Atrophy[‡] | | Deltoid (%) |
		Supraspinatus (%)	Infraspinatus (%)	
Instability	212	8.0	6.2	1.9
RCT	396	13.6	13.6	3.3
Impingement	109	7.3	8.2	3.7
Osteoarthritis	123	29.3	20.3	10.6
AC joint	84	6.0	4.8	0.0

*Source: Data from The Johns Hopkins University shoulder database (unpublished data).

[†]Instability: anterior instability, anterior traumatic instability, multidirectional instability, occult instability, posterior instability. RCT: rotator cuff tendinitis, partial tear, full tear. Impingement: external impingement. Osteoarthritis: glenohumeral osteoarthritis. AC joint: acromioclavicular joint arthritis, separation, osteolysis.

[‡]Percentage of patients with atrophy in each muscle.

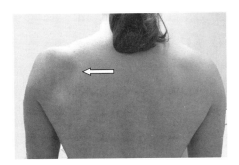

FIGURE 1–15 Infraspinatus muscle atrophy (arrow) can be seen below the scapular spine.

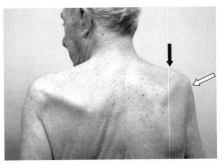

FIGURE 1–16 In this patient, there is infraspinatus atrophy below the spine of the scapula (open arrow) and supraspinatus atrophy above the scapular spine (solid arrow).

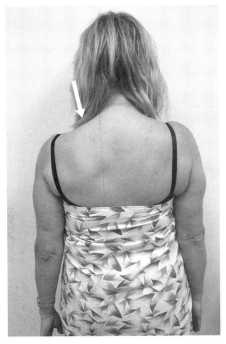

FIGURE 1–17 Trapezius atrophy (arrow) is seen in a patient with a spinal accessory nerve palsy.

It is important to look for isolated atrophy of the infraspinatus muscle (**Fig. 1–15**) or of the supraspinatus and infraspinatus (**Fig. 1–16**). Our studies have shown that 30.5% of rotator cuff tears have atrophy (**Table 1–9**). Trapezius atrophy is rare, but it can be an isolated injury or secondary to lymph node biopsies or radical neck dissections (**Fig. 1–17**). Pectoralis muscle ruptures will present initially with ecchymosis and swelling (**Fig. 1–18**), but after a week to 10 days they will present with a visible defect in the tendon. Proximal tears of the biceps tendon will present with characteristic swelling in the proximal arm with or without ecchymosis (**Fig. 1–19**). Patients on blood thinners may develop a large degree of swelling with trivial injuries or with tears of tendons or muscles around the shoulder.

The second orthopedic principle is to compare both sides. Subtle differences in muscle size can be accentuated by comparing sides. Deltoid atrophy can be especially difficult to detect, and comparison to the other side is helpful. Patients will sometimes inquire as to why their arm is swollen, when in actuality it is the deltoid that is atrophied. We call this atrophy the "scalloped shoulder" because there is a concavity to the shoulder compared with the other side (**Fig. 1–20**). AC joint pathology can be subtle, but an AC separation (**Fig. 1–21**), an AC cyst (**Fig. 1–22**), and AC arthritis (**Fig. 1–23**) can be

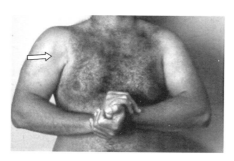

FIGURE 1–18 A deformity due to a pectoralis muscle rupture (arrow) can be seen by having the patient push the hands together in front of the body.

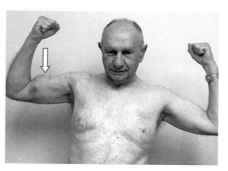

FIGURE 1–19 A tear of the long head of the biceps tendon (arrow) can produce swelling and ecchymosis in the arm.

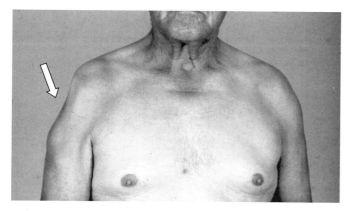

FIGURE 1–20 Deltoid atrophy (arrow) from any etiology can cause a dip or "scalloped shoulder" seen laterally.

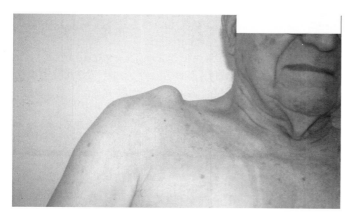

FIGURE 1–21 AC cysts can cause swelling on the top of the shoulder.

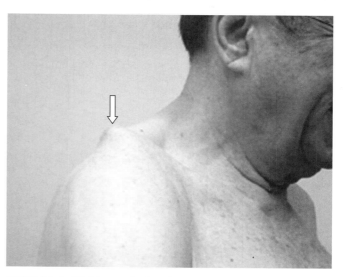

FIGURE 1–22 The typical deformity caused by an acromio-clavicular (AC) separation is seen on the top of the shoulder.

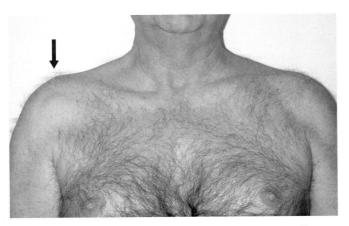

FIGURE 1–23 Arthritis of the AC joint can cause swelling on the top of the shoulder (arrow).

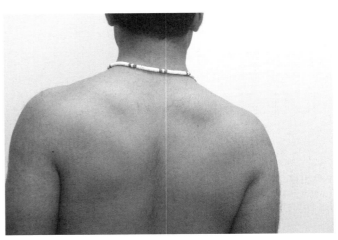

FIGURE 1–24 When viewing the posterior thorax, it is important to look for scapular asymmetry.

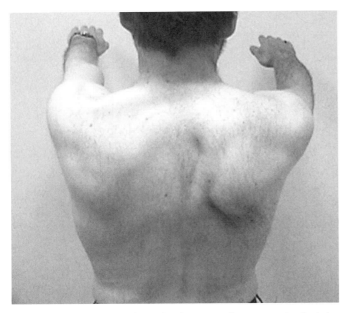

FIGURE 1–25 Scapular winging can be accentuated by having the patient flex his or her arms in front of the body.

accentuated by comparing the deformity to the other side. Atrophy of the arm, forearm, or hand muscles is best detected by side-to-side comparison. The patient should be observed from the back for scapular asymmetry (**Fig. 1–24**) or winging (**Fig. 1–25**).

The third orthopedic principle is to always consider the joint above and below the patient's complaint. For patients with shoulder pain, the joint proximal is the neck. For patients with midhumerus pain, it is the shoulder and neck. The function of the elbow typically can be determined at the time of the shoulder examination.

The fourth orthopedic principle is to do a neurovascular examination as part of the orthopedic evaluation. The examination should be designed so that neurologic or vascular etiologies of the patient's condition can be determined. Range of motion and strength need not be done of every muscle, but selected muscle testing can test each cervical level and peripheral nerve (**Table 1–10**; **Figs. 1–26** through **1–30**). Sensory testing of select areas can provide a simple and quick screen of the upper extremity. This examination can be done so that every dermatome (**Fig. 1–31**) and peripheral nerve (**Fig. 1–32**) can be quickly tested.

Another part of the neurovascular examination is reflex testing, and reflex testing of each cervical spinal

2

Shoulder Range of Motion

Measuring the range of motion of any joint is a basic part of any musculoskeletal evaluation. Although measuring motion is relatively easy for a hinge joint, which has only 1 or 2 degrees of freedom, measuring motion of the shoulder complex presents some unique challenges. These challenges include making a determination of exactly which motions are most clinically important, which components of the shoulder complex are contributing to those motions, and how to measure them. There is increasing appreciation that there is a wide variety of factors that affect shoulder range of motion.

This chapter will discuss traditional methods of measuring shoulder range of motion and critically examine them in light of new biomechanical and clinical knowledge. Advances in the clinical techniques for measuring motion of the shoulder complex will be discussed. In this chapter, new recommendations for measuring shoulder rotations and distinguishing glenohumeral from scapulothoracic motions will be introduced.

■ Nomenclature

A common language regarding shoulder range of motion is important for several reasons. First, accurate measurements of motion is important for making an accurate diagnosis. A stiff shoulder can often simulate rotator cuff tendinitis, or it may aggravate a preexisting rotator cuff condition, and treating the tendinitis alone may not resolve the loss of motion. Second, health care providers need to be able to communicate patient motions to each other reliably and reproducibly. This is important whenever treatment is initiated and specific motion goals are set by the provider. For example, if the surgeon sets a limit of 30 degrees of external rotation as the limit for 4 weeks after a shoulder stabilization, the physical therapist needs to know if that is glenohumeral motion or combined glenohumeral and scapulothoracic motion. Likewise, if a physician thinks that an athlete has lost internal rotation

of the shoulder, the trainer, therapist, and physician should be measuring the same motion.

This system of measurement should allow international communication about motions and comparison of patients. Reproducible measurement of motion is necessary for making the diagnosis and to monitor treatment. Motion of the shoulder complex is an important component of outcome measures, including shoulder scores. Shoulder motion is currently an important part of calculating impairment ratings.[1]

The function of the upper extremity is to position the hand in space, but any measure of hand position will necessarily involve a contribution by the other joints in the upper extremity, including the elbow and wrist. As a result, a standard was needed that all practitioners could use that would have the same reference points and be reproducible. The evolution of the measurement system of the upper extremity motions had its origins in the early 20th century.

The first attempt to provide order to measuring shoulder motion was by Silver in 1923.[2] He proposed a system of zero positions for every joint from which a particular motion would be measured. This was modified by Cave and Roberts in 1936[3] (**Fig. 2–1**), who felt that the best starting position was with the arm at the side with the elbow flexed at 90 degrees. Although they provided a system for measurement of range of motion of the shoulder, they did not provide normative values. The system recommended by Cave and Roberts included exhortations to measure the other extremity for comparison. They also recommended the use of a goniometer and noted that motions of joints above and below the affected joint should be recorded.[3]

In 1958, the American Medical Association (AMA) published "A Guide to the Evaluation of Permanent Impairment of the Extremities and Back." This guide inferred that disability and impairment could be determined by measuring joint motion alone. It provided measures for shoulder range of motion and the disability

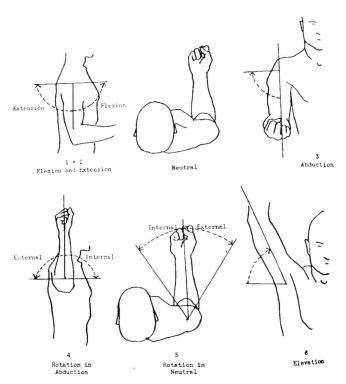

FIGURE 2–1 The zero positions of Cave set the standards still used today. (Adapted with permission from Cave ER, Robert S. A method for measuring and recording joint function. J Bone Joint Surg Am 1936. 18(2):455–465.

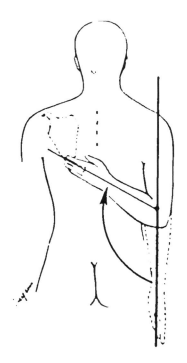

INTERNAL ROTATION POSTERIORLY

FIGURE 2–2 Internal rotation up the back was added by the American Academy of Orthopaedic Surgery as a helpful measurement. (Adapted with permission from the American Academy of Orthopaedic Surgeons. Joint Motion: Method of Measuring and Recording. Chicago: Author; 1965.)

rating for lost motion as a percentage of the extremity (**Table 2–1**).

In 1959, Carter Rowe was appointed by the American Academy of Orthopaedic Surgeons to be the chairman of a committee to study the best way to measure joint motion. The Committee on the Study of Joint Motion published its findings in 1963.[4] The American Academy of Orthopaedic Surgeons (AAOS) adopted the concept of Cave and Roberts[3] for defining a zero position of the joint and published it in pamphlet form in 1965.[5] The recommended system was modified by the AAOS to include internal rotation up the back (**Fig. 2–2**). The AAOS averaged the measures of shoulder motion from four sources (**Table 2–1**), and it should be noted that these values were different from those published by the AMA.

These publications from the AMA[1] and AAOS[5] established the standards for measuring shoulder range of motion utilized for many subsequent generations of clinicians and providers. The important clinical measures were elevation in abduction, elevation in flexion, extension of the arm at the side behind the body, internal and external rotation with the arm at the side, external and internal rotation with the arm at 90 degrees of abduction, and adduction of the arm across the body.[6] The normative values in **Table 2–1** have been the standard since their publication in 1958 and since being accepted by the AAOS in 1964.

It has become increasingly appreciated over time that motion of the upper extremity is a complicated set of

TABLE 2–1 Normal Range of Motion Values for the Shoulder*

Glenohumeral Joint	AMA[1] 1958	AAOS[5] 1965	Boone & Azen[30] 1979	Hoppenfeld [185] 1976
Flexion*	150	180	167	90
Extension*	40	60	62	45
Abduction	150	180	184	180
90° internal rotation†	40	70	69	55
90° external rotation†	90	90	104	45

Source: Adapted with permission from Ellenbecker T. Clinical Examination of the Shoulder, Vol. 1, 1st ed. St. Louis: Elsevier Science; 2004.

*Measurements obtained with the shoulder in 0 degree of abduction.

†Measurements obtained with the arm abducted ninety degrees.

movements by multiple joints, and new knowledge has changed how we think about shoulder motion. As a result, it has become appreciated that there were several problems with the recommended standards promulgated by the AAOS. It should be noted that this system provides a measurement that is the summation of motion of the glenohumeral joint, scapulothoracic joint, and the other joints of the upper extremity. It was not specified whether the patient was to be sitting or supine, nor whether active or passive range of motion was measured. The body references for making the measures were implied by the diagrams, but never really specified. Values for internal and external rotation of the shoulder did not specify if the measures were to be made with the arm in the plane of the body or in the scapular plane.

■ Variables Affecting Range of Motion Measurements

Since the original descriptions, numerous studies have addressed the subject of measuring shoulder range of motion, and there are textbooks devoted to these measurements.[7,8] There are many factors that influence the range of motion measured by health care practitioners. These include the type of measuring device, the complexity of the joint motion being measured, whether the motion is measured actively or passively, the sex of the subject, the age of the subject, the experience of the examiner, the dominance of the extremity, whether the subject has exercised, and what time of the day the measurement is performed.[9,10]

The first dilemma in reporting shoulder motion is what to call motions in certain directions. The nomenclature for describing shoulder motion has a long history, but most sources make a distinction between forward flexion, where the arm is raised in the sagittal plane, and abduction, where the arm is elevated in the coronal plane (**Fig. 2–3**). The scapula sits on the convex thorax and results in an orientation that is ~30 degrees anterior to the coronal plane. This position has been referred to as the plane of the scapula, and elevation occurring in this plane is termed *scaption* or elevation in the scapular plane (**Fig. 2–4**).

Extension of the arm is typically reported as being performed with the arm in an adducted position; however, adduction of the arm can be reported with the arm at the side or with the arm elevated at 90 degrees. When adduction is performed with the arm in elevation, it is typically called horizontal adduction, and it is sometimes referred to as "cross-body adduction" (**Fig. 2–5**). If the arm is elevated 90 degrees and the arm is extended, it is called "horizontal extension."

Rotations of the arm also were sometimes initially described as medial (toward the body) or lateral (away

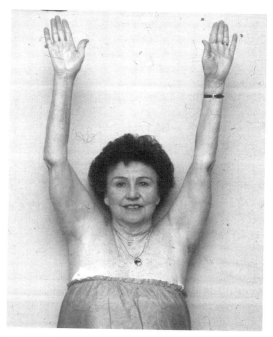

FIGURE 2–3 When the arm is elevated in abduction or in flexion, the end point is the same position where the arm is fully elevated.

from the body). This nomenclature makes sense with the arm in an adducted position at the side of the body but not with the arm elevated. As a result, these arm rotations are typically described now as internal or external rotation. Thus, with the arm adducted at the side, external rotation with the arm at the side is typically measured. Internal rotation up the back has become the standard

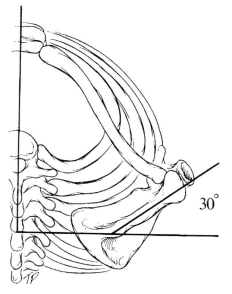

FIGURE 2–4 The plane of the scapula is due to the angled position of the scapula on the thorax and is typically 30 degrees to the plane of the body.

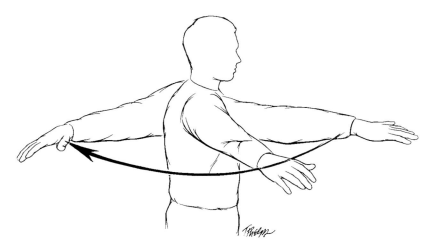

FIGURE 2–5 Horizontal adduction is when the arm is brought across the body in a specified degree of elevation of the arm.

measure of internal rotation in the adducted position. Likewise, rotations with the arm abducted 90 degrees are also described as internal or external rotation.

The complexity and ambiguities of this system prompted some to suggest a global coordinate system to describe shoulder motion[11] (**Fig. 2–6**). This would allow the examiner to describe exactly where the arm could be positioned in space. This system did not gain widespread acceptance, however, because of its complexity and lack of practicality.

■ Validity of Measurements

An important issue in any measurement system is the validity of the measurements.[9] In other words, does a particular system really measure what it says it does? For most joints, the motion measures are supposed to be a representation of the central axis of the limb, which is usually assumed to be roughly the center of the long bones making up that segment. When measuring knee motion, it is assumed that the measure is actually of the femur where it articulates with the tibia, but overlying soft tissue, swelling, or variations in the bony anatomy can significantly affect the measurement.

In the shoulder, the validity of the measure is hampered due to the variability of the bony anatomy and because there are several moving parts that contribute to the motion. Additionally, the motions are often measured in relationship to the thorax, which can have variable size and shape. As will be discussed later, it has always been assumed that the shoulder elevates to 180 degrees in most people, but very accurate studies using sophisticated three-dimensional electronic tracking devices and computed tomography (CT) scans have demonstrated that true elevation of the humeral shaft relative to a vertical line in the thorax is around 150 to 170 degrees.[12–14]

The validity of the traditional measurements of shoulder rotations also has been questioned by these studies: what exactly are we measuring when we measure shoulder internal and external rotation? Are the measures actually measuring the bone movements or the bone and soft tissue movements? Another important issue when measuring shoulder motion is the reliability of the measurements. Reproducibility or intratester reliability refers to the ability of a single examiner to have a repeat measurement that is the same as the first measurement, and it is called test–retest reliability. A second type of reliability is the ability for two examiners to measure the same thing and is known as intertester reliability (see Appendix).

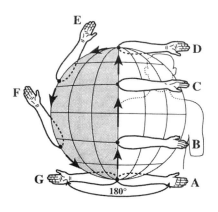

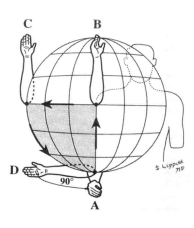

FIGURE 2–6 A global coordinate system was recommended by Matsen et al to define arm position specifically in space. (Adapted with permission from Pearl ML, Jackins S, Lippitt S, Sidles JA, Matsen F. Humeroscapular positions in a shoulder range-of-motion-examination. J Shoulder Elbow Surg 1992;1:296–305.)

In other words, are the measurements going to be the same if repeated by the same examiner or another examiner? The validity, reproducibility, and reliability of the measurements are critical issues when discussing range of motion of the shoulder complex.

■ Techniques of Measurement

An important element of measuring shoulder motion is the technique used for measuring the motion. Upon clinical examination, there are basically three methods that can be used to measure shoulder motion: visual estimation of the motion, goniometric measurement, and measurements obtained using inclinometers.

Visual Estimation

Visual estimation of motion is probably the most commonly used method in the office setting because it is cheap, easy, and quick. Several authors have suggested that visual estimations of range of motion of joints are not as accurate as using instrumented measuring devices, but there are a few studies that actually study this issue. In the lower extremity Watkins et al[15] found that goniometers were better than visual estimates for measuring passive motion of the knee. Williams and Callahan[10] studied the results of measuring a fixed angle of shoulder flexion by 22 physical therapists of a single male model. They found that there was no difference between the visual estimate and the goniometric measure by the therapists and concluded that experienced examiners can reliably estimate some shoulder motions without a goniometer. Most researchers would agree that visual measurement is acceptable in the office evaluation of the shoulder range of motion of patients, but goniometric measurements are necessary for studies or other special applications.

Use of Handheld Goniometers

The standard handheld goniometer with a stationary and a movable arm remains the most frequently used device for measuring shoulder motion because it is inexpensive, portable, and reliable and has been extensively studied.[16,17] The handheld goniometer comes in many models and shapes, with long arms, short arms, telescoping arms, and metal or plastic arms, and may measure in 1- or 5-degree increments. There are many variables that affect the use of the hand-held goniometer, but probably the most important is the experience of the examiner. Identification of the "zero position," as advocated by Clark et al[18] and subsequently the AAOS, is important. The ability to identify a reliable bony landmark is another important variable.

Multiple studies have demonstrated that the reproducibility of handheld goniometers for repeat measurement of joint motions is high for a single examiner. Studies have demonstrated that the intertester reliability using handheld goniometers is only fair to moderate (**Table 2–2**). High intratester reliability and low intertester reliability when using handheld goniometers to measure joint motion are common findings of studies of other joints.[19,20] As a result, when reading the literature regarding shoulder range of motion measurements, it is important to note both "how" the motions are measured as well as "who" performed the measurements. Studies that employ multiple examiners are likely to have some error due to this variable, which should be taken into account when assessing their results.

TABLE 2–2 Comparison of Reliability between Published Studies of Shoulder Motion

	Boon[38]	Riddle[186]	Walker[32]	Bovens[99]	Ellenbecker[84]	Fiebert[187]	Andrews[188]	Green[189]	Clarke[190]	Hoving[115]
Population	High school athletes	Healthy M/F	Healthy M/F	Healthy M/F	Elite tennis players	Healthy M/F	Stroke patients	Shoulder pain	Healthy females	Shoulder pain
Type of motion	Passive	Passive	Active	Active	Active	Active	Passive	Active	Passive	Passive
Age range, years	12–18	19–77	60–84	24–36	11–17	61–93	33–84	45–66	20–28	54–82
N	50	100	60	8	46	26	28	6	12	6
Instrument	UG	UG	UG	UG	UG	UG	HG†	HG	HG	Inc†
Movement	ER, IR (SS)	ER, IR	ER, IR	ER	ER, IR (SS)	ER, IR	ER	ER	ER	ER, IR
Intrarater ICC	ER = 0.78, IR = 0.38	ER = 0.98, IR = 0.93	ER = 0.78, IR > 0.81	ER = 0.76	ER = 0.39, IR = 0.34	ER > 0.88	ER > 0.93, IR > 0.88	ER = 0.75, IR = 0.82	ER = 0.45	ER = 0.75, IR = 0.32
Interrater ICC	ER = 0.58, IR = 0.60	ER = 0.88, IR = 0.43	ER = 5–10 IR > 10	ER = 0.63	Not tested	> 0.88	> 0.86	ER = 0.65, IR = 0.44	NR	ER = 0.11, IR = 0.06
Time between measurements	5 days	Immediately	Same day	8 times in 3 months	48 hours	NR	1 minute	1 hour	NR	1 hour

Source: Adapted with permission from Boon AJ, Smith J. Manual scapular stabilization: its effect on shoulder rotational range of motion. Arch Phys Med Rehabil 2000;81(7):978–983.

ER, external rotation; F, female; HG, hydrogoniometer; ICC, Intra Class Correlation Coefficients; Inc, inclinometer; IR, internal rotation; M, male; NR, not reported; SS, scapular-stabilized measurement; UG, universal goniometer.

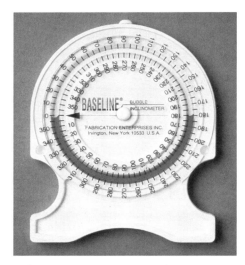

FIGURE 2–7 An example of a mechanical inclinometer available on the market. (Courtesy of Sammons Preston Rolyan.)

Use of Inclinometers

Another technique for measuring shoulder range of motion involves the use of inclinometers. These are basically leveling devices that are commonly used by engineers to determine the relationship of a structure to the horizontal plane. These devices were initially designed for use in the spine to determine the amount of deformity present in the coronal and sagittal planes.[21–23]

Two types of inclinometers have been described: mechanical and digital (**Figs. 2–7, 2–8**). Mechanical arthrometers use a weighted pendulum or a fluid-level indicator (hydrogoniometers) to measure the range of motion. These inclinometers work like a plumb line, using gravity as the mechanism for determining the relationship to a horizontal position. Technically, inclinometers must be firmly applied to the skin so that there is no

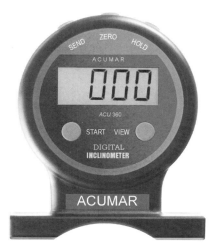

FIGURE 2–8 An example of a digital inclinometer available on the market. (Courtesy of Acumar Technology.)

motion or tilting of the device while the measurement is taken.

Clarke et al[18] in 1975 were the first to report the use of a based inclinometer to measure glenohumeral and scapular range of motion. They reported satisfactory results by using this method, with less than 7% interobserver error. Dover et al[24] used a mechanical inclinometer with a needle to measure the range of motion in 100 female athletes to measure the external and internal rotation and the flexion extension of the shoulder. They calculated the reliability of this device for measuring range of motion and obtained an Intra Class Correlation Coefficients (ICC) value of a mean of 0.99. These devices generally have relatively good reliability for both intraobserver and interobserver reliability (**Table 2–2**).

Digital inclinometers have been used more recently by many authors for measuring shoulder range of motion.[25–29] These inclinometers have internal gravity sensors that indicate the range of motion by calculating the angle from the vertical. Johnson et al[28] studied the reliability and validity of a digital inclinometer to assess scapular motion. They compared the data taken by a two-dimensional digital inclinometer to those taken by a three-dimensional magnetic tracking device. The digital inclinometer demonstrated good to excellent reliability and validity for the measurement of scapular motion with ICC, which varied from 0.89 to 9.96.

■ Factors Affecting Measurements

Age and Range of Motion

Another factor influencing the results of the measurements of shoulder motion is the age of the patients. Several studies have addressed this issue and reported that there is decreasing shoulder range of motion with age.[18,30] Murray et al[31] measured shoulder range of motion in younger men and women (range 25–36 years old) and older men and women (range 55–66 years old) using handheld goniometers. They did not find differences between the two age groups, but they did find differences between men and women for several measures.

Boone and Azen[30] divided their cohort of 109 healthy males into two groups: 53 subjects under age 19 and 56 subjects over age 19. They found the biggest changes between the two groups were with horizontal extension, forward flexion, backward extension, and both internal and external rotation of the shoulder with the arm elevated 90 degrees.

Walker et al[32] evaluated 60 subjects between the ages of 60 and 84. They found that measurements were significantly different from those reported by the AAOS, and suggested that older individuals required revised standards for range of motion. Boone and Azen[30] examined 50 high school athletes and found that that age was a factor in external rotation only, with the younger age group (age 12–15) having more external rotation than the older group (age 16–18).

The most comprehensive study of the relationship of age to shoulder motion was reported by Barnes et al,[33] who measured shoulder motion in 280 subjects, with 40 subjects in each decade from 0 to 70 years of age. They found a nonlinear decline in motion with age for both passive and active motions measured except for internal rotation, which seemed to increase with age. The amount of change per year was the greatest for abduction and external rotation with the arm adducted at the side. Loss of flexion over time was not linear; the researchers thus concluded that a loss of forward elevation in subjects under age 40 should not be attributed to the aging process alone.

Gender and Range of Motion

Another factor influencing measurement of shoulder motion is the gender of the subjects. Allander et al[34] examined a general population and found that women had significantly increased shoulder motion compared with males for most age groups. Clarke et al[18] reported that, in general, males had 92% less motion than females, and that this difference was most marked in abduction (females 85.6 degree vs 77.4 degree for males) as compared with internal and external rotation. Walker et al[32] found significant differences between men and women for all measures except internal rotation (**Table 2–3**). Murray et al[31] found that women had a greater total arc of internal and external rotation of the shoulder compared with men, but their study examined only two age groups, with a large discrepancy in ages between the two groups. Barnes et al[33] found significant differences between all motions measured between men and women for both passive and active range of motion.

Dominance of the Extremity and Range of Motion

Another factor influencing the shoulder range of motion is the dominance of the extremity. Clarke et al[18] found no

difference based on arm dominance between males and females for any age group or any measure of shoulder motion. Boone and Azen[30] found variable differences between right and left extremities depending on age, but they did not make note of the dominance of the extremity. They concluded that overall, both extremities were similar and that, in general, the opposite side could be used for comparison for most joints.

Kronberg et al[35,36] found no difference in range of motion between the dominant and nondominant shoulders for both males and females. Barnes et al[33] found that the nondominant shoulder had statistically significantly greater active internal rotation, passive internal rotation, active extension, and passive extension compared with the dominant side; however, the dominant arm had significantly more external rotation both passively and actively with the arm abducted and at the side compared with the nondominant shoulder. The researchers found no relationship between shoulder range of motion and sports participation, and they concluded that using the opposite shoulder for comparison of rotations was questionable.

Patient Positioning and Range of Motion

There is increasing evidence that body position can affect range of motion measurements, particularly in the shoulder. The main practical concern is whether the examination may be different if the patient is in a sitting or standing position. Another issue is whether the scapular motion is influenced by contact to a rigid surface, such as when lying on a flat surface or when sitting with the thorax against the back of a chair. It is possible that patients who have pain will obtain better range of motion supine if the effects of gravity are eliminated. Some patients in wheelchairs may find examination in the supine position difficult.

Studies support the idea that measures of shoulder range of motion are influenced by whether the patient is supine or sitting. Sabari et al[37] studied flexion and abduction of the shoulder in 30 normal volunteers using handheld goniometers by one examiner with the subjects

TABLE 2–3 Shoulder Range of Motion by Sex

Shoulder Motion	Men*		Women*		Difference Between M/W	Sexes Combined		
	Mean	SD	Mean	SD		p	Mean	SD
Abduction	155	22	175	16	−20	< .001	165	21
Flexion	160	11	169	9	−9	< .001	165	11
Extension	38	11	49	13	−11	< .001	44	13
Internal rotation	59	16	66	13	−7	NS	62	15
External rotation	76	13	85	16	−9	0.02	81	15

Source: Adapted with permission from Walker JM, et al. Active mobility of the extremities in older subjects. Phys Ther 1984;64(6):919–923.
*Age groups were combined.
NS, not significant; SD, standard deviation.

supine and then sitting. They found that the intrarater reliability between trials was high (0.94–0.99) for the measures, so there was good reproducibility of the measures whether they were done with the patient sitting or supine when done by one person.

There were significant differences in the measures obtained supine versus standing, however, even when measurements were done by just one examiner. Sabari et al found that with patients sitting, the examiner had to be diligent to watch that the patients did not use compensatory motions of the thorax or pelvis to influence motion. They concluded that either position was useful for measuring motion, but that the exact position of the subject should be noted when reporting or studying shoulder motion.

There have been several studies that have evaluated the effect of positioning on the measurement of shoulder rotational movements.[38,39] These studies will be discussed in detail later in this chapter because the measurement of shoulder rotations is a controversial and important subject; however, there are indications that shoulder rotational movements can be significantly influenced by whether the patient is supine or standing. We believe that this is due in part to the difficulty in stabilizing the scapula with the patient supine versus using visual and tactile cues with the patient standing.

Active or Passive Motion

Another important variable to consider when measuring shoulder range of motion is whether active or passive motion or both should be measured. In the clinical setting, it is important to measure if the patient has deficits in motion in any one direction. Whether the motion is active or passive, pain can influence the ability of the patient to move the shoulder. The variables that affect passive motion are discussed later in this chapter.

The influence of active versus passive motion of the shoulder was studied by Sabari et al[37] using the same cohort as reviewed earlier. The researchers found that there were no significant differences in shoulder flexion or abduction with active or passive motion. They examined only normal volunteers, however, so this finding may not be capable of extrapolation to abnormal subjects. The experience of most clinicians is that active and passive motions can be significantly different depending on the pathology of the patient.

■ Clinically Relevant Biomechanics of Shoulder Motion

New knowledge of shoulder biomechanics and shoulder motion challenge the previously held misconceptions about how the shoulder moves and functions. Biomechanical studies have shown that shoulder motion is infinitely more complicated than previously appreciated. This is especially true for evaluating glenohumeral and scapulothoracic motions where there are movements in three dimensions that may have clinical importance.

Shoulder motion is a complex interaction of the bony anatomy, the ligamentous laxity, and the activity of the muscles. This interaction of static and dynamic components makes the shoulder motion highly variable and difficult to study. Each shoulder motion and translation places a different portion of the ligaments under stress, and pathological conditions may affect some parts of the ligaments but not others. It is our position that glenohumeral motions can be distinguished from scapulothoracic motions in rotation but not in elevation. The next section will present the biomechanical rationale for these conclusions and clinical support for a new method of measuring and reporting shoulder motions.

> Measurement of shoulder range of motion in rotation can distinguish between glenohumeral and scapulothoracic measurements.

When the arm is moved in space, it is a combination of motion at the glenohumeral joint and the scapulothoracic joint. Although the resulting motion of the humerus is relatively easy to determine, the contribution of the individual components to the motion is more difficult. Early observational studies of shoulder motion estimated that glenohumeral motion occurred in the first 90 degrees of shoulder elevation and that scapular motion occurred after that.[40,41] The 1964 AAOS handbook for range of motion suggested that by stabilizing the scapula, isolated glenohumeral elevation would be only 90 degrees.[40] Subsequent authors have suggested that, with elevation, glenohumeral motion can be distinguished from scapulothoracic motion. We believe that this distinction is very difficult to make, however, and that its clinical utility is yet to be determined.

Radiographic Studies of Shoulder Elevation

Subsequent studies using radiological methods established the relationship of scapulothoracic motion to glenohumeral motion.[14,42] These studies were performed by having the subject elevate the arm from the side to full elevation. These were semi-static studies, where the arm was held actively by the subject in one position, and radiographs were then taken. The contributions of glenohumeral motion and scapulothoracic motion to each level of elevation were measured from the radiographs (**Table 2–4**).

Inman and Abbott[14] were the first to use this technique. They noted that over the entire arc of motion, the ratio of glenohumeral motion to scapulothoracic motion was 2:1; however, the ratio of glenohumeral to scapulothoracic

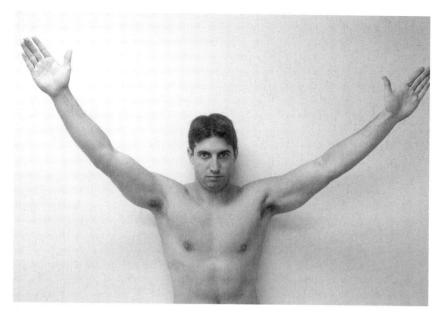

FIGURE 2–12 Full elevation in the scapular plane is best accomplished with the thumb in an up so that the humerus is externally rotated as the arm elevates.

Once the patient has reached the highest level that he or she can reach, the examiner can passively assist the arm to see if further motion is available. This is necessary only if the patient does not reach full elevation. If the patient has full motion with passive motion but not with active, then it is possible that the shoulder is weak. If the active and passive motions are the same, then it is possible that the shoulder is stiff or that the patient is splinting from too much pain. When patients complain of pain with range of motion, it is advisable not to push too hard and to cause further pain. If it cannot be determined whether the patient is stiff or just experiencing pain, then

consideration should be given to injections to decrease the pain. In some instances, the degree of stiffness cannot be determined without an examination under anesthesia.

When measuring elevation of the shoulder, some patients place their arms in a position that will automatically handicap their ability to elevate. The two most common maneuvers will be to try to elevate the arm in the plane of the body (coronal plane) or behind it (**Fig. 2–14**). Physiologically it is very difficult to lift

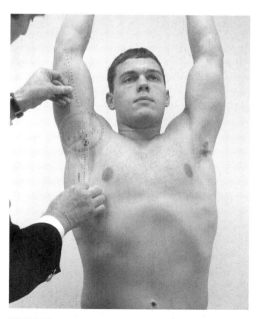

FIGURE 2–13 Abduction is measured with the goniometer centered over the glenohumeral joint.

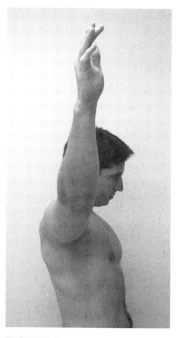

FIGURE 2–14 The arm can be elevated in the plane of the body (coronal plane), which is more constrained than elevating the arm in the scapular plane.

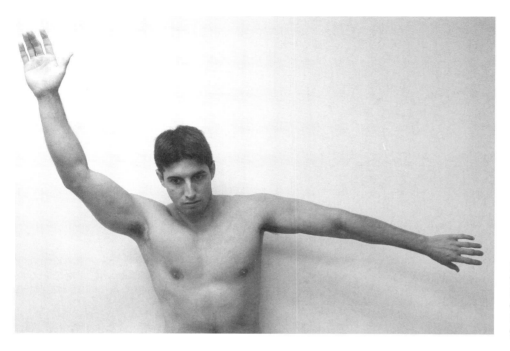

FIGURE 2–15 Full elevation in the plane of the scapula cannot be accomplished with the thumb down because greater tuberosity is restrained by the superior glenoid.

one's arm in this position even if the shoulder is normal. The second maneuver that will prevent elevation is attempting to raise the arm in abduction with the thumb or hand down (**Fig. 2–15**). In abduction, the arm must be in external rotation, or it will not move due to the greater tuberosity contacting the superior glenoid. Sometimes patients with secondary gain issues will attempt to elevate the arm behind the body with the thumb or hand down. It is important to make sure that the arm is brought forward and externally rotated to obtain full appreciation of the ability to elevate the extremity.

Measuring Elevation in Flexion

Elevation of the arm in flexion can be helpful because it typically is not as stressful to the shoulder as elevation in abduction. This is probably because it does not require much external rotation of the arm. When evaluating flexion of the arm, typically the examiner stands at the side and asks the patient to elevate his or her arm with the palm down (**Fig. 2–16**). When the patient has gone as far as possible, the goniometer is placed vertically related to the floor, and the center of the goniometer is placed over the lateral aspect of the shoulder joint. The second arm of the goniometer is placed down the center of the arm.

Once this has been done, if full elevation has not been reached, then the arm can be pushed passively into more flexion. This should be done with care, particularly if the patient is experiencing pain. The ability to push the arm into more flexion passively than actively may indicate weakness. If the arm cannot be elevated further passively, then a stiff joint may be the

cause. If the pain is severe, then injections may help decrease the pain to see the effect upon motion. In some instances it may be necessary to do an examination under anesthesia to determine if the shoulder is stiff or frozen.

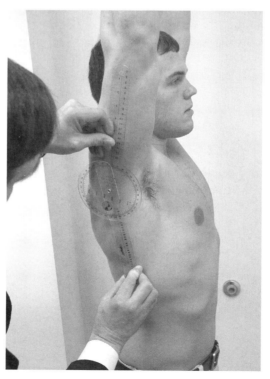

FIGURE 2–16 Flexion of the arm is measured from the side with the goniometer centered as much as possible over the glenohumeral joint.

■ Measuring Rotational Motions of the Shoulder

Rotational movements typically are measured separately from measures of elevation, but both of these components of shoulder motion have clinical significance. Rotational movements are the result of a complex interaction of the scapulae on the thorax and of the humerus on the scapulae. These interactions between the scapulae and the humerus have important implications for the normal and the impaired shoulder. Rotation of the humerus is necessary not only for placing the arm behind the head but also for placing the arm in a cocked position for sports activities. The relationship between the scapula and humerus also has implications for how we measure motion, how we communicate humeral position relative to the scapula, how we express capsular tightness after surgical procedures, and how we measure the results of surgery.

There has been an explosion of information in the past several years on shoulder rotational movements, primarily as they relate to pain in the shoulder of the overhead athlete. Most patients are not involved in overhead sports, however, and it is important to understand the concepts of measurement of shoulder rotation for individuals from all occupations, avocations, and age groups. This section will address the controversy over measuring rotational movements of the shoulders in athletes, the importance of distinguishing total shoulder complex rotations from purely glenohumeral rotations, and techniques for measuring shoulder rotation.

Rotational Range of Motion and the Overhead Athlete

The issue of the effect of arm dominance on range of motion is important for several reasons, but one of the more salient reasons is that it has been postulated that shoulder pathologies in athletes involved in unilateral overhead sports (e.g., baseball, tennis, and javelin throwing) may be due to alterations in shoulder rotations, particularly rotations in which the arm is elevated 90 degrees. Numerous studies have demonstrated that in overhead athletes there is an increased external rotation compared with the nondominant side, with a concomitant loss of internal rotation (**Table 2–6**).

This loss of internal rotation in the dominant arm was termed glenohumeral internal rotation deficit (GIRD). It has been speculated that this altered arc of rotation motion resulting in greater external rotation and diminished internal rotation causes abnormal shoulder motions and translations that predispose or contribute to pathological processes in the shoulder of the overhead athlete.[53,54] These pathological problems include superior labrum anterior to posterior (SLAP) lesions,

secondary impingement, partial rotator cuff tears, internal impingement, and pain.[55]

There are basically three theories on how these abnormal motions contribute to shoulder pathology in the athlete. The first theory was promulgated by Jobe and colleagues,[56–59] who found that baseball players often not only had increased external rotation of the shoulder upon examination but also tended to be loose jointed. This looseness was manifested as increased translation of the shoulder. Jobe et al hypothesized that this increased laxity was exacerbated by placing the extremity in the extreme position of abduction and external rotation, as seen in the throwing motion, or using the arm over shoulder level in some sports.

This position of the shoulder and the forces generated by throwing-type motions of the shoulder contributed to the gradual stretching of the ligaments of the shoulder, particularly the anterior band of the inferior glenohumeral ligament. This caused an occult form of anteroinferior instability, as the humeral head would move too far forward on the socket or glenoid.

This shoulder joint instability was postulated to place extra stress on the rotator cuff and contributed to partial tears of the supraspinatus. This stress also resulted in superior labrum lesions, particularly SLAP lesions. Jobe et al suggested that this contact may be accentuated in patients who have increased laxity of the glenohumeral ligaments. This would result in a "hyperangulation" of the proximal humerus, which was manifested by increased external rotation upon physical examination. The authors recommended a capsular shift to tighten the anteroinferior capsule in patients who demonstrated this combination of findings.[60]

Another theory of how abnormal motions of the shoulder contribute to pain and dysfunction in the overhead athlete relates to contact of the bones of the proximal humerus with the posterosuperior glenoid when the arm is elevated. This theory is called internal impingement, based on observations by Walch et al[61,62] at the time of arthroscopic surgery on the shoulders of patients with pain. While the patient was under anesthesia and with the arthroscope in the shoulder, they noted that with the arm in abduction and external rotation, the greater tuberosity of the humerus and the rotator cuff would make contact with the posterior and superior labrum.

Walch et al suggested that this contact between the humerus and posterosuperior glenoid may contribute to posterior and superior labrum tears and potentially to tears of the rotator cuff, particularly if the contact was frequent, as seen in an overhead athlete. They suggested that this contact would be increased in patients with too much external rotation of the proximal humerus and attempted humeral osteotomies to try to prevent this malady. Unfortunately, the results of this surgical

TABLE 2–6 Summary Table for Shoulder Rotation Range of Motion Studies

Study	N	Population	Pathology	Age (Years)	Gender	Test Position	Measurement Technique
Sauers et al, JAT, 2003[86]	28	Professional baseball pitchers	Non-impaired	22.6 ± 3.4	Male	Supine	Goniometer
	28	Professional baseball pitchers	Non-impaired	22.6 ± 3.4	Male	Supine	Goniometer
Sauers et al, AANA, 2004[74]	49	Professional baseball pitchers	Non-impaired	23 ± 3.3	Male	Supine	Goniometer
	54	Professional baseball position players	Non-impaired	23 ± 3.3	Male	Supine	Goniometer
Crocket et al, AJSM, 2002[81]	25	Professional baseball pitchers	Non-impaired	18 – 35	Male	Supine	Goniometer
	25	Non-overhead athlete controls	Non-impaired	18 – 35	Male	Supine	Goniometer
Downar et al, JAT, 2002[194]	27	Professional baseball players	Non-impaired	20.4 ± 1.6	Male	Supine	Goniometer
Brown et al, AJSM, 1988[71]	18	Professional baseball pitchers	Non-impaired	27.02 ± 4.25	Male	Supine	Goniometer
	23	Professional baseball position players	Non-impaired	27.02 ± 4.25	Male	Supine	Goniometer
Bigliani et al, AJSM, 1997[75]	148	Professional baseball players	Non-impaired	22.8 (16–28)	Male	Standing & supine	Goniometer
	72	Professional baseball pitchers	Non-impaired	22.8 (16–28)	Male	Standing & supine	Goniometer
	76	Professional baseball position players	Non-impaired	22.8 (16–28)	Male	Standing & supine	Goniometer
Baltaci et al, JSMPF, 2001[195]	9	Right handed college baseball pitchers	Non-impaired	20.9 (18–22)	Male	Supine	Goniometer
	6	Left handed college baseball pitchers	Non-impaired	20.9 (18–22)	Male	Supine	Goniometer
	23	College baseball non-pitchers	Non-impaired	20.9 (18–22)	Male	Supine	Goniometer
Osbahr et al, AJSM, 2002[80]	19	College baseball pitchers	Non-impaired	19.1(18–21)	Male	Supine	Goniometer with 3.5 kg force
Reagan et al, AJSM, 2002[79]	54	College baseball players	Non-impaired	19.3 (18–23)	Male	Supine	Goniometer
Johnson, JAT, 1992[196]	9	College baseball pitchers	Non-impaired	20.4 ± 1.4	Male	Supine	Goniometer
	9	College baseball outfielders	Non-impaired	20.4 ± 1.4	Male	Supine	Goniometer
	8	College baseball infielders	Non-impaired	20.4 ± 1.4	Male	Supine	Goniometer
Mourtacos et al, JAT, 2003[178]	15	Youth baseball players age 10 to 12	Non-impaired	10–12	Male	Supine	Goniometer
	13	Youth baseball players age 13 to 14	Non-impaired	13–14	Male	Supine	Goniometer
Ellenbecker et al, MSSE, 2002[197]	46	Professional baseball pitchers	Non-impaired	22.6 ± 2.0	Male	Supine	Goniometer
	117	Elite junior tennis players	Non-impaired	16.4 ± 1.6	Male	Supine	Goniometer
Kibler et al, AJSM, 1996[73]	20	Elite male tennis players	Non-impaired	18 (14–21)	Male	Supine	Goniometer
	19	Elite female tennis players	Non-impaired	18 (14–21)	Female	Supine	Goniometer
Ellenbecker & Roetert, JSCR, 2002[198]	11	Division 1 college tennis players	Non-impaired	Not reported	Female	Supine	Goniometer
Ellenbecker et al, JOSPT, 1996[84]	113	Elite male junior tennis players	Non-impaired	11–17	Male	Supine	Goniometer
	90	Elite female junior tennis players	Non-impaired	11–17	Female	Supine	Goniometer

Active/ Passive	Scapula	Shoulder	90 Abd/ER	90 Abd/IR	90 Abd/ Total Arc	0 Abd/ER	ASES IR	Abduction	Flexion	Extension
Passive	Stabilized	Dominant	101.3 ± 6.9	43.7 ± 10.0	144.9 ± 9.5	N/A	N/A	N/A	N/A	N/A
		Non-Dominant	90.7 ± 7.6	53.2 ± 11.1	143.9 ± 12.4	N/A	N/A	N/A	N/A	N/A
Passive	Unstabilized	Dominant	127.7 ± 11.7	65.4 ± 13.3	193.1 ± 16.7	N/A	N/A	N/A	N/A	N/A
		Non-Dominant	114.2 ± 9.8	77.5 ± 13.6	191.7 ± 12.8	N/A	N/A	N/A	N/A	N/A
Passive	Stabilized	Dominant	99.4 ± 7.8	44.4 ± 9.3	142.1 ± 10.1	N/A	N/A	N/A	N/A	N/A
		Non-Dominant	88.8 ± 10.0	54.5 ± 9.5	142.6 ± 12.8	N/A	N/A	N/A	N/A	N/A
Passive	Stabilized	Dominant	94.2 ± 8.6	40.8 ± 7.7	135.2 ± 10.2	N/A	N/A	N/A	N/A	N/A
		Non-Dominant	84.2 ± 9.2	53.2 ± 7.5	137.6 ± 10.8	N/A	N/A	N/A	N/A	N/A
Passive	Not reported	Dominant	128 ± 9.2	62 ± 7.4	189 ± 12.6	N/A	N/A	N/A	N/A	N/A
		Non-Dominant	119 ± 7.2	71 ± 9.3	189 ± 12.7	N/A	N/A	N/A	N/A	N/A
Passive	Not reported	Dominant	113 ± 14.6	65 ± 8.9	179 + 17.7	N/A	N/A	N/A	N/A	N/A
		Non-Dominant	112 ± 13.9	69 + 7.1	181 + 15.3	N/A	N/A	N/A	N/A	N/A
Passive	Stabilized	Dominant	108.9 ± 9.0	56.6 ± 12.5	165.5 ± 14.4	N/A	N/A	N/A	N/A	N/A
		Non-Dominant	101.9 ± 5.9	68.6 ± 12.6	170.4 ± 10.5	N/A	N/A	N/A	N/A	N/A
Passive	Not reported	Dominant	141 ± 14.7	83 ± 13.9	N/A	71 ± 6.9	N/A	98 ± 10.8	163 ± 7.9	72 ± 15.5
		Non-Dominant	132 ± 14.6	98 ± 13.2	N/A	71 ± 9.4	N/A	105 ± 10.3	168 ± 6.3	78 ± 13.3
Passive	Not reported	Dominant	132 ± 9.8	85 ± 11.9	N/A	67 ± 11.3	N/A	100 ± 11.0	164 ± 10.2	81 ± 11.3
		Non-Dominant	124 ± 12.7	91 ± 13.0	N/A	69 + 9.7	N/A	101 ± 8.0	168 ± 8.7	81 + 11.8
Not reported	Not reported	Dominant	113.5	N/A	N/A	79.5	15.4	N/A	173.3	N/A
		Non-Dominant	99.9	N/A	N/A	78.3	17.5	N/A	175.1	N/A
Not reported	Not reported	Dominant	118.0	N/A	N/A	80.9	15.5	N/A	174.9	N/A
		Non-Dominant	102.8	N/A	N/A	79.7	17.6	N/A	177.3	N/A
Not reported	Not reported	Dominant	109.3	N/A	N/A	78.2	15.4	N/A	171.8	N/A
		Non-Dominant	97.1	N/A	N/A	76.9	17.4	N/A	173.1	N/A
Passive	Not reported	Dominant-R	131.5 ± 11.5	55.8 ± 7.1	187.4 ± 15.8	N/A	N/A	N/A	N/A	N/A
		Non-Dominant	116.6 ± 11.3	69.2 ± 4.8	185.8 ± 14.6	N/A	N/A	N/A	N/A	N/A
Passive	Not reported	Dominant-L	127.0 ± 6.1	62.6 ± 3.6	185.7 ± 7.9	N/A	N/A	N/A	N/A	N/A
		Non-Dominant	114.0 ± 5.7	71.6 ± 3.4	189.2 ± 6.9	N/A	N/A	N/A	N/A	N/A
Passive	Not reported	Dominant-R	122.4 ± 10.9	58.2 ± 7.1	180.6 ± 12.5	N/A	N/A	N/A	N/A	N/A
		Non-Dominant	114.6 ± 11.6	68.7 ± 6.8	183.4 ± 10.5	N/A	N/A	N/A	N/A	N/A
Passive	Unstabilized	Dominant	126.8 ± 12.0	79.3 ± 13.3	N/A	90.1 ± 10.8	N/A	N/A	N/A	N/A
		Non-Dominant	114.5 ± 9.1	91.4 ± 13.6	N/A	81.0 + 10.7	N/A	N/A	N/A	N/A
Passive	Stabilized	Dominant	116.3 ± 11.4	43.0 ± 7.4	159.5 ± 12.4	77.1 ± 10.9	14 ± 2	N/A	175.1 ± 7.0	N/A
		Non-Dominant	106.6 ± 1.2	51.2 ± 7.3	157.8 ± 11.5	76.3 ± 10.4	16 ± 2	N/A	175.6 ± 5.5	N/A
Passive	Not reported	Dominant	136 ± 14.6	111 ± 15.2	N/A	N/A	N/A	N/A	209 ± 10.7	96 ± 10.0
		Non-Dominant	128 ± 12.9	116 ± 12.2	N/A	N/A	N/A	N/A	202 ± 6.6	98 ± 12.2
Passive	Not reported	Dominant	120 ± 19.2	106 ± 12.8	N/A	N/A	N/A	N/A	192 ± 7.2	90 ± 8.7
		Non-Dominant	114 ± 8.0	106 ± 10.6	N/A	N/A	N/A	N/A	195 ± 6.5	90 ± 9.1
Passive	Not reported	Dominant	115 ± 5.8	110 ± 11.8	N/A	N/A	N/A	N/A	187 ± 10.1	92 ± 21.1
		Non-Dominant	109 ± 7.8	114 ± 11.9	N/A	N/A	N/A	N/A	192 ± 10.3	87 ± 16.6
Passive	Stabilized	Dominant	94.6 ± 6.3	56.6 ± 11.5	151.2 ± 14.2	N/A	N/A	N/A	N/A	N/A
		Non-Dominant	90.3 ± 6.7	65.6 ± 9.6	155.9 ± 12.1	N/A	N/A	N/A	N/A	N/A
Passive	Stabilized	Dominant	100.3 ± 5.4	49.7 ± 9.4	150.1 ± 11.1	N/A	N/A	N/A	N/A	N/A
		Non-Dominant	96.1 ± 5.6	59.9 ± 10.7	156.0 ± 12.1	N/A	N/A	N/A	N/A	N/A
Active	Stabilized	Dominant	103.2 ± 9.1	42.4 ± 15.8	145.7 ± 18.0	N/A	N/A	N/A	N/A	N/A
		Non-Dominant	94.5 ± 8.1	52.4 ± 16.4	146.9 ± 17.5	N/A	N/A	N/A	N/A	N/A
Active	Stabilized	Dominant	103.7 ± 10.9	45.4 ± 13.6	149.1 ± 18.4	N/A	N/A	N/A	N/A	N/A
		Non-Dominant	101.8 ± 10.8	56.3 ± 11.5	158.2 ± 15.9	N/A	N/A	N/A	N/A	N/A
Passive	Stabilized	Dominant	124	41.7	165.3	N/A	N/A	N/A	N/A	N/A
		Non-Dominant	111.7	68	178.7	N/A	N/A	N/A	N/A	N/A
Passive	Stabilized	Dominant	126.5	43.3	168.9	N/A	N/A	N/A	N/A	N/A
		Non-Dominant	120.7	72.8	193.5	N/A	N/A	N/A	N/A	N/A
Active	Stabilized	Dominant	101 ± 9	49 + 10	150	N/A	N/A	N/A	N/A	N/A
		Non-Dominant	95 + 6	61 + 8	156	N/A	N/A	N/A	N/A	N/A
Active	Stabilized	Dominant	103.7 ± 10.9	45.4 ± 13.6	149.1 ± 18.4	N/A	N/A	N/A	N/A	N/A
		Non-Dominant	101.9 ± 10.8	56.3 ± 11.5	158.2 ± 15.9	N/A	N/A	N/A	N/A	N/A
Active	Stabilized	Dominant	105.2 ± 10.2	52.2 ± 10.7	157.4 ± 14.9	N/A	N/A	N/A	N/A	N/A
		Non-Dominant	104.0 + 10.3	60.3 + 9.8	164.4 ± 13.6	N/A	N/A	N/A	N/A	N/A

(Continued)

TABLE 2–6 *(Continued)*

Study	N	Population	Pathology	Age (Years)	Gender	Test Position	Measurement Technique
Roetert et al, JSCR, 2000[199]	44	Youth tennis players age 14	Non-impaired	14	Mixed	Supine	Goniometer
		Youth tennis players age 15	Non-impaired	15	Mixed	Supine	Goniometer
		Youth tennis players age 16	Non-impaired	16	Mixed	Supine	Goniometer
		Youth tennis players age 17	Non-impaired	17	Mixed	Supine	Goniometer
Chandler et al, AJSM, 1990[72]	86	Elite junior tennis players	Non-impaired	15.4 (12–21)	66 Males, 20 Females	Supine	Goniometer
	139	Athletes in non-overhead dominant sports	Non-impaired	15.9 (13–22)	95 Males, 44 Females	Supine	Goniometer
Beach et al, JOSPT, 1992[77]	32	Competitive swimmers	31% pain-free, 69% painful	19 (15–21)	Mixed	Supine	Goniometer
Bak & Magnusson, AJSM, 1997[76]	7	Danish National Team swimmers	Injured	18 (16–19)	4 Males, 3 Females	Not reported	Not reported
	8	Danish National Team swimmers	Non-impaired	19 (15–25)	5 Males, 3 Females	Not reported	Not reported
Rupp et al, IJSM, 1995[85]	22	Elite swimmers	Shoulder pain	17.7 (14–26)	10 Males, 12 Females	Not reported	Not reported
	22	Non-overhead athlete controls	Non-impaired	17.7 (14–26)	10 Males, 12 Females	Not reported	Not reported
Lintner et al, AJSM, 1996[114]	76	Mixed athlete population	Non-impaired	19	32 Males, 44 Females	Supine	Goniometer
Boon & Smith, APMR, 2000[38]	50	High school athletes	Non-impaired	12–18	18 Males, 32 Females	Supine	Goniometer
Awan et al, APMR, 2002[27]	56	High school athletes	Non-impaired	13–18	32 Males, 24 Females	Supine	Inclinometer
							Inclinometer
							Visual Inspection
Sauers et al, AJSM, 2001[78]	51	Non-overhead recreational athletes	Healthy	22 ± 2.8	28 Female, 23 Male	Supine, prone, & standing	Goniometer
Barnes et al, JSES, 2001[33]	280	General population	Healthy	4–70	Male	Supine & prone	Goniometer
					Female	Supine & prone	Goniometer
					Male	Supine & prone	Goniometer
					Female	Supine & prone	Goniometer
Warner et al, AJSM, 1990[109]	10	Patients	Impingement	31 (17–47)	8 Males, 2 females	Supine	Goniometer
	28	Patients	Instability	24 (16–43)	20 Males, 8 females	Supine	Goniometer
Tyler et al, AJSM, 2000[176]	19	Patients with dominant shoulder injury	Subacromial Impingement	44 ± 16.5	Mixed	Supine	Not reported
	12	Patients with non-dominant shoulder injury	Subacromial Impingement	44 ± 16.5	Mixed	Supine	Not reported
	33	Volunteer controls	Non-impaired	33 ± 9.3	20 Males, 13 females	Supine	Not reported

Active/ Passive	Scapula	Shoulder	90 Abd/ER	90 Abd/IR	90 Abd/ Total Arc	0 Abd/ER	ASES IR	Abduction	Flexion	Extension
Passive	Stabilized	Dominant	N/A	44	N/A	N/A	N/A	N/A	N/A	N/A
		Non-Dominant	N/A	55	153	N/A	N/A	N/A	N/A	N/A
Passive	Stabilized	Dominant	N/A	53	N/A	N/A	N/A	N/A	N/A	N/A
		Non-Dominant	N/A	62	173	N/A	N/A	N/A	N/A	N/A
Passive	Stabilized	Dominant	N/A	53	N/A	N/A	N/A	N/A	N/A	N/A
		Non-Dominant	N/A	66	172	N/A	N/A	N/A	N/A	N/A
Passive	Stabilized	Dominant	N/A	50	N/A	N/A	N/A	N/A	N/A	N/A
		Non-Dominant	N/A	68	162	N/A	N/A	N/A	N/A	N/A
Passive	Stabilized	Dominant	110 ± 11	65 + 19	N/A	N/A	N/A	N/A	N/A	N/A
		Non-Dominant	103 ± 11	76 ± 12	N/A	N/A	N/A	N/A	N/A	N/A
Passive	Stabilized	Dominant	96 ± 14	74 ± 14	N/A	N/A	N/A	N/A	N/A	N/A
		Non-Dominant	94 + 11	82 + 13	N/A	N/A	N/A	N/A	N/A	N/A
Active	Unstabilized	Right	101 ± 11	45 ± 12	N/A	N/A	N/A	195 ± 15	187 ± 9	59 ± 14
		Left	100 ± 10	49 ± 14	N/A	N/A	N/A	196 ± 14	188 ± 10	62 ± 16
Not reported	Not reported	Injured	110 ± 10.3	66 ± 9.2	176 ± 11.0	N/A	N/A	N/A	N/A	N/A
		Healthy	110 ± 8.7	68 ± 7.4	177 ± 10.8	N/A	N/A	N/A	N/A	N/A
Not reported	Not reported	Both	106 ± 14.7	73 ± 5.1	179 ± 16.5	N/A	N/A	N/A	N/A	N/A
Passive	Not reported	Right	115 ± 14	74 ± 14	N/A	69 ± 14	N/A	N/A	N/A	N/A
		Left	113 ± 12	74 ± 15	N/A	70 ± 17	N/A	N/A	N/A	N/A
Passive	Not reported	Right	80 ± 12	63 ± 12	N/A	59 ± 14	N/A	N/A	N/A	N/A
		Left	79 ± 13	60 ± 15	N/A	57 ± 16	N/A	N/A	N/A	N/A
Passive	Stabilized	Both	108	70	N/A	72	T-5	N/A	N/A	N/A
Passive	Stabilized	Both	108.1 ± 14.1	62.8 ± 12.7	170.9 ± 19.8	N/A	N/A	N/A	N/A	N/A
	Unstabilized	Both	116.9 ± 12.3	89.1 ± 23.0	206.0 ± 27.4	N/A	N/A	N/A	N/A	N/A
Passive	Unstabilized	Right	115.4 ± 12.0	91.2 ± 15.4	N/A	N/A	N/A	N/A	N/A	N/A
		Left	109.2 ± 12.5	99.5 ± 13.0	N/A	N/A	N/A	N/A	N/A	N/A
Passive	Stabilized	Right	N/A	63.2 ± 11.8	N/A	N/A	N/A	N/A	N/A	N/A
		Left	N/A	70.2 ± 12.3	N/A	N/A	N/A	N/A	N/A	N/A
Passive	Unstabilized	Right	N/A	60.6 ± 10.9	N/A	N/A	N/A	N/A	N/A	N/A
		Left	N/A	70.7 ± 13.0	N/A	N/A	N/A	N/A	N/A	N/A
Passive	Stabilized	Dominant	99 ± 11.9	61 ± 13.3	N/A	N/A	N/A	179 ± 0.4	179 ± 2.3	49 ± 11.3
		Non-Dominant	94 ± 11.8	70 ± 12.5	N/A	N/A	N/A	179 ± 0.3	179 ± 3.1	51 ± 13.6
Active	Unstabilized	Dominant	101.2 ± 11.6	41.2 ± 9.3	N/A	78.3 ± 10.6	N/A	180.1 ± 18.2	173.6 ± 8.0	64.6 + 9.6
		Non-Dominant	91.1 ± 12.0	50.1 ± 10.2	N/A	73.7 ± 11.7	N/A	181.8 ± 17.1	173.5 ± 7.6	67.3 ± 9.2
Active	Unstabilized	Dominant	104.9 ± 12.0	47.5 + 11.2	N/A	81.4 ± 13.0	N/A	187.6 ± 16.1	176.7 ± 5.5	67.3 ± 8.7
		Non-Dominant	97.3 ± 11.3	54.5 ± 11.3	N/A	77.2 ± 12.1	N/A	188.6 ± 15.4	176.2 ± 5.9	68.7 ± 9.3
Passive	Unstabilized	Dominant	113.8 ± 15.7	48.6 ± 7.0	N/A	87.2 ± 12.9	N/A	187.4 ± 18.9	176.2 ± 7.4	77.4 ± 11.8
		Non-Dominant	101.9 ± 15.5	63.5 ± 8.2	N/A	82.2 ± 13.4	N/A	189.0 ± 18.3	176.1 ± 6.6	80.0 ± 10.1
Passive	Unstabilized	Dominant	118.0 ± 15.5	57.5 ± 12.3	N/A	92.3 ± 13.2	N/A	194.6 ± 16.5	178.7 ± 3.5	83.2 ± 11.2
		Non-Dominant	110.2 ± 15.1	65.4 ± 12.2	N/A	87.3 ± 12.5	N/A	195.0 ± 16.6	178.3 ± 4.4	84.6 ± 11.3
Passive	Not Reported	Symptomatic	96	46	N/A	N/A	T-6	N/A	N/A	N/A
Passive	Not Reported	Symptomatic	108	73	N/A	N/A	T-3	N/A	N/A	N/A
Passive	Not Reported	Dominant	96.18 ± 2.02	38.71 ± 2.80	N/A	N/A	N/A	N/A	N/A	N/A
		Non-Dominant	95.82 ± 1.93	61.00 ± 2.64	N/A	N/A	N/A	N/A	N/A	N/A
Passive	Not Reported	Dominant	95.58 ± 2.09	49.58 ± 4.29	N/A	N/A	N/A	N/A	N/A	N/A
		Non-Dominant	84.42 ± 4.64	44.58 ± 5.53	N/A	N/A	N/A	N/A	N/A	N/A
Passive	Not Reported	Dominant	96.09 ± 1.90	47.67 ± 1.49	N/A	N/A	N/A	N/A	N/A	N/A
		Non-Dominant	93.91 ± 2.02	54.36 ± 1.37	N/A	N/A	N/A	N/A	N/A	N/A

procedure were not as good as hoped, and osteotomy is no longer recommended for treatment of internal impingement.[63]

The third theory regarding motion and shoulder pathology in overhead athletes suggests that loss of internal rotation contributes to the development of superior labral lesions. The theory suggests that contracture of the posterior capsule causes an obligatory migration of the humeral head superiorly and posteriorly.[64] As the arm is placed in abduction and external rotation, this increased shift of the humeral head causes increased contact of the rotator cuff and humerus to the superior labrum, resulting in "peeling off" of the superior labrum.[65] This "peel back" is an abnormal movement of the labrum off the glenoid rim and theoretically contributes to the shoulder pain experienced by the athlete.

Once the labrum tears, it has been suggested that a superior instability pattern develops where there is too much laxity in the shoulder.[66] Because this is not a true anterior and inferior laxity pattern as suggested by Jobe et al,[58] this laxity as a result of a SLAP lesion has been called a "pseudolaxity."[53] The postulated treatment of the contracture or loss of motion depends on the degree of pathology. Physical therapy is directed toward increasing external rotation by stretching the posterior capsule. If nonsurgical treatments fail, then surgical treatment includes repair of any SLAP lesions and, in some instances, release of the posterior capsule to increase external rotation.

Several biomechanical studies have been performed in an attempt to see if this postulated sequence of events to the throwing shoulder could actually result in increased forces to the posterior and superior shoulder. Grossman et al[67] conducted a study in which they first stretched the posterior capsule of cadaver shoulders. This resulted in an increase in external rotation, as may be seen in a thrower's shoulder. This also resulted in an increased anterior translation of the shoulders tested. The researchers then performed a plication of the posterior capsule and found that with the arm in a cocked position, there was a posterior and superior shift of the humeral head compared with the normal shoulder.

Koffler et al[68] performed a biomechanical evaluation using electromagnetic sensors in cadavers to compare humeral translations in the late cocking phase of pitching. The cadavers were studied by mounting the scapula to a board and removing all tissues except the rotator cuff and capsule. Three-dimensional kinematics were tested with the humerus in neutral, at 90 degrees of elevation, and in a simulated cocking position of throwing. When 20% of the posterior capsule was tightened, the humeral head moved in an anterosuperior direction compared with controls. When 40% of the capsule was tightened, the humeral head moved in a posterosuperior direction compared with controls. Although these findings

were descriptive, Koffler et al could not demonstrate a statistically significant difference. They concluded that posterior capsular tightness may put other structures at risk, but this was not proven in their study.

Anderson et al[69] also used cadaveric shoulders to induce posterior capsular contracture and reported significant reductions in internal rotation with the arm at the side and at 90 degrees of abduction. This was accompanied by a significant displacement of coupled anteroposterior translation of the humeral head anteriorly (7 mm). Although the head translated differently, the authors did not explicitly comment on the direction, nor did they comment on the effect of force on the shoulder structures of these alterations.

All of these theories depend in some part on accurate measurement of shoulder motion, especially rotations. A recent debate on the amount of diminished internal rotation (GIRD) seen in baseball players and its role in the pathophysiology of shoulder problems suggested that the different measures of arm rotation by different examiners were a critical issue in the evaluation of players, in the development of the theories of what causes the problems in overhead athletes, in the treatment of the problems, and in determining the results of both nonoperative and surgical treatments.[70]

In that debate, Kibler et al[70] suggested that low levels of GIRD (less than 25 degrees) are normal, but that GIRD greater than 25 degrees predisposes the shoulder to injury. In a cohort of baseball players with arthroscopically proven SLAP lesions, Burkhart et al[66] reported the GIRD in that cohort averaged 53 degrees, with a range of 25 to 80 degrees. In an unpublished study of 38 athletes with type II SLAP lesions, Burkhart et al[66] found an average GIRD of 33 degrees, with a range of 26 to 58 degrees. It should be noted that the technique for measuring range of motion was not specified in these two studies. In contrast, Kibler et al[70] reported that, in their evaluation of baseball players, it was rare to have a player with GIRD of over 25 degrees. These differences in opinion between the debaters on the amount of GIRD seen in baseball players may be based on different techniques of measurement of shoulder rotation.

There have been several studies of shoulder motion in overhead athletes that have supported the contention that different methodologies have affected these range of motion measurements. A review of these studies reveals that the results are not consistent between studies. This may be explained by the influence of multiple technical variables, as mentioned in the previous discussion (**Table 2–6**).

Brown et al[71] found that, in 41 asymptomatic baseball players, pitchers had significantly more external rotation with the arm abducted 90 degrees than did position players. They also found that pitchers had decreased internal rotation and increased external rotation of the dominant arm compared with the nondominant arm with the arm abducted 90 degrees. However, in pitchers there was no difference in external rotation between the dominant and nondominant arm with the arm at the side. Chandler et al[72] and Kibler et al[73] observed similar findings in both elite and professional tennis players. They also found increasing loss of internal rotation with the age of the player, which they speculated may contribute to increased shoulder pathologies with tennis players as they age.

Sauers and Keuter[74] studied 103 professional baseball players (49 pitchers and 54 position players) and found that the throwing shoulder exhibited significantly increased external rotation and decreased internal rotation compared with the nonthrowing shoulder. They also found that pitchers exhibited greater external rotation compared with position players.

Bigliani et al[75] studied 148 baseball players and suggested that the active shoulder rotations were the same as passive rotations. They found that both position players and pitchers had increased external rotation and decreased internal rotation compared with the nondominant shoulder. Bak and Magnusson[76] studied a small cohort of injured ($N = 7$) and not in pain ($N = 8$) swimmers and found no significant differences between the two groups in rotations with the arm abducted 90 degrees. They also found no statistically significant difference in rotation between the injured and noninjured shoulders.

Beach and Whitney[77] studied 32 competitive swimmers (31% pain-free, 69% with pain) for internal and external rotation of the shoulder. They found nonsignificant changes in the range of motion of the shoulders in the two groups but did not find any relationship between shoulder flexibility and pain. They also found no significant difference between sides for range of motion in their cohort.

Sauers et al[78] reported that nonoverhead recreational athletes exhibited significant side-to-side asymmetries for both external and internal rotation. Passive measures with the scapula stabilized were obtained with the subjects supine. Dominant shoulder external rotation was ~5 degrees greater and dominant internal rotation was ~9 degrees less than the contralateral, nondominant shoulder. These data cast further doubt on the ability to make reasonable side-to-side comparisons in the general population.

Rotational range of motion adaptations in overhead athletes have received a great deal of attention in the sports medicine literature. The body of evidence demonstrating that overhead athletes exhibit an increase in external rotation with a concomitant decrease in internal rotation is undeniable; however, it remains unclear exactly what causes these rotational range of motion adaptations in overhead athletes.

The current theories of shoulder dysfunction in overhead athletes summarized above are predicated upon the theory that capsular alterations are the cause of these range of motion changes. For example, Jobe et al's microinstability theory suggests that the underlying problem is attenuation of the anteroinferior capsuloligamentous restraints leading to secondary impingement and rotator cuff tears. Burkhart et al's peel back theory conversely maintains that the underlying problem is posterior capsular contracture leading to altered translational kinematics and eventually to a SLAP lesion (see Chapter 6). Increased external rotation range of motion has been cited as supportive of Jobe et al's theory of micro-instability, and reduced internal rotation range of motion has been cited as supportive of Burkhart et al's peel back theory.

There is increasing evidence, however, that some of the alterations in shoulder range of motion seen in athletes may be due to alterations in the shape of the bones. Studies have demonstrated that collegiate and professional baseball players demonstrate changes in both humeral and glenoid retroversion in their throwing shoulder.[79–81] These osseous changes are attributed to proximal humerus physeal changes that are thought to occur during the developmental years of young baseball players. The magnitudes of change in humeral and glenoid retroversion are similar to the observed magnitudes of change in rotational range of motion. These studies would suggest that the throwing shoulder is essentially "spun back" into greater external rotation due to these bone alterations. It has been suggested that the observed alterations of rotational range of motion in the overhead athlete are attributed at least in part to osseous changes and are not the result of anterior capsular attenuation and posterior capsular contracture.[70]

Total Arc of Motion and the Overhead Athlete

Support for the theory that rotational range of motion adaptations are caused at least in part by osseous changes can be found by looking at the total arc of rotational motion. The total arc of motion is the sum of external rotation and internal rotation with the arm at 90 degrees of elevation. Studies of healthy overhead athletes have consistently demonstrated that in spite of the observed changes in motion in the dominant shoulder (i.e., increased external rotation and decreased internal rotation), the total arcs of motion when compared between sides are nearly identical.[74]

Numerous studies have compared the total arc of motion between the throwing and nonthrowing shoulders of baseball players and have consistently reported bilateral symmetry of total motion (**Table 2–6**). These studies have been interpreted by some to mean that for every degree of external rotation gained, there is 1 degree of internal rotation lost, subsequently maintaining a symmetric total arc of motion. According to this idea of a maintenance of total range of motion to 180 degrees, if there were osseous changes such as increased humeral retroversion, then this would create symmetric changes in range of motion based on the mechanics of rotating a rigid bar. Thus, if the humerus is spun back 10 degrees into external rotation, then there would be a mandatory decrease in internal rotation of an identical magnitude in the absence of any soft tissue changes. Unfortunately, this concept that the total arc should be maintained has not been proven, and it is unknown whether reciprocal changes are necessary for normal shoulder function in overhead sports. In addition, it is currently unknown how much of total motion is altered by soft tissue changes and how much by bone changes.

Asymmetry between sides in the total arc of motion has been implicated as a causative factor in the development of shoulder pathology in overhead athletes. Wilk et al[82] stated that the total arc of motion should be symmetric within 10 degrees of motion; that is, the throwing shoulder should not gain or lose more than 10 degrees of total arc of motion. They refer to this as the "total motion concept," whereby side-to-side asymmetry may predispose the throwing shoulder to injury.

Morgan[83] referred to the "180 degree rule," where the shoulder can safely lose 1 degree of internal rotation for every degree of external rotation gained; however, when the shoulder loses more internal rotation than is gained in external rotation, the shoulder is at risk of developing injury. We are not aware of any prospective studies evaluating the relationship between the total arc of motion and injury in the overhead athlete.

It is of interest that not all overhead sports lead to the same changes in rotational range of motion. Studies of the total range of motion in baseball players have repeatedly shown that the healthy throwing shoulder demonstrates increased external rotation, decreased internal rotation, and a symmetric total arc of motion; however, range of motion studies in tennis players have consistently reported a decrease in the total arc of motion in the dominant shoulder. Ellenbecker et al[84] studied pain-free elite male and female junior tennis players and found that both genders exhibited similar range of motion changes. External rotation was similar between the dominant and nondominant shoulders, but the dominant shoulder exhibited a significant decrease in internal rotation. As a result, the dominant shoulder exhibited a significant decrease in the total arc of motion compared with the nondominant shoulder.

Kibler et al[73] reported similar findings in elite male and female tennis players, except they found significantly greater external rotation in the dominant shoulder compared with the nondominant shoulder; however, the deficit in internal rotation exceeded the external rotation gain, and this resulted in a diminished total arc of motion in the dominant shoulder. Both the Ellenbecker et al and Kibler et al studies reported a 10 degree or greater loss of the total arc of motion in the dominant shoulder of tennis players. Similar to baseball players, tennis players are unilateral overhead athletes; that is, their overhead shoulder activity is predominantly performed by their dominant shoulder; however, the range of motion adaptations between these two sports appear quite different. We are not aware of any studies that have reported on the humeral and glenoid version of competitive tennis players. At this time, it is unclear if range of motion in tennis players is the result of osseous changes, soft tissue changes, or both.

In contrast to the unilateral nature of baseball throwing and tennis, swimmers use both arms in their sport, albeit not always symmetrically. It may therefore be expected that swimmers exhibit different range of motion adaptation patterns than athletes in sports where one arm is clearly used more than the other overhead. Like unilateral overhead athletes, swimmers exhibit increased external rotation with a concomitant decrease in internal rotation.[76,77,85]

Studies of range of motion of the shoulders of swimmers, however, have demonstrated that this shift occurs in both shoulders, as opposed to the unilateral change observed in the dominant shoulder of baseball and tennis players. As a result, the total arc of motion is symmetric between shoulders in healthy swimmers. Bak and Magnusson[76] reported a symmetric total arc of motion in elite swimmers with and without shoulder injury. We are unaware of any studies reporting on the normal values of humeral and glenoid versions in swimmers. It is unknown whether the forces in swimming are large enough to result in osseous adaptations and whether the observed motion changes in swimmers are the result of capsular adaptations.

As a result of these studies, rotational range of motion adaptations in the overhead athlete should be considered normal to a certain degree. It is clear that no one factor may be responsible for determining the absence or presence of associated shoulder pathology. Similar to the issue of increased glenohumeral joint laxity, changes in rotational range of motion in the overhead athlete should not be considered problematic unless they are correlated to symptoms.

There are significant differences in the absolute values for shoulder rotations reported in all of these studies (**Table 2–6**). In many of these studies the conditions of the measurements are not defined, such as whether the subject is sitting or supine. Few of the studies mention who performed the measurements, and in many studies the measurements are performed by more than one examiner. Some of the studies stabilize the scapula, but it is not specified if the measurements were performed with or without stabilization of the scapula in all positions studied.

Future studies of shoulder range of motion must clearly identify the conditions under which the measurements

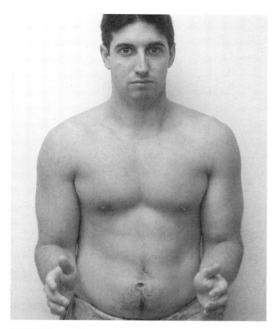

FIGURE 2–17 The starting position for measuring rotations with the arm at the side. It is important that the subject keep the elbows at the side and not be allowed to abduct.

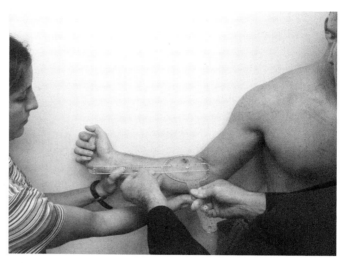

FIGURE 2–19 Passive combined motion of external rotation with arm at side can be measured with one or two examiners.

II. Passive Combined Glenohumeral and Scapulothoracic External Rotation with the Arm at the Side

The second measure of external rotation is a combined passive motion that includes the glenohumeral joint and the scapulothoracic joint. This measurement is performed by the examiner externally rotating the patient's arm until it will not go any further (**Fig. 2–19**). The examiner should not allow the patient to extend the arm behind the plane of the body or to use hyperlordosis to increase this measurement.

III. Active Combined Glenohumeral and Scapulothoracic External Rotation with the Arm at the Side

The last measurement of external rotation that can be performed is active external rotation. This can be used if the examiner is interested in the patient's ability to perform a motion, but typically it is not used for measuring motion in the office or for studies of motion. In this test the patient voluntarily moves the arm in external rotation as far as he or she can (**Fig. 2–20**). It is important to make sure that the patient does not try to increase the measure by extending the arm or by increasing lordosis.

Internal Rotation at 90 Degrees of Shoulder Elevation

With the patient standing, the arm is elevated to 90 degrees and held there by the examiner. There are three different measurements of internal rotation that can be performed with the patient standing.

I. Passive Isolated Glenohumeral Internal Rotation with the Arm at 90 Degrees

Passive, isolated glenohumeral internal rotation in this position is performed by supporting the arm and gradually internally rotating until the scapula is seen to move, the

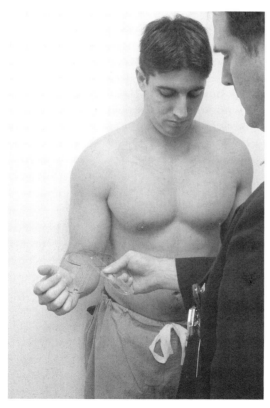

FIGURE 2–18 Passive glenohumeral external rotation with the arm at the side is defined as the first "end feel."

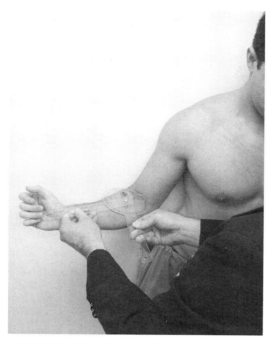

FIGURE 2–20 Active combined external rotation with the arm at the side requires the subject to hold the arm externally rotated as far as possible.

shoulder begins to hike up, or the body begins to turn (**Fig. 2–21**). It is recommended that the starting position be around 45 degrees of external rotation because some patients with severe loss of internal rotation cannot reach the zero position. In this case, the degree of loss of

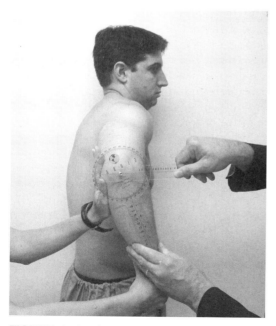

FIGURE 2–22 Combined passive internal rotation with the arm at 90 degrees of abduction can be measured with one or two examiners.

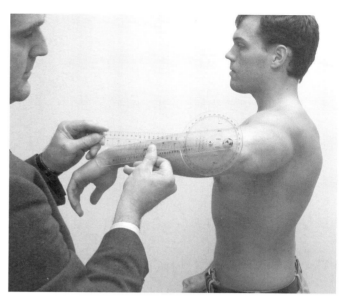

FIGURE 2–21 Passive glenohumeral internal rotation with the arm at 90 degrees of abduction.

motion is written as a negative number. It is important not to push the patient's arm forcefully into internal rotation because this position is quite painful for patients with stiff shoulders, rotator cuff disease, and arthritis of the shoulder.

II. Passive Combined Glenohumeral and Scapulothoracic Internal Rotation with the Arm at 90 Degrees
The next motion to be measured is combined passive internal rotation with the arm elevated 90 degrees. The arm is stabilized and then rotated internally until no further motion is possible (**Fig. 2–22**). The patient is asked to hold this position, and the degrees are measured using the goniometer. It is important not to push the arm into internal rotation because this can be painful.

III. Active Combined Glenohumeral and Scapulothoracic Internal Rotation with the Arm at 90 Degrees
The last type of internal rotation of the shoulder that can be measured with the arm at 90 degrees is active internal rotation. The patient is asked to move the arm in internal rotation as far as possible and hold it there (**Fig. 2–23**). It is common for patients to elevate their elbow and lean their bodies in an attempt to gain more motion, so it is important to stabilize the arm at 90 degrees and to ask the patient to stand up straight.

External Rotation at 90 Degrees of Shoulder Elevation
There are three measures of external rotation that can be measured with the arm at 90 degrees of elevation. The one measured depends upon the goal of the examination.

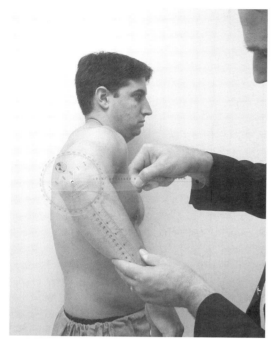

FIGURE 2-23 Combined active internal rotation with the arm at 90 degrees of abduction requires the patient to hold the arm internally rotated.

I. Passive Isolated Glenohumeral External Rotation with the Arm at 90 Degrees

Passive external rotation with the arm in this position is performed by holding the patient's arm in 90 degrees of elevation and gradually externally rotating until the first end point is reached (**Fig. 2–24**). Both visual and tactile cues as described above are used to determine when the glenohumeral motion ceases and when the scapula begins to move. A handheld goniometer is used to

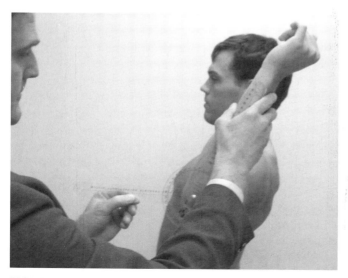

FIGURE 2-25 Passive combined external rotation with the arm at 90 degrees of abduction.

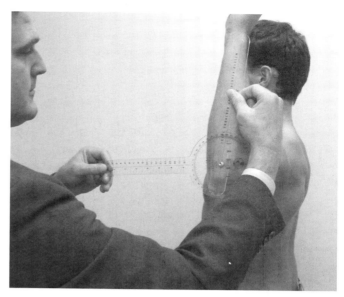

FIGURE 2-24 Passive glenohumeral external rotation with the arm at 90 degrees of abduction.

measure the rotation while having the patient maintain the position. This measure can be difficult in very loose-jointed individuals because the rotation can be so large that it is difficult to measure by one examiner.

II. Passive Combined Glenohumeral and Scapulothoracic External Rotation with the Arm at 90 Degrees

This examination is conducted by having the patient hold the arm elevated, and the examiner then passively pushes the arm into as much external rotation as the patient will allow (**Fig. 2–25**). This is measured using a goniometer with one or two examiners. It is important that the patient not be allowed to use lumbar lordosis to increase the measurement. Also, there is a tendency for patients to rotate their bodies to get more motion. This position of measurement can be painful if the joint is pushed too far, and it is important to watch the patient's face for signs that the motion is uncomfortable. This examination may be painful for patients who have arthritis or a stiff shoulder from any cause.

III. Active Combined Glenohumeral and Scapulothoracic External Rotation with the Arm at 90 Degrees

The examination is performed like the other measures of shoulder motion with the patient in this position. The patient is asked to rotate the arm externally as far as he or she can using his or her muscles (**Fig. 2–26**). This position is then held by the patient and measured using a goniometer. In some instances two examiners may be needed, but this is usually not necessary. It is important to hold the patient's arm in the plane of the body so that he or she does not use arm extension in an attempt to increase the measure.

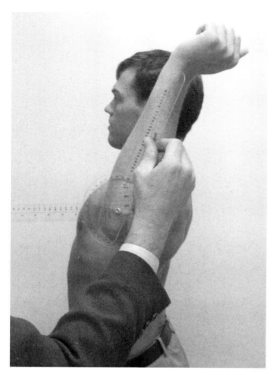

FIGURE 2–26 Active combined external rotation with the arm at 90 degrees of abduction requires the patient to hold the position of external rotation. (Starting position demonstrated here.)

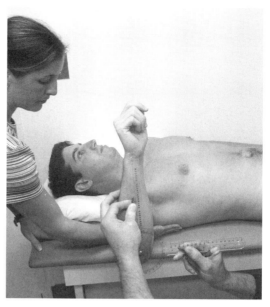

FIGURE 2–27 When measuring isolated glenohumeral motion with the patient supine, one method for detecting scapular movement is to place the hand between the table and the scapula.

Supine Examination

Measuring shoulder rotations traditionally has been performed with the patient in a supine position. The measurements can be performed with one or two examiners, but to our knowledge no study has evaluated the reliability of these measures when one examiner is used versus two examiners. Several studies have examined the reliability and reproducibility of supine measures of shoulder isolated glenohumeral or combined glenohumeral and scapulothoracic measures of shoulder motion (**Table 2–6**).

One source of variation in these studies is the techniques used to detect scapular motion. If the examiner is interested in only glenohumeral motion, then it is critical to be able to determine when scapular motion begins. The first technique is for the examiner to hold one hand between the subject and the table as the humerus is rotated (**Fig. 2–27**). When the examiner feels the scapula begin to move, then the humeral motion is stopped, and the rotation is measured. To our knowledge, this technique for measuring scapular movement has not been validated by independent measures such as a cadaver model, radiographic techniques, or electromagnetic tracking device studies.

Another technique advocated for determining scapular motion with the patient supine is for the exam-iner to place one hand on the anterior shoulder of the subject's shoulder (**Fig. 2–28**). This "scapular stabilization" technique has as its premise that the shoulder will begin to rise off the table in an anterior direction as the scapula begins to move or rotate. As the humerus is rotated, the examiner feels for the shoulder to begin to move anteriorly, which is taken to indicate that the scapula is beginning to move. The measurement of rotation is then noted using a goniometer. To our knowledge this technique for measuring scapular movement has not

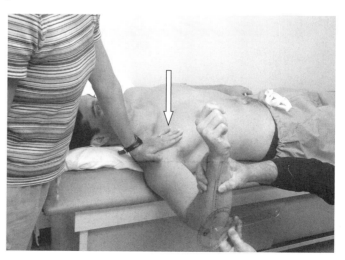

FIGURE 2–28 Another method of detecting scapular motion when measuring isolated glenohumeral motion with the patient supine is to place a hand on the anterior shoulder.

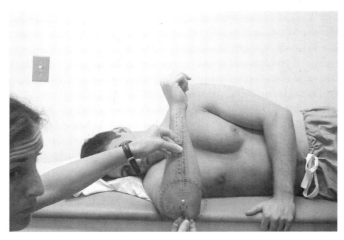

FIGURE 2–29 A technique for measuring isolated glenohumeral motion has been advocated by placing the patient in a lateral decubitus position. (Starting position demonstrated here.)

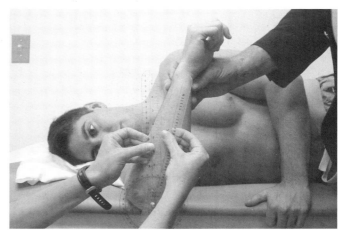

FIGURE 2–30 The technique for measuring isolated glenohumeral internal rotation with the subject in a lateral decubitus position.

been validated by an independent measure such as a cadaver model, radiographic techniques, or electromagnetic tracking device studies.

A third way to determine scapular movement with the subject supine is to visualize the shoulder complex for movement, in addition to feeling when there is resistance or an end feel is first felt. This is similar to the technique suggested previously that is used when the patient is standing. This "visual inspection" technique was studied by Awan et al,[27] who compared it to the scapular stabilization technique and found that the visual inspection technique detected scapular motion earlier than the stabilization technique for both shoulder internal rotation. They also found that the inter- and intraobserver reliability using the visual inspection method was similar to other techniques for measuring shoulder motion.

Lateral Decubitus Examination

A more recent technique for measuring shoulder internal and external rotations has been advocated by Donelly et al (personal communication). They have suggested that this technique is helpful when measuring for GIRD in the shoulders of athletic individuals. In this technique, the subject is placed in a lateral decubitus position with the affected arm on the table side (**Fig. 2–29**). It is important that the patient be stabilized so that he or she does not lean and the patient's body stays perpendicular to the table. This positioning is felt to help stabilize the scapula of the shoulder nearer the table. The down arm should be placed in an elevation of 90 degrees. The examiner then rotates the arm until resistance is felt or the scapula is felt to move. Both internal (**Fig. 2–30**) and external (**Fig. 2–31**) rotations should be performed.

Donelly et al have suggested that both sides be measured to determine if GIRD is present or not. A side-to-side difference of less than 20 degrees of internal rotation is considered normal, whereas more than that is considered a risk for future injury to the shoulder complex with throwing.

To our knowledge this technique for measuring scapular movement has not been validated by such independent measures as a cadaver model, radiographic techniques, or electrogoniometric studies. The results of these tests have not yet been published, so they have not had the advantage of peer review. Although we agree with the intent to measure isolated glenohumeral motion compared with combined motions, these techniques require further study of their overall accuracy, reliability, and relationship to other methods for measuring shoulder motion.

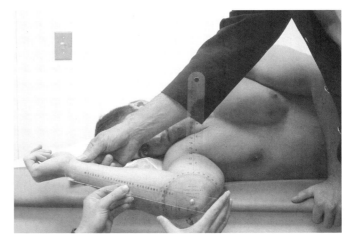

FIGURE 2–31 The technique for measuring isolated glenohumeral external rotation with the subject in a lateral decubitus position.

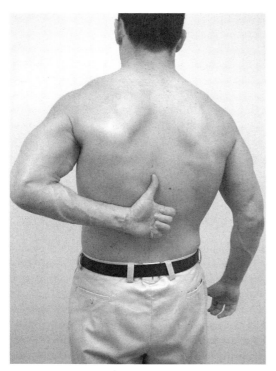

FIGURE 2–32 Technique for measuring internal rotation with the hand up the middle of the back, with the thumb up.

■ Measuring Internal Rotation Up the Back

In 1994 the examination committee of the American Shoulder and Elbow Society recommended a system for measuring shoulder range of motion.[90] The members recommended that shoulder external-internal rotation should be measured with the arm elevated 90 degrees, but they recommended that internal rotation be measured with the hand up the back (**Fig. 2–32**). Their recommendation for using this method for internal rotation was based on the recognition that internal rotation up the back is important for reaching into the back pocket for a wallet, for toilet hygiene, for fastening a bra, putting on a belt, and scratching one's back.

The technique recommended for measuring internal rotation up the back was to instruct the patient to place the thumb up and then reach up the center of the back as far as possible. The examiner was to note how high the tip of the thumb reached up the back. This measure was to be based on the spinal level that the thumb reached. However, normative values for this measure were not reported. The commonly accepted landmarks for internal rotation up the back are roughly the following: back pocket, belt (L4–L5), lower border of scapula (T7), midscapula (T3), and prominence C spine (C7).[91]

Subsequent examiners have noted that internal rotation up the back was not an isolated shoulder movement but that it involved the glenohumeral, scapulothoracic, elbow, wrist, and hand movements. Mallon et al[92] examined the components of upper extremity motion that contributed to internal rotation up the back. They found that internal rotation up the back was primarily a combination of scapulothoracic, glenohumeral, and elbow motion. The scapulothoracic joint contributed more to this motion than the glenohumeral joint at a ratio of ~2:1. Mallon et al also found that elbow flexion contributed a significant amount to the measure, particularly in the portion of the motion from the sacrum to more proximal vertebral levels. They concluded that evaluating internal rotation up the back is a complex motion and cannot be considered a measure of glenohumeral motion alone.

> Although internal rotation up the back is an excellent functional measure, it is not an accurate measure of isolated shoulder motion.

As a result, one might expect the relationship of internal rotation up the back to other measures of shoulder internal rotation to be inexact; however, in clinical practice it often appears in some overhead athletes that a loss of internal rotation at 90 degrees of elevation is accompanied by a corresponding loss of internal rotation up the back. Kibler et al[73] evaluated 57 athletes, with one observer measuring internal rotation up the back using spinal level and one observer measuring passive internal rotation with the subject supine. They found no correlation between the spinal level measures and internal rotation with the arm elevated 90 degrees. They concluded that different portions of the capsule may be stressed by the two measures.

■ Factors Affecting the End Feel When Measuring Joint Motion

When measuring shoulder rotational motions passively in a patient with no pain, the first resistance felt before scapulothoracic motion occurs is the limit of the glenohumeral joint motion. This end feel is due to a host of factors, including the bone geometry in that individual and the length of excursion of the ligaments, tendons, muscles, and other soft tissue.

Others have suggested that this end feel can be affected by several variables, particularly pain. Maitland[93] suggested that pain should be factored into the measurements, so that four measures should be taken when measuring joint range of motion (**Table 2–16**). He also suggested that if pain is the primary problem, the pain (P1 position) will come before resistance is felt (R1). If stiffness is the main problem, the resistance (R1) will occur before pain (P1), and mobilization and stretching would be indicated to treat the stiffness. To our knowledge

TABLE 2-16 Maitland Range of Motion Scheme

		Movement	Definition
R1	Resistance 1		Point in motion where resistance is first detected
R2	Resistance 2		Point in motion where no further motion can be achieved
P1	Pain 1		Point in range of motion where pain is first reported by patient
P2	Pain 2		Point in range where no further motion can be achieved due to pain

Modified from Maitland, GD, Vertebral Manipulation. 5 ed. 1986, London: Butterworth.

this schema has not been independently studied, and it has not gained widespread acceptance.

> When measuring range of motion in a patient with pain, reexamination at a time when there is less pain may be beneficial to obtain a more complete examination.

Another schema for measuring end feel was promulgated by Cyriax[94] in his textbook first published in 1947. He divided the tissues that restrict motion into contractile elements (i.e., muscle) and noncontractile elements (i.e., ligaments, capsule, bone). When passively examining a joint, the examiner feels different sensations at the extreme of joint motion. Cyriax suggested that there were six of these end feels: bone to bone, spasm, capsular feel, springy block, tissue approximation, and empty feel.[94]

A bone-to-bone end feel is an abrupt end point when two hard surfaces meet, such as in terminal extension of the elbow. Spasm also can have a hard end feel, but it is characterized by a "vibrant twang" felt by the examiner. Capsular feel typically is felt prior to full range of motion and is as if a piece of thick leather were being stretched. Cyriax suggested that this end feel may indicate a nonacute arthritis. A springy block is when there is rebound after the extreme of motion, such as might be felt when a meniscus is trapped in the knee joint and the joint springs back from movement. Tissue approximation is a normal sensation due to passive motion, such as that seen with full passive motion of the normal joint. An empty feel occurs when there is considerable pain before full motion is reached, yet there is no mechanical resistance to further motion. This gives the examiner an "empty" feel, as if more motion would be possible if the pain could be eliminated.

Paris and Loubert[95] have suggested that there are 15 end feels, with 5 normal and 10 abnormal. Donatelli[96] says in his text that this system may be difficult to use and that it is sufficient to limit the variables in the assessment of end feel to pain or no pain when resistance is felt.

These systems of end feel do suggest that measuring range of motion in patients who are symptomatic may be more difficult than in normal subjects. It is suggested that patients who are being treated for painful conditions be examined more than once and that they be measured before and after any intervention. In many patients motion will be improved once they have pain relief. It is not uncommon to demonstrate more motion in patients under anesthesia than when they are awake.

> Systems of various types of end feel have not been validated and need further study.

The utility of the use of a variety of end feels in clinical practice for shoulder conditions has not been validated. Although there are many proponents of the Cyriax system, it is cumbersome and difficult to use clinically. Special training has been recommended for those interested in this system or similar systems. Rothstein[97] agreed in an editorial, maintaining that we "have no evidence for the use of capsular patterns. The patterns represent a concept widely accepted and widely used, but one never validated." The reality is that an end point is due to a variety of anatomic structures that cannot be divided by feel alone. When the limit of movement of a joint is obtained, it is a summation of the bony anatomy, the soft tissue, and the muscular components. The onus is on those who advocate this system to validate it against cadaveric or pathological studies.

One study by Pellecchia et al[98] evaluated 21 painful shoulders with two therapists who had training in the Cyriax method of evaluation of musculoskeletal complaints. Using the history, examination, and assessment forms of Cyriax, they were able to agree on the type of lesion present in the Cyriax system in 19 of 21 patients. They also were able to agree on such diagnoses as capsulitis, suprascapular neuritis, and subscapular tendinitis. Although the examiners agreed with each other, there was no independent assessment of their diagnoses using examination by a physician or with radiographs. In addition, the validity of the Cyriax system against a gold standard was not evaluated. We recommend significantly more study of this system before it can be suggested for routine clinical evaluation of the shoulder.

■ Clinically Significant Motions versus Goniometric Measurements

These studies that question the accuracy of measuring shoulder motion have caused some observers to suggest that the measurement of motion is not as important as the ability of the subjects to achieve function. The relationship of motion to function has been studied only in a limited manner. How much motion must be lost before it affects function? Similarly, using standard measures of motion with a goniometer, how much motion change must there be for an examiner to know that there has really been a change in the patient motion? If the measures are sensitive for motion change, but the change does not reflect shoulder function, why bother with measuring motion at all?

Studies of interobserver reliability suggest that a handheld goniometer can clinically detect a significant difference of only 5 to 10 degrees.[99,100] In other words, a variability of 5 to 10 degrees may not indicate any real change in the status of the shoulder range of motion. For repeat measurements by one examiner, a minimum change of 3 to 5 degrees has been suggested as necessary to define a clinically significant change.[100]

One must question, however, which motions are clinically significant to measure. Outcome measurements have been developed that inquire about a variety of functional motions, such as the ability to reach the back of one's head, to comb one's hair, to reach into the back pocket, to do perineal care, and to reach a cabinet. The patient's responses to these questions are typically incorporated into a score that is used to measure clinical impairment or clinical improvement after procedures.[90,101–104]

Triffett[105] studied the relationship of shoulder motion to function in a cohort of patients with a variety of diagnoses. He found that range of motion in certain directions correlated well with specific activities of daily living. Internal rotation correlated best with the ability to wash the back, whereas elevation was best correlated with the ability to comb the hair. He noted that few functional motions of the shoulder require elevation over 90 degrees. There was no correlation between range of motion and the ability to perform work or sports, but Triffett did not specifically evaluate an athletic population.

This discussion of the relationship between range of motion and function is important for treating athletes who present with shoulder pain that prevents full participation in their sport. It has been argued that accurate measurement of shoulder motion may allow one to predict which athlete is at risk for the development of shoulder problems.[106] Although it may be important to measure accurately their range of motion and flexibility, the ultimate functional question is whether they can participate in their sport or not. Attempts have been made to develop sport-related outcome measures for the upper extremity,[107] but it is unknown if the scores or the examination findings predict the ability to perform a sport or not.

Pearl suggests that we should really ask the patient to demonstrate three pertinent motions in external rotation and four in internal rotation that more accurately reflect their function (Dr. Michael Pearl, personal communication). Motion analysis studies have demonstrated the degree of motion needed to achieve activities of daily living (**Table 2–17; Figs. 2–33, 2–34**).

TABLE 2–17 Range of Motion Needed for Activities of Daily Living

Activity	Range of Motion
Eating	70–100° horizontal adduction 45–60° abduction
Combing hair	30–70° horizontal adduction 105–120° abduction 90° external rotation
Reach perineum	75–90° horizontal adduction 30–45° abduction 90°+ internal rotation
Tuck in shirt	50–60° horizontal adduction 55–65° abduction 90° external rotation
Hand behind head	10–15° horizontal adduction 110–125° forward flexion 90° external rotation
Put something on shelf	70–80° horizontal adduction 70–80° forward flexion 45° external rotation
Wash opposite shoulder	60–90° forward flexion 60–120° horizontal adduction

Source: Adapted with permission from Magee D. Orthopedic physical examination, Vol. 1. Philadelphia: Saunders; 2002:1020.

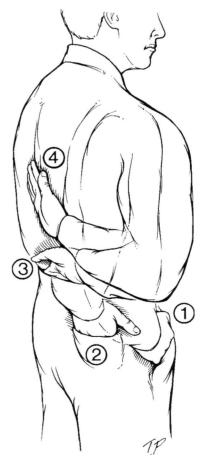

FIGURE 2–33 Four functional positions of internal rotation advocated by Pearl to be recorded in the examination (Dr. Michael Pearl, personal communication).

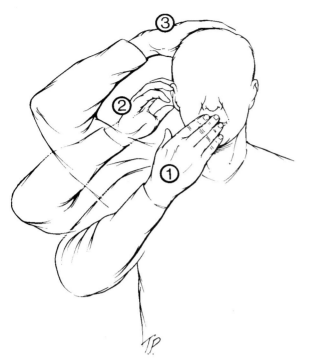

FIGURE 2–34 Three functional positions of external rotation advocated by Pearl to be recorded in the examination (Dr. Michael Pearl, personal communication).

■ Scapular Motions and Examination

The role of the scapula in shoulder motion has received increasing attention due to its central role in supporting the arm and its role in transferring forces from the trunk and lower extremities to the arm in throwing or overhead sports.[108] Scapular motions are also considered to be important because some authors have suggested that abnormal scapular positioning may contribute to impingement of the rotator cuff or to symptoms of instability.[109–111] Scapular malpositioning has been suggested to be a contributing factor in the development of shoulder problems in athletes.[106]

Kibler and McMullen[112] have promoted the concept that it is important to evaluate the scapula, and they suggest that it has four roles in upper extremity function. The first role was mentioned above and includes its role in moving in an integrated way with the humerus for upper extremity motion. The second role is to provide motion along the thorax, where it provides a stable base for the upper extremity to generate force and power. The third role is to allow elevation of the acromion so that the rotator cuff can glide beneath it without causing contact or impingement of the tendons against the acromion. The fourth role of the scapula is to provide a conduit for the transfer of energy from the trunk to the hand during athletic activities that involve overhead or ballistic movements. Overhead athletic activities, such as throwing a ball, hitting a tennis ball, and

swimming, require a sequential transfer of force from the legs to the hips and torso and eventually to the upper extremity. Kibler and McMullen have called alterations in these synchronized motions "scapular dyskinesis."

Scapular motion is one of the most complex aspects of the shoulder, however, and the examination requires study and practice. Isolated scapular motion has been difficult to study for several reasons. First, the motions are complex and occur in three dimensions. The nomenclature for describing these motions is not easily comprehended, nor is it easy to use in everyday discussion. Words like *protraction*, *retraction*, and *tilt* are not everyday words for most of us and can be difficult to conceptualize. Second, the scapula has a peculiar shape, with curves and angles that are variable from patient to patient. This curved bone moves on another curved surface of the thorax, so the motions of two curved surfaces on each other can be very complex. Abnormalities of the thorax theoretically could affect those motions, as seen in patients with scoliosis, but fortunately this has proven not to be the case.

Another reason scapular motions are difficult to assess is that the scapula is largely covered by muscle, making it hard to visualize the underlying motion of the scapula. Also, the interaction of the scapular position with the glenohumeral joint is nearly impossible to deduce because the glenohumeral joint is deep to the surface. It is virtually impossible on physical examination to deduce the position of the glenoid due to these factors. Finally, it is difficult to know if changes in scapular position or movement are due to intrinsic problems with the scapula, or if they are compensatory for other shoulder pathologies. Despite this cautionary tone, progress has been made in developing techniques to measure scapula motion in clinical practice. The goal of this chapter is to unravel some of the mystery regarding scapular motion and function.

Scapular Motion versus Glenohumeral Motion in Elevation

Some studies have attempted to divide physical examination of the upper extremity into two separate, identifiable component parts: humeral motion and scapular motion. The AAOS manual for motion suggests that if the scapula is stabilized as one elevates the arm, then the glenohumeral motion occurs first and with arm elevation can be measured to be around 90 degrees.[40] Clarke et al[18] suggested passive abduction in a cohort of patients ages 20 to 40 was 85.6 in females and 77.4 in males.

Gagey and Gagey[113] reported that humeral elevation before scapular motion occurs if the scapula is stabilized at less than 90 degrees; 95% of the subjects with normal shoulders had glenohumeral motion in elevation between 85 and 90 degrees. These studies each report values less than those reported by Lintner et al[114] and Sauers et al,[78] who reported passive, isolated glenohumeral shoulder elevation in the scapular plane to be ~109 degrees and 112 degrees, respectively.

There has been one study evaluating the reliability of measuring isolated glenohumeral motion in elevation. Hoving et al[115] had six rheumatologists measure elevation of the shoulder using an inclinometer. They measured glenohumeral abduction (or isolated glenohumeral motion) and then total shoulder elevation (combined glenohumeral and scapulothoracic) in six patients who had varying degrees of shoulder pain and stiffness. The rheumatologists reexamined the patients 1 hour later to determine test–retest reliability. In this cohort of patients, they found glenohumeral abduction to be a range of 47 to 108 degrees and total shoulder abduction of 68 to 140 degrees; however, they found the intrarater reliability on average for glenohumeral abduction to be 0.35 and for total shoulder abduction 0.35. Hoving et al[115] concluded that the results may have been better if the examiners were more familiar with the measuring devices and if the patient population was more homogeneous. They also questioned the need to measure isolated motions of the glenohumeral joint if time was an issue.

> It is difficult to determine isolated glenohumeral motion in elevation due to a variety of factors that call into question the clinical usefulness of this measure.

Subsequent biomechanical studies have demonstrated that it is difficult to stabilize the shoulder so that only glenohumeral motion can be measured with elevation. When elevating the arm actively, although a majority of scapular movement occurs above 90 degrees in most studies, there is some scapular motion below this level. Saha[116] noted that the first phase of arm elevation occurs in the first 30 to 60 degrees and is highly variable. He referred to this portion of upper extremity elevation as the "setting phase of the scapula."

The concept that the scapula "sets" and then glenohumeral motion occurs is not supported by biomechanical studies using live subjects. Instead, the scapular position changes depending on the need to place the arm in space and on the demands placed upon the upper extremity. Although the ratio of movement of the scapulothoracic joint to the glenohumeral joint may remain constant over a certain range, both are still moving throughout that range. The finding that the scapula and humerus movements were sometimes independent of each other opened the door for further study of scapular motion and its relationship to normal and abnormal shoulder movements.

The Resting Position of the Scapula

The assessment of scapular position begins with defining its position with the arm at rest. The scapula rests at an angle to the coronal plane of the body, so that a line drawn through the scapula demonstrates that the "scapular plane" compared with the coronal plane is ~30 degrees (**Fig. 2–4**). This position has been reported to be the plane that allows the humerus the optimum rotation for elevation of the arm. This has been referred to as the plane of the scapula when the arm is placed 30 to 40 degrees anterior to the plane of the body (or the coronal plane).

It should be noted that the plane of the scapula refers to only one plane of the relationship of the scapula to the thorax and not to the relationship of the amount of tilt in the scapula to the thorax. In the other planes, the scapula at rest is rotated so that its medial border is about 3 degrees from the midline.[117] It is also slightly tilted forward so that the superior edge is closer to the thorax than the lower edge. Fung et al,[12] in a study of cadavers, found that relative to the spine the scapular positions were 3 degrees of lateral rotation, minus 2 degrees for backward tilt, and 40 degrees of internal rotation.

Scapular position at rest has been considered important by some investigators because it may disclose the presence of other abnormalities. The static position of the scapula with the arm at rest can be influenced by posture and curvature of the spine. Culham and Peat[118] reported that the scapula became more retracted with age in a cohort of 91 women between the ages of 20 and 85. They postulated that this retraction was due to increasing thoracic kyphosis with aging. They found that forward tilt of the scapula when viewed from the side (sagittal plane) was ~9 degrees and that it increased with age as the subjects became more kyphotic.

Resting Scapular Position and the Lennie Test

Sobush et al[119] took the measurement of the resting position of the scapula to new levels with a study in which they attempted to quantify the resting position of the scapula with the so-called Lennie test. In that study they measured multiple landmarks of the scapula (**Fig. 2–35**) and calculated the angular position on the thorax (**Fig. 2–36**). These measures were then validated using radiographs taken of each subject. Sobush et al found that the superior angle of the scapula was at the level of the second rib, that the medial border of the scapular spine approximated the spinous process of the third thoracic vertebrae, and that the scapula on the dominant side tends to be farther from the midline than the nondominant arm. This test took less than 15 minutes to perform, had moderate to high intertester reliability, and was found to measure accurately scapular position compared with the radiographic measures as a standard.

The three-dimensional position of the scapula with the arm at rest was determined using three-dimensional spatial tracking sensors by Pearl et al.[11] They demonstrated that with the arm at the side, "the average humeroscapular position was 25 degrees of elevation in the 62 degree plane with 47 degrees external rotation relative to the sagittal plane of the scapula." Although this description

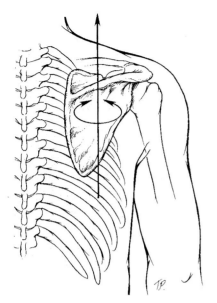

FIGURE 2–45 Scapular internal or external rotation occurs along its vertical or long axis, as viewed from above.

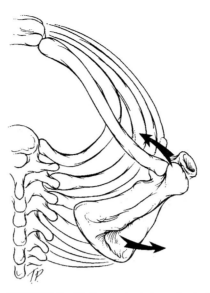

FIGURE 2–47 Scapular internal rotation along its vertical axis from behind.

scapula on the thorax. Rotation of the scapula is one of the more difficult movements of the scapula to understand and visualize. It is also one of the most difficult to see when elevating the arm due to the muscle covering the scapula and due to the complexity of the motion.

There have been numerous studies evaluating scapular motion with elevation in flexion and abduction (**Table 2–18**). When the arm is elevated, the scapula moves laterally or upwardly rotates in a linear fashion (i.e., as elevation increases, the scapula moves laterally at a similar rate). The magnitude of upward rotation of the

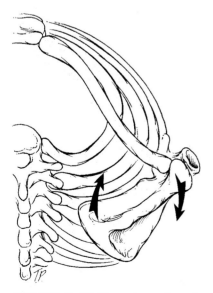

FIGURE 2–46 Scapular external rotation along its vertical axis, as viewed from behind.

scapula is not very different when the arm is elevated in the plane of the body (abduction in the coronal plane), the scapular plane (abduction in the scapular plane), and the frontal plane (forward flexion). When lifting the arm in the plane of the body, however, the scapular upward rotation increases faster from 40 to 90 degrees of elevation than when elevating the arm in other planes. This can be felt when you lift your arm in this plane where your arms are even with your body or slightly behind.[12]

The tilt of the scapula that occurs as the arm is elevated has also been studied by several researchers. The amount of tilt that occurs with full arm elevation is around 10 degrees. Several studies have verified that the most scapular tilt occurs at the extreme of elevation. In our passive model the amount of tilt increased the most above 90 degrees of elevation. The amount of tilt seen at lower levels of elevation was the same for the three movements (elevation plane of the body, elevation in the scapular plane, and elevation in flexion), but there was more tilt at lower levels of flexion when the arm was lifted in front of the body (forward flexed).

Because scapular internal and external rotation is the most difficult to conceptualize and to evaluate upon examination, there have been no clinical studies of this motion and its relationship to disease. The only studies of this motion are biomechanical studies using radiographs or three-dimensional electromagnetic sensors. As the arm is raised and the scapula moves laterally, the amount of scapular internal rotation decreases as the arm is elevated (in other words, the scapula externally rotates). Most of the internal and external rotation occurs with the arm elevated greater than 90 degrees.[12]

The scapular internal and external rotation was the scapular motion most influenced by the direction the arm was elevated in a passive cadaver model.[12] The greatest external rotation was seen with elevation of the arm in the coronal plane, followed by elevation in the scapular plane elevation and elevation in flexion (sagittal plane). The amount of scapular internal and external rotation retraction reported in the literature varies widely, with the studies using radiographic techniques reporting less retraction than studies that used more sophisticated three-dimensional techniques (**Table 2–18**). When the arm is elevated 90 degrees and externally rotated, this external rotation of the scapula does not occur until the extreme of humerus external rotation.[13]

■ Clinicial Evaluation of Scapular Motions

Scapular motion measurements in clinical practice initially were subjective evaluations by an examiner where the subject was observed from the back, and abnormal or "asynchronous" scapular motions were noted by the examiner.[121] The presence of a "hitch" or a shrug with elevation was felt to be indicative of some underlying shoulder problem. This asynchronous movement of the scapula on the shoulder blade was described as "scapular dyskinesis."

Measurement of scapular motion in clinical practice has taken several forms since the observations of Pappas et al[121] that scapular motion is important in athletic performance. The first records movement of the medial scapular border away from the thoracic spine. The second involves the use of inclinometers that can be utilized to measure the movement of the scapular spine. The third describes patterns of scapulothoracic motion and relates them to specific pathologies of the shoulder complex.

This section will concentrate on the clinical evaluation of scapula positioning and scapular motion. Scapular winging is covered in Chapter 3. It should be noted, however, that there are a variety of conditions that can result in scapular winging or scapular movement disorders. Scapular winging is most commonly caused by injury to the long thoracic nerve with resulting weakness in the serratus anterior muscle (**Fig. 2–48**). This can sometimes be seen at rest in more severe cases, but mere forward flexion of the arms can make it more prominent (**Fig. 2–49**).

The first challenge when examining the posterior thorax is to determine the scapular position, then determine if it is within the limits of normal. This can be done by simple observation, but there have been several attempts to make this evaluation more scientific.

Lateral Scapular Slide Test

The first clinical study of scapular positioning was performed by DiVeta et al,[122] who measured the distance from

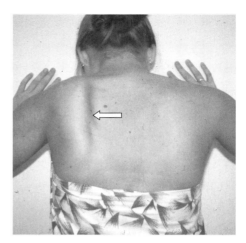

FIGURE 2–48 Scapular winging due to long thoracic nerve palsy may be visible with the arms at the side in severe cases.

the posterolateral edge of the acromion to the spinous process of the third thoracic vertebra (**Fig. 2–50**). They called this the "scapular distance." To normalize for scapular size, the scapular width was measured from the same point on the acromion to the medial border of the scapula. To normalize for subject size, the two measures were used as a ratio, referred to as scapular abduction. The measures were performed by one examiner for two trials after a 1-minute rest period. DiVeta et al reported excellent reliability for one examiner for scapular distance (ICC = 0.94), scapular size (ICC = 0.85), and scapular abduction (ICC = 0.78).

Subsequent study by Neiers and Worrel[123] found scapular distance and scapular size had good-to-high reliability (ICC = 0.80 and 0.96, respectively), but that scapular abduction had an ICC of only 0.34. They suggested that inaccuracies of the first two measures were compounded when they were used as a ratio. They also suggested that these measures, particularly the ratio, should be interpreted with caution.

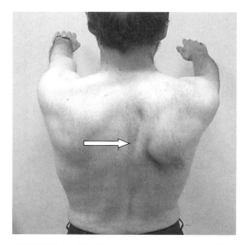

FIGURE 2–49 Scapular winging can be accentuated simply by asking the subject to forward flex the arms.

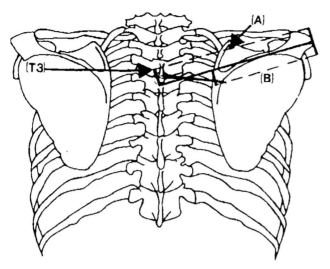

FIGURE 2–50 The scapular distance is a ratio of two measures, as suggested by DiVeta et al. (Adapted with permission from DiVeta J, Walker ML, Skibinski B. Relationship between performance of selected scapular muscles and scapular abduction in standing subjects. Phys Ther 1990;70(8):470–476; discussion 476–479.)

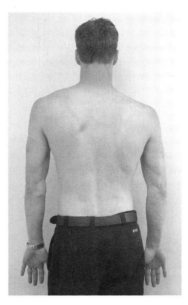

FIGURE 2–51 The first position recommended by Kibler et al for measuring the scapula is with the arm at the side.

Kibler[124] described a modification of this technique with the arm in different degrees of abduction: with the arm at the side (position 1), the arm abducted with the hand resting on the hip (position 2), and with the arm abducted 90 degrees (position 3) (**Figs. 2–51, 2–52, 2–53**). He measured from the medial border of the scapula to the nearest vertebral spinous process. Although the results were never published in a peer review journal, Kibler suggested that intratester ICC was between 0.84 and 0.88, and that intertester reliability was between 0.77 and 0.85.[108]

Kibler reported that a difference in any measure of scapular slide of 1.5 cm between the symptomatic and asymptomatic extremities was abnormal. He and his colleagues postulated that this measure was clinically helpful in determining the presence of scapular dyskinesia and that it could be useful in the assessment and treatment of patients with shoulder pain.[108,112,125–127] They also suggested that the lateral slide test was more diagnostic of type I and II scapular dyskinesis patterns[112] (see below). To date these findings have not been substantiated by any

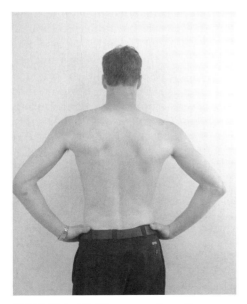

FIGURE 2–52 The second position recommended by Kibler et al for measuring the scapular position is with the hands on the hips.

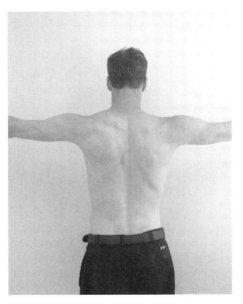

FIGURE 2–53 The third position recommended by Kibler et al for measuring the scapular position is with the arms abducted 90 degrees.

other studies in the literature, and one study suggests that this correlation is inexact.[128]

Daniels et al[129] evaluated the validity of the lateral scapular slide test in all three positions in nine subjects seeking medical evaluation for shoulder pain. They compared the clinical measures obtained on the skin surface to the actual distances between the spinous process and the scapula as seen on radiographs. They found that the lateral scapular slide test was valid in the first two test positions (0 and 45 degrees of abduction, $r \geq 0.80$), but not in the third test position (90 degrees of abduction). They therefore recommended caution when interpreting the lateral scapular slide test at the 90-degree position.

Gibson et al[130] evaluated the intratester and intertester reliability of DiVeta's scapular distance measurement and all three of Kibler's scapular slide measures using 32 subjects. They found that the DiVeta measure had excellent intratester and intertester reliability, with ICCs greater than 0.90. The ICC for intratester reliability for the Kibler measures was generally greater than 0.81 for all measures, but there were several measures where there were significant differences between the trials for one examiner despite this. The intertester reliabilities revealed decreasing ICC with increasing abduction, so that the ICC for position 1 was 0.67 to 0.69, for position 2 0.52 to 0.53, and for position 3 0.18 to 0.28. Gibson et al felt that palpating and measuring to the inferior border of the scapula was difficult, and they concluded that further study of these measurements to improve the reliability was warranted.

> Tests of scapular mobility based on measurements to the thoracic spine are accurate only at lower degrees of elevation and not greater than 60 degrees of arm elevation.

A second study was performed by Odom et al,[128] who used the scapular slide to determine if the measurements could be employed to distinguish patients with shoulder symptoms from those who do not have shoulder impairments They found that the ICCs were poor for all three arm positions between observers for patients with or without symptoms. They also found that the sensitivity and specificity of the measures based on a side-to-side difference of 1.5 cm were 28% and 53%, respectively, with the arm at the side, 50% and 58%, respectively, for the arm in position 2, and 34% and 52%, respectively, with the arm abducted 90 degrees. Odom et al concluded that the lateral slide was not reliable and was not accurate for distinguishing shoulders with dysfunction from those without.

Koslow et al[131] evaluated the specificity of the lateral scapular slide test in asymptomatic competitive athletes who had no shoulder symptoms or history of shoulder problems. They found that 52 of the 71 subjects (73%) displayed a difference of at least 1.5 cm in one or more of the three positions. They also found overall specificity of the test to be 26.8% for asymmetry. Koslow et al concluded that asymmetry is common in noninjured athletes and that this test frequently fails to determine a negative result in asymptomatic individuals. They concluded that the presence of variances in scapular position did not seem to indicate shoulder dysfunction.

Daniels et al[129] also studied the intrarater and interobserver reliability of the lateral scapular slide test in 18 shoulders of 9 patients with shoulder pathology. Three athletic trainers tested the subjects, with the arms of the subjects abducted 0, 45, and 90 degrees. One examiner who repeated the measures reported excellent intrarater reliability for all three test positions (ICC = 0.91 − 0.97). Among the three observers interrater reliability was excellent for the first position (ICC = 0.87) and the second position (ICC = 0.83), but decreased to fair to good for the third test position (ICC = 0.71).

A study by Crotty and Smith[132] from the Mayo Clinic verified that the ICC were acceptable for the DiVeta measurement and for the measurement of the Kibler 1 position, but in that study they did not measure other scapular positions, nor did they measure patients with shoulder pathology. They found that intertester ICCs were lower than intratester ICCs for all measures; however, they found that the three measures did not record any significant change in scapular positioning in a cohort of swimmers when checked before and after practice.

Although Sobush et al[119] reported that the Lennie test described earlier had moderate-to-high accuracy when compared with radiographs, they performed only a measure of static scapular position with the arm at the side. Also, although Sobush et al concluded that these measures could be helpful in measuring scapular position at rest, the measures were validated for only one position with the arm at the side. We are not aware of any further study of the Lennie test, and its use in clinical practice has been limited. Burkhart et al[66] suggest, however, that static malpositioning of the scapula is a contributing factor to shoulder problems in athletes, so further study is warranted.

> The scapular slide test has not been demonstrated to be diagnostic for any one shoulder pathology, and its exact place in the shoulder examination has yet to be defined.

Scapular Positioning with Inclinometers

A second technique for measuring scapular position has been reported by Johnson et al[28] and involves the use of an inclinometer. This device is a modified digital protractor that can be attached to the scapular spine and used to measure scapular upward rotation. Scapular upward rotation measures are obtained with the arm positioned at four separate positions of humeral elevation (rest, 60, 90, and 120 degrees) in the scapular plane.

The validity of this device was evaluated by comparing measures obtained using the inclinometer to measures obtained using a previously validated method that incorporated three-dimensional electromagnetic sensors attached to the skin with plastic mounting devices and tape. Johnson et al[28] found a difference in reported values between the two techniques of 10 to 13 degrees, and for each degree measured by the inclinometer, there was a change of 0.9 to 1.2 degrees registered by the electromagnetic sensors. Only one tester made the measures, and no intertester reliability was performed, but the intratester reliability was excellent for all between-trial measures at each of the four test positions (ICC = 0.89 – 0.96).

A subsequent study by Borsa et al[26] took an additional measurement of scapular upward rotation at 30 degrees of humeral elevation. They reported excellent intraobserver or between-trial reliability when comparing three separate repeated measures during one testing session (ICC = 0.97 – 0.99). They reported the between-session reliability between measures obtained 1 week apart to be excellent at the lower positions with decreasing reliability at the later test positions (ICC at rest or 0 degree elevation was 0.94, ICC at 30 degrees was 83, ICC at 60 degrees was 0.73, ICC at 90 degrees was 0.70, and ICC at 120 degrees was 0.56). The intertester reliability and diagnostic value of this device need further study before its widespread use can be recommended.

Barnett et al[133] studied a similar inclinometer with legs that rested on specific bony landmarks on the scapula. This device was called the "locator," and the researchers compared the measures obtained with the device to measures using electromagnetic sensors. They applied the device at 10-degree increments of elevation up to 90 degrees of elevation. Barnett et al found that reproducibility of the measures by two examiners varied according to which angle of the scapula was being measured. They suggested that the device could be accurate for lateral scapular motion to around 3 to 4 degrees. They also suggested that the device could measure scapular tip with an accuracy of 2.5 degrees and rotation to 3.6 degrees. This device was not validated for measure over 90 degrees of abduction. To our knowledge this device has not been used in a widespread manner in clinical practice.

In summary, inclinometers may have some usefulness for research purposes when measuring scapular motion but their usefulness for the clinician is currently limited. This conclusion is due in part to two observations. The first is that some of the measures that are obtained more accurately with inclinometers, particularly upward scapular rotation, have not been proven to have distinct clinical significance. The effort needed to use an inclinometer may not translate into a clinically relevant measurement. The second observation is that, although inclinometers may be capable of measuring small differences in scapular motion, it is not known if these differences are clinically significant. Inclinometers reinforce the findings using other methods of measuring scapular motion, specifically that scapular motion above 60 degrees of elevation is difficult to measure accurately and reproducibly. Further study of the clinical utility of inclinometers is warranted.

■ Scapular Dyskinesis

Kibler[112] defined scapular dyskinesis as "observable alterations in the position of the scapula and the patterns of scapular motion in relation to the thoracic cage." These abnormalities could be caused by bony posture, such as excessive thoracic kyphosis or increased cervical lordosis. Kibler suggested that it could also be seen secondary to malunited clavicle fractures with shortening or angulation. Acromioclavicular (AC) joint injuries that were painful or that did not provide a support for the shoulder could result in scapular dyskinesis.

The most common cause of scapular dyskinesis occurs, however, as a result of abnormal muscle firing patterns or due to altered muscle activation and coordination with extremity elevation and rotation. The muscle injury could be the result of injury to the nerves due to direct trauma or traction, due to chronic strain from repetitive activities or overuse, and from painful conditions around the shoulder that cause muscle inhibition and weakness. Scapular dyskinesis also could be the result of inflexibility or contracture due to any cause, such as the loss of internal rotation as seen in baseball throwers (also known as GIRD). It has been postulated that this loss of internal rotation causes the scapula to over-rotate in the follow-through phase of a throw or a swing. This leads to increased scapula protraction as the arm is adducted. This position of the scapula increases its vulnerability to lesions of the superior labrum and rotator cuff.

Types of Scapular Dyskinesis

Kibler and McMullen[112] described three patterns of scapular dyskinesis based on which part of the scapula becomes prominent with movement. The evaluation begins by observing the patient with the arm at the side, and any asymmetry or winging is noted (**Fig. 2–51**). Next, the patient is instructed to elevate his or her arms to 90 degrees (**Fig. 2–53**). The scapular motion is observed for any abnormalities as the arm is elevated.

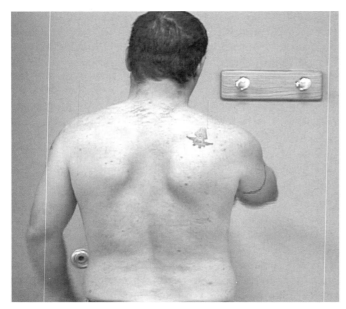

FIGURE 2–54 Type I scapular dyskinesis. (Courtesy of T. Uhl, PhD, ATC.)

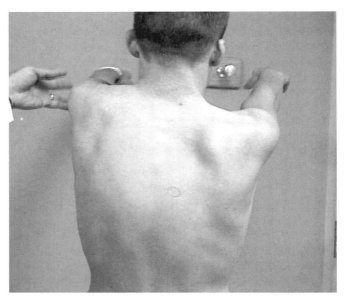

FIGURE 2–56 Type III scapular dyskinesis. (Courtesy of T. Uhl, PhD, ATC.)

Type I scapular dyskinesis is characterized by a prominence of the inferior medial scapular border with elevation of the arm (**Fig. 2–54**). This prominence is due to tilting of the inferior margin of the scapula. At rest the inferior and medial border may be prominent. The axis of rotation of the scapula with elevation is in the horizontal plane, according to Kibler et al.[127]

Type II scapular dyskinesis appears as a prominence of the entire medial border of the scapula, particularly with forward elevation of the arm (**Fig. 2–55**). At rest the entire border is prominent. The axis of rotation of the scapula is vertical in the frontal plane.[127]

Type III scapular dyskinesis demonstrates a superior translation of the whole scapula with a prominence of the medial superior border (**Fig. 2–56**). With elevation

the shrug of the trapezius elevates the superior border of the scapula. At rest the superior border is prominent and may be elevated, and the entire scapula may seem displaced anteriorly. The axis of rotation is in the sagittal plane for this type of dyskinesia.

Type IV, or "symmetric," scapular dyskinesis is characterized at rest by symmetric scapula positioning, although the dominant arm may be slightly lower than the other side. Type IV essentially looks normal with the arms at the side. As the arms are elevated, there is a symmetric translation of the inferior angles away from the thorax, but the medial borders stay flush against the thorax.[127]

The validity of these patterns has not been established concerning their pathophysiology and relationship to specific shoulder pathologies. The inter- and intrarater reliability of this schema of scapular dyskinesis was studied by Kibler et al.[127] They studied 26 subjects, 6 of whom had no shoulder pathology or problems. All were videotaped from the back, and the videotapes were observed by two physicians and two physical therapists. In their study the intertester agreement between the two physicians ($k = 0.31$) was poor to fair, and the agreement between the two physical therapists ($k = 0.42$) was moderate. Intratester agreement was reported to be moderate for one physician ($k = 0.59$) and one physical therapist ($k = 0.49$). Although Kibler et al concluded that agreement on the classification of scapular dyskinesis patterns was moderate, many clinicians find the distinctions between the types difficult. Further study and education of providers will be needed for the use of this schema in clinical practice.

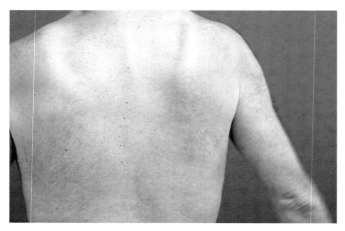

FIGURE 2–55 Type II scapular dyskinesis. (Courtesy of T. Uhl, PhD, ATC.)

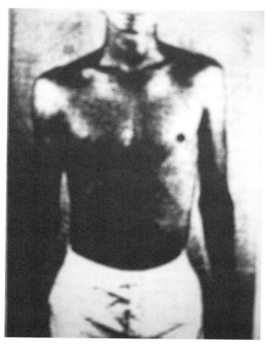

FIGURE 2–57 Tennis shoulder was described as depression of the dominant arm with hypertrophy of the muscles of the dominant upper extremity.

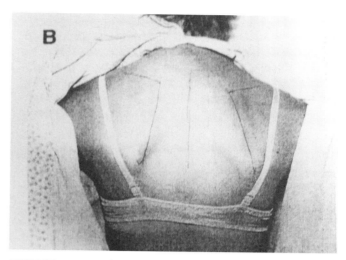

FIGURE 2–58 Scapular landmarks used by Morgan et al for measurement of scapular malpositioning in subjects. (Adapted with permission from Burkhart SS, Morgan CD, Kibler WB. The disabled throwing shoulder: spectrum of pathology. Part 1: Pathoanatomy and biomechanics. Arthroscopy 2003;19(4): 404–420.)

"Tennis Shoulder"

Priest and Nagel[54] described "tennis shoulder" in 1976 as a combination of postural changes seen in tennis players and baseball players. This syndrome was described as depression or "drooping" of the dominant shoulder, dominant arm muscular hypertrophy, and "apparent scoliosis" (**Fig. 2–57**). The dominant arm hypertrophy was known as "King Kong's arm" or "Rod Laver arm," after the famous left-handed tennis player who had one arm markedly larger than the other.

Priest and Nagel[54] studied 84 world-ranked tennis players and found that these asymmetries were more noticeable in men than women, but they were present to varying degrees in more than 50% of the players. They noted that tennis shoulder can occur in athletes involved in other sports and reported it in an athlete who was a shot putter and javelin thrower. They also noted these changes in a worker who used his dominant extremity to carry heavy glass plates for years.

The researchers speculated that this position would result in malpositioning of the scapula, so that it could increase rotator cuff symptoms. They suggested that with the scapula rotated downward, there would not be enough space for the rotator cuff to clear the acromion, and this would result in impingement. They also suggested that the "droop" was due to stretching of the suspensory muscles of the shoulder.

The validity of the supposition that scapular malpositioning results in impingement has not been established. The prevalence of these changes and the relationship to injury have never been studied. In an editorial accompanying the article by Priest and Nagel,[54] the commentator questioned whether the changes they noticed were a cause of the rotator cuff tendinitis symptoms or if other factors were at work. The debate over these issues continues to this day.

The SICK Scapula

Scapular malpositioning at rest has been postulated by many authors as a sign of shoulder dysfunction. The theory is that the scapula is in a position to contribute to the development of rotator cuff problems or SLAP lesions. The SICK scapula has several components; these include static asymmetry with the arms at the side (*S*capular malpositioning, *I*nferior medial prominence), *C*oracoid pain and malpositioning, and scapular dys*K*inesis with movement.[106]

According to Burkhart et al,[106] the static scapular malpositioning at rest can be measured with the arm at the side (**Fig. 2–58**). The three measurements are the inferior position of the scapula compared with the opposite side, the lateral displacement, and the abduction of the scapula. Scapular abduction was measured as the difference in degrees of tilt of the scapula from the vertical between the dominant and nondominant arm (**Fig. 2–59**). The authors suggest that this is a rotatory problem with the scapula tilted forward and rotated.

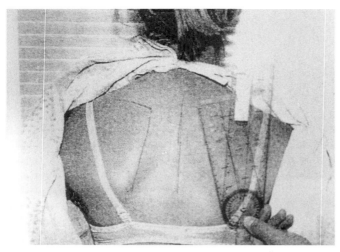

FIGURE 2–59 Measurements employing the technique used by Morgan et al for measurement of scapular malpositioning in subjects. (Adapted with permission from Burkhart, SS, Morgan CD, and Kibler WB, The disabled throwing shoulder: spectrum of pathology Part III: the SICK scapula, scapular dyskinesis, the kinetic chain, and rehabilitation. Arthroscopy 2003;19(6):641–661.)

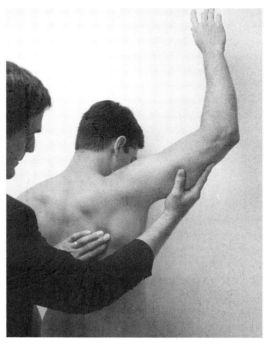

FIGURE 2–60 The scapular assistance test is performed by stabilizing the scapula to allow it to move more normally as the subject elevates the arm.

The exact method for measuring these parameters was not presented by the authors, and no results were reported. To our knowledge the scapular abduction angle as measured by Burkhart et al[106] has not been validated or statistically studied. Scapular motions in three dimensions can be difficult and subject to wide variability. The clinical and diagnostic accuracy of these measures of scapular motion and positioning are discussed below.

Scapular Dysfunction Tests Related to Scapular Dyskinesis

There are three tests that have been described that relate scapular malpositioning to shoulder pathologies. The first is the lateral scapular slide test, which is described above. The other two tests are designed to assist with the evaluation of patients with scapular dyskinesias when they are diagnosed.

Scapular Assistance Test

The scapular assistance test (SAT) was described by Kibler and McMullen[112] and is used for evaluating patients with rotator cuff tendinitis symptoms. This test is performed with the patient standing and the examiner standing behind the patient on the affected side (**Fig. 2–60**). The patient then elevates the arm in the scapular plane, and the examiner stabilizes the inferior border of the scapula as the arm moves. This force by the examiner simulates muscle activity from the lower trapezius and serratus anterior. A positive test is when the stabilization of the

shoulder blade relieves or diminishes the impingement symptoms.

The validity of this test has not been proven, in the sense that no independent biomechanical or anatomic study has validated that stabilization of the scapula significantly alters scapulothoracic mechanics; however, patients can clinically have improvement of their symptoms with this test. The relationship of this test to specific pathologies and its place in the assessment and management of the symptomatic shoulder remain to be determined.

Scapular Flip Sign

The scapular flip sign was developed by Kelly et al[134] as a means for detecting spinal accessory nerve palsy. This test is performed with the patient standing, with the examiner behind the subject (**Fig. 2–61**). The patient holds his or her arms adducted at the side of the body, with the arm in neutral rotation and with the elbow flexed 90 degrees. The patient is asked to externally rotate, and this motion is resisted by the examiner.

A positive test is observed when the medial border of the scapula of the affected extremity becomes more prominent medially than the other extremity (**Fig. 2–62**). In other words, there is medial border winging of the scapula. This test is an observational sign (i.e., positive or negative) only and is not quantitated by the examiner. Likewise, no attempt is made to subdivide the scapular movements into different types.

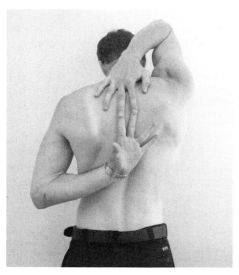

FIGURE 2–69 The second part of the Apley scratch test.

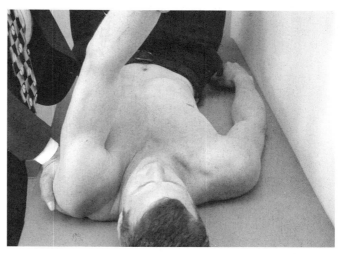

FIGURE 2–71 The horizontal flexion test is completed by adducting the arm across the body to measure posterior shoulder tightness.

Horizontal Flexion Test (Posterior Shoulder Flexibility Test)

The first test described by Pappas et al[121] was a measure of horizontal flexion, which they suggested measured tightness in the posterior shoulder. The test was performed with the patient supine and the arm flexed at 90 degrees (**Fig. 2–70**). The arm was placed in adduction and then across the body (**Fig. 2–71**). The examiner would check for when resistance was felt and measure the angle from the vertical. If the angle was less than 45 degrees, the patient had decreased posterior shoulder flexibility.

Warner et al[109] used a modification of this test by determining in degrees how much adduction was seen in subjects with normal shoulder, impingement, and glenohumeral instability. They found that patients with impingement had significantly less adduction (20 degrees crossed-arm adduction) than patients with instability (52 degrees). The patient was examined supine, but Warner et al did not specify who made the measures, what the intratester or intertester reliability was, or how the goniometric measures were performed.

No validity study is available that defines the anatomic structures that are limited with the horizontal flexion test, and no study has evaluated the intra- or intertester reliability of this measure. Likewise, there is no study that suggests eliminating this particular inflexibility is necessary to prevent injury or to eliminate certain injuries in patients. Although it may have some anecdotal usefulness in clinical practice, further study is needed before its exact role can be defined.

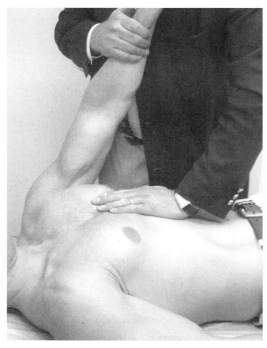

FIGURE 2–70 The horizontal flexion test is performed with the patient supine and the arm forward flexed to 90 degrees.

Crossed-Arm Test

The origin of the crossed-arm test is unknown, but it is meant to be a general measure of shoulder flexibility. It is also known as the coracoantecubital distance test. It is performed with the patient sitting or supine and the examiner standing in front of the patient. The arm is flexed 90 degrees and then adducted across the body, as in the horizontal flexion test. Once maximum adduction is achieved, a ruler is used to measure from the lateral epicondyle of the flexed arm to the AC joint of the

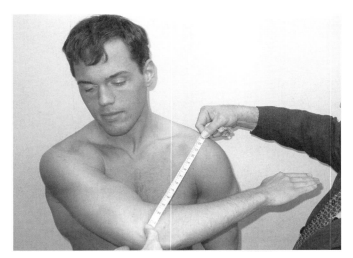

FIGURE 2–72 The use of a ruler to measure posterior shoulder tightness.

opposite shoulder (**Fig. 2–72**). This measurement is then repeated with the other arm elevated, and the two sides are compared with each other. This test measures the flexibility of the entire shoulder complex and can be affected by numerous factors. There are no studies evaluating its validity or clinical usefulness.

Combined Abduction Test

The second test described by Pappas et al[121] was the combined abduction test, which is performed with the patient supine (**Fig. 2–73**). The examiner stands to the side of the patient and feels for scapular movement, but the scapular motion is not restricted in any way. The arm is then elevated in a combination of abduction and flexion until the arm reaches the table behind the subject. If the arm cannot reach the table, then inflexibility was present. Pappas et al suggested that this motion is necessary to reach the "cocking" position of throwing fully.

Kendall et al[174] suggested that another way to perform this test was to have the supine subject raise his or her arm until the arm was on the table over his or her head and parallel to the floor. If the subject had to raise his or her spine, thereby increasing lordosis, to have the arm reach the table, then the subject was judged to have shortened shoulder adductor and internal rotator muscles. Kendall et al found that an inability to place the arm flat indicated shortness of the latissimus dorsi, pectoralis major, and teres major.

This test has not been validated, in that it is not known exactly which structures limit this motion. It is likely that the combined abduction test measures a motion that is a summary of muscle tightness, ligament tightness, and bone conformation. The inter- and intrarater reliability of this test has never been reported. Its clinical usefulness in the treatment of any specific condition has not been reported.

Posterior Shoulder Tightness Test

Another test that measures posterior shoulder tightness has been described by Tyler et al.[175,176] This was a modification of the Pappas et al[121] test, which also had been used by Warner et al[109] when measuring shoulder tightness. Both Warner et al and Pappas et al performed this test with the patient supine, whereas Tyler et al placed the patient on the unaffected side so that scapular motion could be reduced more easily through manual stabilization by the examiner (**Fig. 2–74**). The nontested arm was placed beneath the subject's head, and the knees and hips were flexed so that the patient would be comfortable. The medial epicondyle of the elbow of the affected

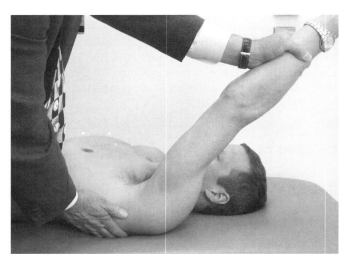

FIGURE 2–73 Another general measure of shoulder complex flexibility is the combined abduction test, where the scapula is stabilized and the arm elevated as far as possible.

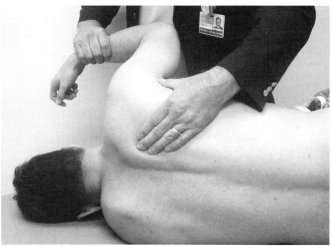

FIGURE 2–74 The posterior shoulder tightness test is done with the patient in a lateral position and the scapula stabilized to prevent motion.

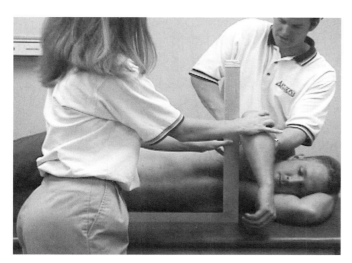

FIGURE 2–75 The degree of posterior shoulder tightness can be determined by measuring the distance from the medial epicondyle to the table.

extremity was marked with a pen, because that would be the reference for making the measurement. The examiner stood facing the subject.

The affected arm was then elevated to 90 degrees of flexion, and the scapula was manually retracted on the thorax and stabilized with one hand of the examiner. With the other hand the examiner would move the arm into adduction (crossed-body adduction) slowly across the body. Care was taken to make sure that the arm stayed in neutral rotation, with no external or internal rotation. The arm adduction was continued until the shoulder motion ceased or rotation of the humerus occurred. This movement of the shoulder blade could be determined by placing one hand on the shoulder blade as the arm was brought across the table. At this point the distance from the medial epicondyle to the surface of the table was measured using a standard carpenter's square (**Fig. 2–75**). A second examiner would perform the measurement while one examiner held the arm in the test position. The examination was then performed on the opposite extremity, and the two values measured were compared.

Tyler et al first performed a study of the intra- and intertester reliability.[175] They studied the intraobserver reproducibility by measuring 21 subjects on 5 consecutive days. Tyler et al found that the intratester reproducibility was high, with a correlation coefficient of 0.92 for the measure of the dominant extremity and 0.95 for the nondominant extremity. Next, they measured the interobserver agreement on 28 normal subjects, with the measures made within 5 minutes of each other. The interobserver reliability between the two testers was in a good range, with a correlation coefficient of 0.80.

The researchers then used this technique to measure the posterior shoulder tightness in 22 Division I National Collegiate Athletic Association (NCAA) collegiate baseball pitchers. They measured shoulder range of motion in the players and in normal subjects, but it should be noted that the two groups were not age matched. Tyler et al found that the baseball players had statistically significantly more shoulder external rotation, less shoulder internal rotation, and increased posterior shoulder tightness than the control subjects. They found in pitchers an inverse relationship between lower shoulder internal rotation and the measure of posterior shoulder tightness; that is, a pitcher with a larger value on the posterior shoulder tightness scale (the elbow is farther away from the table) will also be likely to have a greater loss of internal rotation.

Tyler et al[176] then evaluated this measure in 31 patients with secondary subacromial impingement syndrome. This diagnosis was made based on the patient's having full shoulder flexion and a positive Neer impingement sign (see Chapter 4). They excluded patients with frozen shoulders, rotator cuff tears, or signs of cervical spine arthritis. They found that patients with impingement had increased loss of internal rotation of the shoulder compared with controls with the arm abducted 90 degrees, and that the impingement group had significantly greater posterior shoulder tighter tightness with this measure compared with controls.[177] Tyler et al found a strong correlation between loss of internal rotation of the shoulder and a tight posterior shoulder using this test. They suggested that for every 4 degrees of loss of internal rotation with the arm abducted, there was a loss of 1 cm of the distance to the table. Although the researchers demonstrated a relationship between loss of internal rotation and a tighter posterior shoulder, they admitted that whether the shoulder tendinitis caused the tightness or whether the tightness caused the tendinitis was unclear.

Other studies have used this test to evaluate the posterior shoulder tightness in the throwing shoulder of baseball players. A study in baseball players ages 10 to 14 years demonstrated that the throwing shoulder exhibited significantly greater posterior shoulder tightness (3.5 cm) compared with the contralateral nonthrowing shoulder that was increased with age and years of play.[178] A comparison of 103 professional baseball players (49 pitchers and 54 position players) revealed that the throwing shoulder exhibited an average of 4.4 cm more posterior shoulder tightness compared with the nonthrowing extremity. A comparison of pitchers to position players demonstrated that pitchers exhibited an average of 2.4 cm more posterior shoulder tightness than position players.[74] Neither of these studies correlated the findings with a history of a previous, current, or future injury.

The validity of the posterior shoulder tightness test has not been fully established by anatomic or biomechanical studies. It has not yet been fully elucidated what anatomic structures contribute to a positive posterior capsular tightness test, and it is possible that a combination of bony, tendinous, and muscle components may be involved. In addition, although there is a correlation between their test and loss of range of shoulder motion, the authors have found an association between the findings but have not proven a causal relationship. Further study will elucidate the pathological mechanisms that create these findings on physical examination.

> These tests of posterior shoulder tightness are not practical and are labor intensive, and further study is needed before they can be recommended for routine use.

Subscapularis Muscle Tightness Test

Donatelli[173] describes a test for subscapularis tightness. The test is performed with the arm in 45 degrees and 90 degrees of elevation. If external rotation is limited more with the arm in 45 degrees of abduction than in 90 degrees of abduction, then there is presumed tightness of the subscapularis muscle–tendon complex.[179] There has been no study to establish the validity of this test. It is unlikely that this position tests subscapularis tightness alone.

Pectoralis Minor Muscle Contracture Test

Pectoralis minor muscle and tendon tightness have been described as a contributor of pain in the shoulder.[174] The theory is that if the scapula is held forward (or protracted), the acromion is tilted downward on the anterior side of the shoulder. It is postulated that when the arm is raised, the scapula cannot adjust due to the tightness of the pectoralis minor muscle. As the arm is lifted, the rotator cuff hits the acromion earlier, which this causes rotator cuff pain. Pectoralis minor tightness has been suggested as a problem in overhead athletes who have a SICK scapula.[66]

In their book, Kendall et al[174] described a test of shoulder mobility that measures tightness of the pectoralis minor muscle. The test is performed with the patient supine (**Fig. 2–76**). The examiner stands at the head of the table and places his or her hands on the patient's anterior shoulder. The examiner then pushes the shoulder toward the table, and the distance from the posterior shoulder to the table is noted. Asymmetry with an inability to push the affected shoulder down to the table indicates that the pectoralis minor muscle is tight.

Other methods have been described to test pectoralis muscle tightness (Dr. G. Malanga, personal communication). The patient can be seated or supine and the arm placed in abduction and external rotation. The scapula is stabilized and the arm brought posteriorly (**Fig. 2–77**).

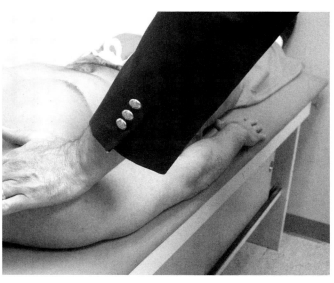

FIGURE 2–76 One measure of pectoralis minor muscle tightness was recommended by Kendall[164] and involves trying to push the shoulder toward the table.

The degree of tightness is subjectively observed and compared with the other extremity.

A third way of observing pectoralis minor muscle strength has been described (**Fig. 2–78**). With the patient supine, the patient is asked to place his or her arms behind the head and to let them drop toward the table. The difference between the two sides is noted.

None of these measures have been validated using cadaver, radiographic, or kinematic studies. It is unlikely that loss of motion with any of these positions or tests is due to weakness of the the pectoralis minor alone, and the exact contributors to restriction of this motion need further study. Likewise, the clinical utility of this study

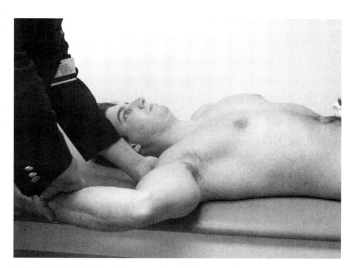

FIGURE 2–77 Another method of measuring pectoralis minor tightness, as described by Malanga (Dr. G. Malanga, personal communication).

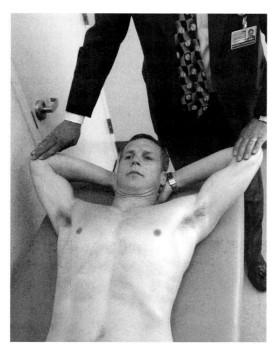

FIGURE 2–78 Another technique for measuring pectoralis minor tightness, as described by Malanga (Dr. G. Malanga, personal communication).

and its relationship to performance, any disease states, or results of treatment have not been studied.

The Quadrant Position and Test

The quadrant position and test were described by Mullen and summarized by Magee.[142,180] The quadrant test is designed to detect subtle changes in shoulder motion due to pain or shoulder pathology. It is based on Codman's paradox, which is an interesting phenomenon of the shoulder that occurs due to rotations of the shoulder in different positions.

Codman's paradox is the observation that if you lift your arm in flexion above shoulder level with your palm facing backward initially, then let the arm down in the plane of the body until the arm is where it began, the hand in the final resting position will be with the palm forward (**Fig. 2–79**). In other words, as the arm is elevated in flexion and returned in abduction, the arm appears to rotate 180 degrees. This is explained by the necessary rotation of the humerus that must occur as the arm moves from one plane to another.

The quadrant test is designed to determine if this rotation occurs easily and without impediment. The test is performed with the patient supine and the examiner standing at the head of the table. The examiner places one hand behind the patient's shoulder, with the hand on the scapula and the clavicle. The goal is to prevent the scapula from shrugging up with motion.

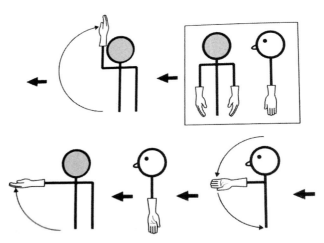

FIGURE 2–79 In Codman's paradox, the arm is elevated in abduction with the palms forward; when the arms are brought down in the front, the hands end up with the palms pointing posteriorly. (Adapted with permission from Nobuhara K. The Shoulder: Its Function and Clinical Aspects, Vol. 1. Singapore: World Scientific Publishing; 2003.)

The arm is then elevated in the plane of the body to 90 degrees of elevation, with the arm in 90 degrees of external rotation (**Fig. 2–80**). The arm is then adducted across the body until it is seen to move from the coronal plane (**Fig. 2–81**). The point at which the arm moves slightly from the coronal plane is the quadrant position. It indicates the point at which the arm is internally rotating as it goes from one position to another. This typically occurs around 60 degrees of adduction and 120 degrees of abduction.

The clinical usefulness of this test has not been established.[180] There is no way to quantitate it, and the reproducibility of the test has not been established.

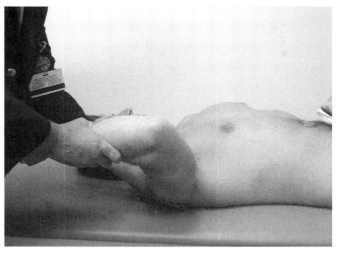

FIGURE 2–80 The quadrant test is performed by first elevating the arm to 90 degrees, then externally rotating the arm to 90 degrees with the arm elevated.

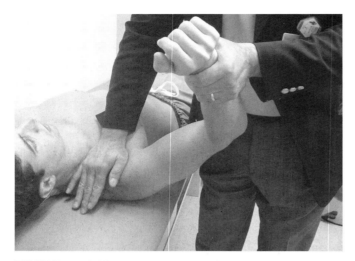

FIGURE 2–81 The second portion of the quadrant test is to adduct the arm until resistance is felt.

The Locked Quadrant Position

The locked quadrant position is the point at which the shoulder will no longer elevate due to the greater tuberosity of the humerus hitting the superior glenoid.[142,180] It is demonstrated by elevating the arm in the plane of the body with the arm in internal rotation (**Fig. 2–82**). If the arm is allowed to move forward from the plane of the body and externally rotated, more elevation can be accomplished.

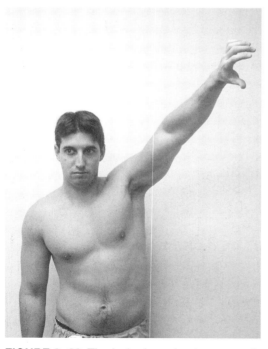

FIGURE 2–82 The locked quadrant supposedly represents a position where the shoulder is most stable and there is no translation due to the bony restraints of the shoulder.

The locked quadrant position will typically be around 80 to 120 degrees of elevation, depending on the patient's flexibility.

This concept was supported by biomechanical studies by An et al,[42] who demonstrated that maximum elevation of the arm occurs in the coronal plane (in the plane of the body) or in the plane of the scapula only if the arm is externally rotated[181]; however, maximum elevation with the arm in flexion can occur with the arm in internal rotation.[12]

Although the clinical utility of the locked quadrant position has not been established, it is relevant when examining patients who may demonstrate loss of motion for no apparent reason. We have noticed in some patients who have secondary gain that abduction will be limited if they attempt to elevate their arm with their thumb down. It is important that the examiner note the rotation of the arm as the patient attempts to elevate it. When elevating in the plane of the body or in the plane of the scapula, the patient should rotate the arm so that the thumb is up (i.e., the arm is in external rotation). If the patient elevates the arm in flexion, the arm must be in internal rotation.

> The quadrant and locked quadrant positions have not been shown to have any clinical relevance.

The Zero Position of Saha

In 1950 Saha[116] described a position of the shoulder that he said was clinically important for several reasons. The first was based on his observation that for the shoulder to move from this position, rotation had to occur. Second, this position was best for treating proximal humerus fractures or when reducing shoulder dislocations. The zero position was roughly 165 degrees of elevation in the plane of the scapula, which Saha described as 45 degrees in front of the coronal plane (**Fig. 2–83**).

This position represented to Saha the point at which the humerus was in neutral with no rotation. He also suggested that this was the position where there was minimal glenohumeral gliding or rolling and where the mechanical axis of the humerus was aligned with its anatomic axis.

The clinical usefulness of this position has not been substantiated by subsequent authors; however, Saha's analysis of shoulder motion and function served as a base for future investigators.

The Hammock Position of Codman and the Pivotal Position

Codman[182] described a position of the shoulder that was similar to the position of the arms when lying in a

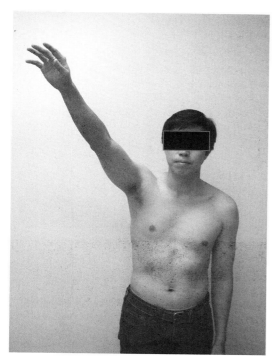

FIGURE 2–83 The "zero position" of Saha was described as a stable position of the shoulder; only the arm is in external rotation.

hammock with the hands behind the head (**Fig. 2–84**). In this position, the shoulder is elevated and externally rotated, but some external rotation is still possible. As a result, the humerus is not entirely locked into the glenoid.

When the arm is elevated in abduction far enough, a position is achieved where the arm is entirely locked so that no rotation is possible. This has been called the pivotal

position of the shoulder. The pivotal position occurs when the arm is elevated in the plane of the body until it is stopped due to the ligaments and conformation of the joint. This occurs around 120 degrees of elevation, and for further elevation to occur the humerus must be externally rotated.[183]

In the hammock, position, the arm is not entirely locked, and some motion can occur. This position has also been called the subordinate pivotal position by Codman because some rotation is still possible.

This nomenclature has not received widespread use for a variety of reasons. First, the clinical significance of these positions has not been convincingly demonstrated. Second, the biomechanics of these positions and the relationships of the various structures to each other are complicated and difficult to understand. Although these concepts help challenge us to better understand shoulder positioning and biomechanics, further study is needed to determine their clinical utility.

The Pivotal Area

Nobuhara[183] noted that there is no one pivotal position of the shoulder, but rather that there is an area where the shoulder has maximum joint play. He referred to this as the zero position. According to Nobuhara, this is the point at which the coracoid and acromion are in the same plane and the arm cannot rotate or elevate. This location is typically around 120 degrees of elevation in the scapular plane (**Fig. 2–85**). It is important to note that

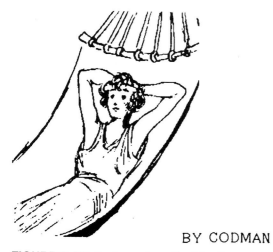

BY CODMAN

FIGURE 2–84 Codman described the "hammock position" as an inherently stable position of the shoulder. (Adapted with permission from Nobuhara K. The Shoulder: Its Function and Clinical Aspects, Vol. 1. Singapore: World Scientific Publishing; 2003.)

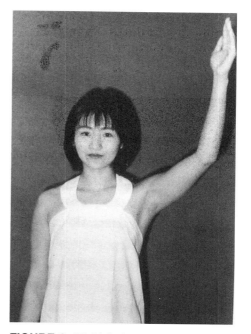

FIGURE 2–85 Nobuhara described a pivotal area where the shoulder was most stable. (Adapted with permission from Nobuhara K. The Shoulder: Its Function and Clinical Aspects, Vol. 1. Singapore: World Scientific Publishing; 2003.)

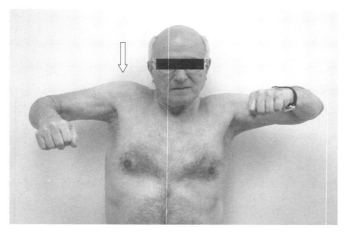

FIGURE 2–86 The shrug sign (arrow) is a nonspecific sign of shoulder dysfunction that is performed by asking the subject to elevate both arms to 90 degrees.

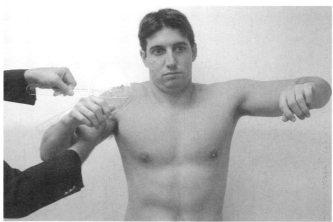

FIGURE 2–87 The shrug sign can be quantitated by measuring how far the arm falls short of 90 degrees.

the arm is in external rotation with the hand pointing toward the head. This hand position distinguishes it from the Neer impingement sign, where the hand faces forward. The zero position is important because it forms the basis of Nobuhara's zero position test for shoulder laxity and instability.

The Shrug Sign

The origin of the shrug sign cannot be established. This test is a nonspecific sign of shoulder dysfunction, and it can be seen with weakness due to any cause, stiffness due to any cause, and due to pain alone (**Fig. 2–86**). We have observed that when it is due to contracture, the tightness is in the glenohumeral joint for any reason. As a result, it can be seen in patients with a variety of diagnoses (**Table 2–19**). This test is performed simply by asking the patient to elevate his or her arms to 90 degrees. If the patient is weak or stiff, then to make the arm reach so that it is parallel to the ground, the patient has to shrug the shoulder girdle up using the scapular muscles,

particularly the trapezius muscle. Some patients will be so weak that the arm will not be capable of staying in that position. The shrug sign test has some utility postoperatively in patients who appear to have normal motion and function, but the test may detect subtle stiffness.

This test can be semiquantified by eliminating the shrug, then measuring how far from the horizontal the patient's arm is located (**Fig. 2–87**). Usually the higher the degree of lag from 90 degrees, the more severe the pathological process preventing the patient from having normal motion. A study of our patients demonstrated that the shrug sign most likely is a semiquantitative measure of shoulder tightness because the two groups with the highest degrees of loss of motion included patients with degenerative arthritis and frozen shoulder (**Table 2–19**).

The shrug sign has not been studied in a rigorous way by us or in any other study. It is currently an abnormality that can be used to alert the observer that the shoulder is not functioning normally.

Anterior and Superior Subluxation

This observation is not a specific test of the shoulder and will be discussed in more detail in Chapter 5. Anterior and superior subluxation is due to a loss of the static restraints of the humeral head when the patient attempts to elevate the arm (**Fig. 2–88**). Although the exact combination of structures that have to be deficient to cause this to occur is not entirely known, the structures that are typically deficient for this to occur are the supraspinatus tendon and the coracoacromial ligament. Other structures that may be absent include the infraspinatus tendon, the subscapularis tendon, and portions of the acromion if a partial acromioplasty has been done.

The test can be done by asking the sitting or standing patient to elevate his or her arms as high as possible.

TABLE 2–19 Shrug Sign Positives According to Diagnosis

		Shrug Sign	
Diagnosis	N	Positive (%)	Negative (%)
Impingement	123	32.2	67.7
RTC	584	58.0	42.0
SLAP lesion	30	26.7	73.3
Instability	361	15.9	83.5
Osteoarthritis[†]	132	92.4	7.6
Frozen shoulder	16	94.0	6.0

Source: Data from The Johns Hopkins University Shoulder Database.

Frozen shoulder, adhesive capsulitis; Impingement, external impingement; Instability, anterior instability, anterior traumatic instability, multidirectional instability, occult instability, and posterior instability; Osteoarthritis, glenohumeral osteoarthritis; RCT, rotator cuff tendinitis, partial tear, and full tear; SLAP, superior labrum anterior to posterior.

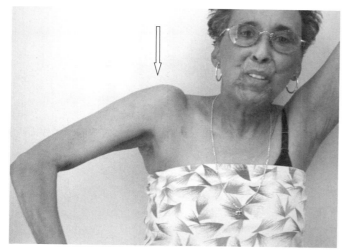

FIGURE 2–88 In patients with massive rotator cuff tears, anterior and superior subluxation of the humeral head occurs such that the head (arrow) can be seen protruding in the anterior shoulder with attempted elevation.

The arm typically will not elevate more than 80 to 100 degrees, and there will be a prominence on the upper anterior shoulder. This movement often will be accompanied by a shrug sign as the patient attempts to elevate the arm with the trapezius and scapular muscles.

> Anterior and superior subluxation of the shoulder with elevation is a sign of significant shoulder pathology, usually extensive rotator cuff disease.

Reverse Scapulothoracic Rhythm

Reverse scapulothoracic rhythm is used to describe the shoulder complex when the glenohumeral joint moves less than the scapulothoracic joint with elevation of the shoulder.[184] The hallmark of this phenomenon is hiking of the shoulder, which is another term for shrugging of the shoulder complex. This could be caused by conditions that can result in severe dysfunction of the glenohumeral joint but not the scapulothoracic articulation. The condition includes severe contracture of the glenohumeral joint, a flail shoulder, anterior and superior subluxation, and severe paralysis of the deltoid and rotator cuff.

This term has not been used on a widespread basis because it is confusing and does not accurately describe exactly what is happening to the shoulder. It is very difficult upon physical examination to measure accurately the exact contributions of the glenohumeral and scapulothoracic joints to elevation or to bringing the arm down from an elevated position. The observation that the patient cannot elevate the arm is nonspecific; this observation alone indicates severe dysfunction of the shoulder complex that should be carefully investigated.

■ Snapping Scapula Syndrome

Crepitus with motion of the scapula is common and often does not cause symptoms. Many patients present primarily for reassurance that it is nothing serious. There is sometimes a history of overuse of the extremity such as due to repetitive motion in the workplace or with a sporting activity. The crepitus is sometimes palpable by the examiner and frequently is audible.

When examining for this entity, it is important to be able to view the patient's thorax and posterior shoulder. Deformity or malpositioning of the scapula or cervical or thoracic spine may indicate a congenital or acquired abnormality that may be contributing to the crepitus. The patient should be examined for winging of the scapula at rest or when pushing off a wall. The patient should be asked to lean forward to evaluate for the presence of scoliosis, which may be contributing to rib prominence (**Fig. 2–89**). The patient should be asked to replicate the crepitus by moving the extremity through space. The examiner can place a hand on the scapula to palpate the scapula, but the examiner should not inhibit the motion producing the crepitus.

When palpating the scapula, it is often helpful to have the patient move the scapula by placing the arms in front of the body in flexion. The examiner should first

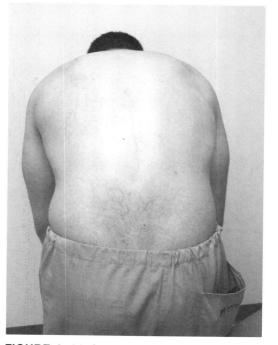

FIGURE 2–89 Scoliosis can produce scapular asymmetry, which is typically asymptomatic.

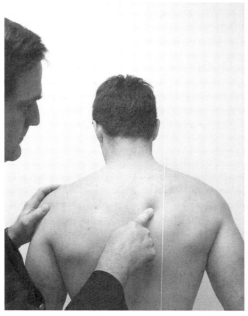

FIGURE 2–90 When examining the posterior thorax, it is important to distinguish rib pain from scapular pain.

palpate the location of the pain on the posterior thorax (**Fig. 2–90**). The patient then is asked to protract the scapula by placing the arms in front of the body. If the location of the pain changes with the position of the scapula, it may indicate that the source of pain is not the ribs but rather the edge of the scapula (**Fig. 2–91**). In our experience the subscapularis bursa does not

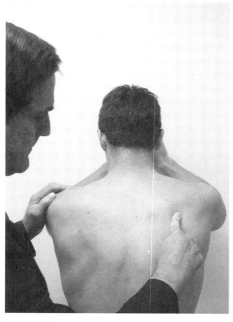

FIGURE 2–91 If the scapula is tender, the painful area will move with scapular protraction.

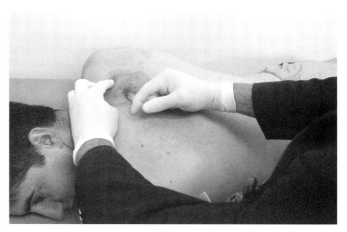

FIGURE 2–92 Injection of subscapular bursa can be performed with the patient supine.

become palpably inflamed or thickened upon physical examination.

■ Subscapular Bursitis

The diagnosis of subscapular bursitis may be assisted by a cortisone shot into the subscapular area (**Fig. 2–92**). This should be done under sterile conditions, and we recommend that a large volume of anesthetic agent be used (i.e., ~10 cc). The patient should be prone, but the head should not be extended by a pillow. The subscapular space should be entered in the upper one half of the scapula from medial to lateral. It sometimes helps to have the patient bring the arm anteriorly to increase the space between the scapula and the thorax.

Care must be taken to aim the needle parallel to the thorax and not to penetrate into the intercostals space or into the lung. These complications are typically not seen with an injection into the subscapular space, but they can be seen when injecting trigger points on the posterior thorax. Patients after the injection should be warned of the possibility of some winging if the long thoracic nerve should become affected by the anesthetic agent, but we have not seen this complication. It is important to ascertain from the patient if the anesthetic has relieved any of the pain within 5 to 10 minutes after the injection. This helps the examiner to localize the location of the pain; if necessary, the patient should be reexamined after the injection.

REFERENCES

1. American Medical Association, "Committee of medical rating and physical impairment," *A guide to the evaluation of permanent impairment of the extremities and back.* J Am Med Assn, 1958. special, (15):p.1–109.
2. Silver, D., *Measurement of range of motion in joints.* J Bone Joint Surg Am, 1923. 5:p.569.

3. Cave, E.F., Robert, S., *A method for measuring and recording joint function.* J Bone Joint Surg Am, 1936. 18(2):p.455–465.

4. Rowe, C.R., *The Surgical Management of Recurrent Anterior Dislocations of the Shoulder Using a Modified Bankart Procedure.* Surg Clin North Am, 1963. 43:p.1663–1666.

5. American Academy of Orthopaedic Surgeons, *Joint Motion: Method of Measuring and Recording.* 1965, Chicago: American Academy of Orthopaedic Surgeons.

6. American Medical Association, Cocchiavella, L, Gunner, BJ, eds. *Practical application of the guides,* in *Guides to the evaluation of permanent impairement,* American Medical Association. 2001.

7. Russe, O.G., and J.J. Gerhardt in *International SFTR Method of measurement and recording joint motion,.* 1975. Hans Huber, Bern.

8. Gerhardt, J., *Documentation of joint measurement.* 1992, Portland, Oregon, Isomed.

9. Gajdosik, R., Simpson, R., Smith, R., and DonTigny, R.L., *Pelvic tilt. Intratester reliability of measuring the standing position and range of motion.* Phys Ther, 1985. 65(2):p.169–174.

10. Williams, J.G., Callaghan, M., *Comparison of visual estimation and goniometry in determination of a shoulder joint angle.* Physiotherapy, 1990. 76(10):p.655–657.

11. Pearl, L., Jackin, S., Lippit, S., Sidle, J., Matsen, F., *Humeroscapular positions in a shoulder range-of-motion-examination.* J Shoulder Elbow Surg, 1992. 1:p. 296–305.

12. Fung, M., Kato, S., Barrance, P.J., Elias, J.J., McFarland, E.G., Nobuhara, K., and Chao, E.Y., *Scapular and clavicular kinematics during humeral elevation: a study with cadavers.* J Shoulder Elbow Surg, 2001. 10(3):p.278–285.

13. McClure, P.W., Michener, L.A., Sennett, B.J., and Karduna, A.R., *Direct 3-dimensional measurement of scapular kinematics during dynamic movements in vivo.* J Shoulder Elbow Surg, 2001. 10(3):p.269–277.

14. Inman, V.T., Saunders, J.B., Abbott, L.C., *Observations on Function of shoulder motion.* J Bone Joint Surg Am, 1944. 26:p.1–30.

15. Watkins, M.A., Riddle, D.L., Lamb, R.L., and Personius, W.J., *Reliability of goniometric measurements and visual estimates of knee range of motion obtained in a clinical setting.* Phys Ther, 1991. 71(2):p.90–96; discussion 96–97.

16. Gajdosik, R.L. and Bohannon, R.W., *Clinical measurement of range of motion. Review of goniometry emphasizing reliability and validity.* Phys Ther, 1987. 67(12):p.1867–1872.

17. Lea, R.D., and Gerhardt, J.J., *Range-of-motion measurements.* J Bone Joint Surg Am, 1995. 77(5):p.784–798.

18. Clarke, G.R., Willis, L.A., Fish, W.W., and Nichols, P.J., *Preliminary studies in measuring range of motion in normal and painful stiff shoulders.* Rheumatol Rehabil, 1975. 14(1):p.39–46.

19. Ekstrand, J., Wiktorsson, M., Oberg, B., and Gillquist, J., *Lower extremity goniometric measurements: a study to determine their reliability.* Arch Phys Med Rehabil, 1982. 63(4):p.171–175.

20. Tomsich, D.A., Nitz, A.J., Threlkeld, A.J., and Shapiro, R., *Patellofemoral alignment: reliability.* J Orthop Sports Phys Ther, 1996. 23(3):p.200–208.

21. Mellin, G., *Measurement of thoracolumbar posture and mobility with a Myrin inclinometer.* Spine, 1986. 11(7):p.759–762.

22. Rondinelli, R., Murphy, J., Esler, A., Marciano, T., and Cholmakjian, C., *Estimation of normal lumbar flexion with surface inclinometry. A comparison of three methods.* Am J Phys Med Rehabil, 1992. 71(4):p.219–224.

23. Boline, P.D., Keating Jr., J.C., Haas, M., and Anderson, A.V., *Interexaminer reliability and discriminant validity of inclinometric measurement of lumbar rotation in chronic low-back pain patients and subjects without low-back pain.* Spine, 1992. 17(3):p.335–338.

24. Dover, G.C., Kaminski, T.W., Meister, K., Powers, M.E., and Horodyski, M., *Assessment of shoulder proprioception in the female softball athlete.* Am J Sports Med, 2003. 31(3):p.431–437.

25. de Winter, A.F., Heemskerk, M.A., Terwee, C.B., Jans, M.P., Deville, W., van Schaardenburg, D.J., Scholten, R.J., and Bouter, L.M., *Interobserver reproducibility of measurements of range of motion in patients with shoulder pain using a digital inclinometer.* BMC Musculoskelet Disord, 2004. 5(1):p.18.

26. Borsa, P.A., M.K. Timmons, and E.L. Sauers, *Scapular-Positioning Patterns During Humeral Elevation in Unimpaired Shoulders.* J Athl Train, 2003. 38(1):p.12–17.

27. Awan, R., J. Smith, and A.J. Boon, *Measuring shoulder internal rotation range of motion: a comparison of 3 techniques.* Arch Phys Med Rehabil, 2002. 83(9):p.1229–1234.

28. Johnson, M.P., P.W. McClure, and A.R. Karduna, *New method to assess scapular upward rotation in subjects with shoulder pathology.* J Orthop Sports Phys Ther, 2001. 31(2):p.81–89.

29. van Royen, B.J. and P.W. Pavlov, *Treatment of frozen shoulder by distension and manipulation under local anaesthesia.* Int Orthop, 1996. 20(4):p.207–210.

30. Boone, D.C. and S.P. Azen, *Normal range of motion of joints in male subjects.* J Bone Joint Surg Am, 1979. 61(5):p.756–759.

31. Murray, M.P., D.R. Gore, G.M. Gardner, and L.A. Mollinger, *Shoulder motion and muscle strength of normal men and women in two age groups.* Clin Orthop, 1985(192):p.268–273.

32. Walker, J.M., D. Sue, N. Miles-Elkousy, G. Ford, and H. Trevelyan, *Active mobility of the extremities in older subjects.* Phys Ther, 1984. 64(6):p.919–923.

33. Barnes, C.J., S.J. Van Steyn, and R.A. Fischer, *The effects of age, sex, and shoulder dominance on range of motion of the shoulder.* J Shoulder Elbow Surg, 2001. 10(3):p.242–246.

34. Allander, E., O.J. Bjornsson, O. Olafsson, N. Sigfusson, and J. Thorsteinsson, *Normal range of joint movements in shoulder, hip, wrist and thumb with special reference to side: a comparison between two populations.* Int J Epidemiol, 1974. 3(3):p.253–261.

35. Kronberg, M., L.A. Brostrom, and V. Soderlund, *Retroversion of the humeral head in the normal shoulder and its relationship to the normal range of motion.* Clin Orthop, 1990(253):p.113–117.

36. Kronberg, M., G. Nemeth, and L.A. Brostrom, *Muscle activity and coordination in the normal shoulder. An electromyographic study.* Clin Orthop, 1990(257):p.76–85.

37. Sabari, J.S., I. Maltzev, D. Lubarsky, E. Liszkay, and P. Homel, *Goniometric assessment of shoulder range of motion: comparison of testing in supine and sitting positions.* Arch Phys Med Rehabil, 1998. 79(6):p.647–651.

38. Boon, A.J. and J. Smith, *Manual scapular stabilization: its effect on shoulder rotational range of motion.* Arch Phys Med Rehabil, 2000. 81(7):p.978–983.

39. McKuen, J., S. France, and E.G. McFarland. *Reproducibility and Reliability of Measuring Glenohumeral versus Scapulothoracic Motion Upon Physical Examination.* in *American College of Sports Medicine.* 1998. Orlando, FL.

40. Rowe, C.R., *Joint measurement in disability evaluation.* Clin Orthop Relat Res, 1964. 32:p.43–53.

41. Freedman, L. and R.R. Munro, *Abduction of the arm in the scapular plane: scapular and glenohumeral movements. A roentgenographic study.* J Bone Joint Surg Am, 1966. 48(8):p.1503–1510.

42. An, K.N., A.O. Browne, S. Korinek, S. Tanaka, and B.F. Morrey, *Three-dimensional kinematics of glenohumeral elevation.* J Orthop Res, 1991. 9(1):p.143–149.

43. Fung, M., *Visualization and Quantification of the Coupled Passive Shoulder Motion in vitro,* in *Biomedical Engineering.* 1997, Johns Hopkins University: Baltimore.p.84.

44. Mandalidis, D.G., B.S. Mc Glone, R.F. Quigley, D. McInerney, and M. O'Brien, *Digital fluoroscopic assessment of the scapulohumeral rhythm.* Surg Radiol Anat, 1999. 21(4):p.241–246.

45. Lease, K., E.G. McFarland, P.J. Barrance, J.J. Elias, K. Nobuhara, and E.Y.S. Chao. *Application of Kinematic Chain Theory in Passive Motion of the Shoulder.* in *Presented at the orthopaedics research society meeting.* 2000. Orlando, Fl, March 12–15 2000.

46. Hebert, L.J., H. Moffet, B.J. McFadyen, and C.E. Dionne, *Scapular behavior in shoulder impingement syndrome.* Arch Phys Med Rehabil, 2002. 83(1):p.60–69.

47. Sugamoto, K., T. Harada, A. Machida, H. Inui, T. Miyamoto, E. Takeuchi, H. Yoshikawa, and T. Ochi, *Scapulohumeral rhythm: relationship between motion velocity and rhythm.* Clin Orthop, 2002(401): p.119–124.

48. McQuade, K.J. and A.M. Murthi, *Anterior glenohumeral force/translation behavior with and without rotator cuff contraction during clinical stability testing.* Clin Biomech (Bristol, Avon), 2004. 19(1):p.10–15.

49. Warner, J.J., L.J. Micheli, L.E. Arslanian, J. Kennedy, and R. Kennedy, *Scapulothoracic motion in normal shoulders and shoulders with glenohumeral instability and impingement syndrome. A study using Moire topographic analysis.* Clin Orthop Relat Res, 1992(285): p.191–199.

50. McQuade, K.J., S. Hwa Wei, and G.L. Smidt, *Effects of local muscle fatigue on three-dimensional scapulohumeral rhythm.* Clin Biomech (Bristol, Avon), 1995. 10(3):p.144–148.

51. McQuade, K.J., J. Dawson, and G.L. Smidt, *Scapulothoracic muscle fatigue associated with alterations in scapulohumeral rhythm kinematics during maximum resistive shoulder elevation.* J Orthop Sports Phys Ther, 1998. 28(2):p.74–80.

52. Fayard, L., Merolla, E., Brilhault, J., Lautmann, S., *Dynamic Assessment of Arm Elevation in the Scapular Plane with and without Weight Bearing.* Journal of Bone and Joint Surgery British, 2001. 83-B(Suppl I): p. 36.

53. Burkhart, S.S., C.D. Morgan, and W.B. Kibler, *Shoulder injuries in overhead athletes. The "dead arm" revisited.* Clin Sports Med, 2000. 19(1):p.125–158.

54. Priest, J.D. and D.A. Nagel, *Tennis shoulder.* Am J Sports Med, 1976. 4(1):p.28–42.

55. Jobe, F.W., *Operative Techniques in Upper Extremity Sports Injury.* 1996, St Louis: Mosby.

56. Jobe, F.W. and M. Pink, *The athlete's shoulder.* J Hand Ther, 1994. 7(2):p.107–110.

57. Jobe, F.W. and M. Pink, *Classification and treatment of shoulder dysfunction in the overhead athlete.* J Orthop Sports Phys Ther, 1993. 18(2):p.427–432.

58. Jobe, F.W., R.S. Kvitne, and C.E. Giangarra, *Shoulder pain in the overhand or throwing athlete. The relationship of anterior instability and rotator cuff impingement.* Orthop Rev, 1989. 18(9):p.963–975.

59. Jobe, F.W. and J.P. Bradley, *Rotator cuff injuries in baseball. Prevention and rehabilitation.* Sports Med, 1988. 6(6):p.378–387.

60. Jobe, F.W., C.E. Giangarra, R.S. Kvitne, and R.E. Glousman, *Anterior capsulolabral reconstruction of the shoulder in athletes in overhand sports.* Am J Sports Med, 1991. 19(5):p.428–434.

61. Walch, G., J.P. Liotard, P. Boileau, and E. Noel, *[Postero-superior glenoid impingement. Another shoulder impingement].* Rev Chir Orthop Reparatrice Appar Mot, 1991. 77(8):p.571–574.

62. Walch, G., J.P. Liotard, P. Boileau, and E. Noel, *[Postero-superior glenoid impingement. Another impingement of the shoulder].* J Radiol, 1993. 74(1):p.47–50.

63. Riand, N., C. Levigne, E. Renaud, and G. Walch, *Results of derotational humeral osteotomy in posterosuperior glenoid impingement.* Am J Sports Med, 1998. 26(3):p.453–459.

64. Vaitl, T., A. Burkart, E. Steinhauser, E. Hohmann, and A. Imhoff, *[Biomechanical investigations for the development of a SLAP-II-lesion].* Orthopade, 2003. 32(7):p.608–615.

65. Morgan, C.D., S.S. Burkhart, M. Palmeri, and M. Gillespie, *Type II SLAP lesions: three subtypes and their relationships to superior instability and rotator cuff tears.* Arthroscopy, 1998. 14(6):p.553–565.

66. Burkhart, S.S., C.D. Morgan, and W.B. Kibler, *The disabled throwing shoulder: spectrum of pathology Part I: pathoanatomy and biomechanics.* Arthroscopy, 2003. 19(4):p.404–420.

67. Grossman, M.G., J.E. Tibone, M.H. McGarry, D.J. Schneider, S. Veneziani, and T.Q. Lee, *A cadaveric model of the throwing shoulder: a possible etiology of superior labrum anterior-to-posterior lesions.* J Bone Joint Surg Am, 2005. 87(4):p.824–831.

68. Koffler, K.B., D. Eager, M. *The effect of posterior capsule tightness on glenohumeral translation in the late cocking phase of pitching: A cadaveric*

stuy. in The 21st Annual Meeting of the Arthroscopy Association of North America, Washington, DC. April 25–28, 2002.

69. Anderson, K., Xian-Hua, D., Johnson, T., Altcheck, D.W. *Biomechanical analysis of a posterior capsular contracutre of the shoulder.* in *The American Orthopaedic Society for Sports Medicine 27th Annual Meeting, Keystone, CO.* June 30-July 1, 2001.

70. Kibler, W.B., Andrews, J.R., Morgan, C.D. *The painful throwing shoulder anterior instability versus posterior tightness.* in *The American Orthopaedic Society for Sports Medicine annual meeting.* Quebec, Canada. June 24–27, 2004.

71. Brown, L.P., S.L. Niehues, A. Harrah, P. Yavorsky, and H.P. Hirshman, *Upper extremity range of motion and isokinetic strength of the internal and external shoulder rotators in major league baseball players.* Am J Sports Med, 1988. 16(6):p.577–585.

72. Chandler, T.J., W.B. Kibler, T.L. Uhl, B. Wooten, A. Kiser, and E. Stone, *Flexibility comparisons of junior elite tennis players to other athletes.* Am J Sports Med, 1990. 18(2):p.134–136.

73. Kibler, W.B., T.J. Chandler, B.P. Livingston, and E.P. Roetert, *Shoulder range of motion in elite tennis players. Effect of age and years of tournament play.* Am J Sports Med, 1996. 24(3):p.279–285.

74. Sauers, E.L., Koh, J.L., Keuter, G. *Scapular and glenohumeral motion in professional baseball players: effects of position and arm dominance.* in *Arthroscopy Association of North America Annual Meeting.* 2004. Orlando, FL.

75. Bigliani, L.U., T.P. Codd, P.M. Connor, W.N. Levine, M.A. Littlefield, and S.J. Hershon, *Shoulder motion and laxity in the professional baseball player.* Am J Sports Med, 1997. 25(5):p.609–613.

76. Bak, K. and S.P. Magnusson, *Shoulder strength and range of motion in symptomatic and pain-free elite swimmers.* Am J Sports Med, 1997. 25(4):p.454–459.

77. Beach, M.L., S.L. Whitney, and S.A. Dickoff-Hoffman, *Relationship of shoulder flexibility, strength, and endurance to shoulder pain in competitive swimmers.* J Orthop Sports Phys Ther, 1992. 16(6):p.262–268.

78. Sauers, E.L., P.A. Borsa, D.E. Herling, and R.D. Stanley, *Instrumented measurement of glenohumeral joint laxity and its relationship to passive range of motion and generalized joint laxity.* Am J Sports Med, 2001. 29(2):p.143–150.

79. Reagan, K.M., K. Meister, M.B. Horodyski, D.W. Werner, C. Carruthers, and K. Wilk, *Humeral retroversion and its relationship to glenohumeral rotation in the shoulder of college baseball players.* Am J Sports Med, 2002. 30(3):p.354–360.

80. Osbahr, D.C., D.L. Cannon, and K.P. Speer, *Retroversion of the humerus in the throwing shoulder of college baseball pitchers.* Am J Sports Med, 2002. 30(3):p.347–353.

81. Crockett, H.C., L.B. Gross, K.E. Wilk, M.L. Schwartz, J. Reed, J. O'Mara, M.T. Reilly, J.R. Dugas, K. Meister, S. Lyman, and J.R. Andrews, *Osseous adaptation and range of motion at the glenohumeral joint in professional baseball pitchers.* Am J Sports Med, 2002. 30(1): p.20–26.

82. Wilk, K.E., K. Meister, and J.R. Andrews, *Current concepts in the rehabilitation of the overhead throwing athlete.* Am J Sports Med, 2002. 30(1):p.136–151.

83. Morgan, C.D. *SLAP Lesions in Throwing Athletes.* in *American Academy of Orthopaedic Surgeons Annual Meeting.* Orlando, FL. March 15–19, 2000.

84. Ellenbecker, T.S., E.P. Roetert, P.A. Piorkowski, and D.A. Schulz, *Glenohumeral joint internal and external rotation range of motion in elite junior tennis players.* J Orthop Sports Phys Ther, 1996. 24(6): p.336–341.

85. Rupp, S., K. Berninger, and T. Hopf, *Shoulder problems in high level swimmers—impingement, anterior instability, muscular imbalance?* Int J Sports Med, 1995. 16(8):p.557–562.

86. Sauers, E.L., G. Keuter, M.F. Schafer, and J.L. Koh, *A comparison between passive shoulder complex and isolated glenohumeral joint rotation range of motion in professional baseball pitchers.* Journal of Athletic Training, 2003. 38(2):p.72.

87. O'Brien, S.J., R.S. Schwartz, R.F. Warren, and P.A. Torzilli, *Capsular restraints to anterior-posterior motion of the abducted shoulder: a biomechanical study.* J Shoulder Elbow Surg, 1995. 4(4):p.298–308.

88. Harryman, D.T., 2nd, J.A. Sidles, J.M. Clark, K.J. McQuade, T.D. Gibb, and F.A. Matsen, 3rd, *Translation of the humeral head on the glenoid with passive glenohumeral motion.* J Bone Joint Surg Am, 1990. 72(9):p.1334–1343.

89. McFarland, E.G., M. Fung, S. Kato, J.D. DesJardins, and E.Y.S. Chao. *Glenohumeral motion can be distinguished from scapulothoracic motion in rotation.* Proceedings of the Orthopedic Research Society, 1998. Vol. 23:266.

90. Richards, R.R., K. An, L.U. Bigliani, R.J. Friedman, G.M. Gartsman, A.G. Gristina, J.P. Iannotti, V.C. Mow, J.A. Sidles, and J.D. Zuckerman, *A standardized method for the assessment of shoulder function.* Journal of Shoulder and Elbow Surgery, 1994. 3(6):p.347–352.

91. Matsen, F.A., S.B. Lippitt, J.A. Sidles, and D.T. Harryman, *Practical Evaluation and management of the Shoulder.* 1994, Philadelphia: W.B.Saunders.

92. Mallon, W.J., C.L. Herring, P.I. Sallay, C.T. Moorman, and J.R. Crim, *Use of vertebral levels to measure presumed internal rotation at the shoulder: a radiographic analysis.* J Shoulder Elbow Surg, 1996. 5(4):p.299–306.

93. Maitland, G.D., *Vertebral Manipulation.* 5 ed. 1986, London: Butterworth.

94. Cyriax, J., *Textbook of Orthopaedic Medicine.* 7 ed. 1978, London: Bailliere Tindall.

95. Paris, S.V. and P.V. Loubert, *Foundations of clinical orthopaedics.* 1990, St.Augustine institutional press.

96. Donatelli, R.A., *Physical Therapy of the Shoulder.* 4 ed. 2004, St. Louis, MO: Churchill Livingstone. 98–99.

97. Rothstein, J.M., *Editorial response.* Physical Therapy, 1994. 74: p. 1075.

98. Pellecchia, G.L., J. Paolino, and J. Connell, *Intertester reliability of the cyriax evaluation in assessing patients with shoulder pain.* J Orthop Sports Phys Ther, 1996. 23(1):p.34–38.

99. Bovens, A.M., van Baak, M.A., Vrencken, J.G., Wijen, J.A., Verstappen, F.T., *Variability and reliability of joint measurements.* Am J Sports Med, 1990. 18:p.58–63.

100. Boone, D.C., Azen, S.P., Lin, C.M., Spence, C., Baron, C., Lee, K., *Reliability of goniometric measurements.* Phys Ther, 1978. 58(11): p.1355–1390.

101. Iannotti, J.P., Williams, G.R., *Disorders of the Shoulder: Diagnosis and Management.* 1999, Philadelphia: Lippincott Williams & Wilkins.

102. Constant, C.R. and A.H. Murley, *A clinical method of functional assessment of the shoulder.* Clin Orthop Relat Res, 1987(214): p.160–164.

103. Beaton, D.E. and R.R. Richards, *Measuring function of the shoulder. A cross-sectional comparison of five questionnaires.* J Bone Joint Surg Am, 1996. 78(6):p.882–890.

104. Kirkley, A., S. Griffin, H. McLintock, and L. Ng, *The development and evaluation of a disease-specific quality of life measurement tool for shoulder instability. The Western Ontario Shoulder Instability Index (WOSI).* Am J Sports Med, 1998. 26(6):p.764–772.

105. Triffitt, P.D., C. Wildin, and D. Hajioff, *The reproducibility of measurement of shoulder movement.* Acta Orthop Scand, 1999. 70(4): p.322–324.

106. Burkhart, S.S., C.D. Morgan, and W.B. Kibler, *The disabled throwing shoulder: spectrum of pathology Part III: The SICK scapula, scapular dyskinesis, the kinetic chain, and rehabilitation.* Arthroscopy, 2003. 19(6):p.641–661.

107. Kuhn, J.E., *The Assessment of outcomes for the treatment of overhead athlete.,* in *The Shoulder and the Overhead Athlete.,* S.G. Krishman, R.K. Hawkins, and R.F. Warren, Editors. 2004, Lippincott: Philadelphia.

108. Kibler, W.B., *The role of the scapula in athletic shoulder function.* Am J Sports Med, 1998. 26(2):p.325–337.

109. Warner, J.J., L.J. Micheli, L.E. Arslanian, J. Kennedy, and R. Kennedy, *Patterns of flexibility, laxity, and strength in normal shoulders and shoulders with instability and impingement.* Am J Sports Med, 1990. 18(4):p.366–375.

110. Kibler, W.B., *Clinical aspects of muscle injury.* Med Sci Sports Exerc, 1990. 22(4):p.450–452.

111. Lukasiewicz, A.C., P. McClure, L. Michener, N. Pratt, and B. Sennett, *Comparison of 3-dimensional scapular position and orientation between subjects with and without shoulder impingement.* J Orthop Sports Phys Ther, 1999. 29(10):p.574–583; discussion 584–576.

112. Kibler, W.B. and J. McMullen, *Scapular dyskinesis and its relation to shoulder pain.* J Am Acad Orthop Surg, 2003. 11(2):p.142–151.

113. Gagey, O.J. and N. Gagey, *The hyperabduction test.* J Bone Joint Surg Br, 2001. 83(1):p.69–74.

114. Lintner, S.A., A. Levy, K. Kenter, and K.P. Speer, *Glenohumeral translation in the asymptomatic athlete's shoulder and its relationship to other clinically measurable anthropometric variables.* Am J Sports Med, 1996. 24(6):p.716–720.

115. Hoving, J.L., R. Buchbinder, S. Green, A. Forbes, N. Bellamy, C. Brand, R. Buchanan, S. Hall, M. Patrick, P. Ryan, and A. Stockman, *How reliably do rheumatologists measure shoulder movement?* Ann Rheum Dis, 2002. 61(7):p.612–616.

116. Saha, A.K., *Mechanism of shoulder movements and a plea for the recognition of "zero position" of glenohumeral joint.* Indian J Surg, 1950. 12(2):p.153–165.

117. Itoi, E., B.F. Morrey, and K.N. An, *Biomechanics of the shoulder.,* in *The Shoulder,* C.A. Rockwood, et al., Editors. 2004, Elsevier: Philadelphia.p.223–267.

118. Culham, E. and M. Peat, *Functional anatomy of the shoulder complex.* J Orthop Sports Phys Ther, 1993. 18(1):p.342–350.

119. Sobush, D.C., G.G. Simoneau, K.E. Dietz, J.A. Levene, R.E. Grossman, and W.B. Smith, *The lennie test for measuring scapular position in healthy young adult females: a reliability and validity study.* J Orthop Sports Phys Ther, 1996. 23(1):p.39–50.

120. Borstad, J.D. and P.M. Ludewig, *Comparison of scapular kinematics between elevation and lowering of the arm in the scapular plane.* Clin Biomech (Bristol, Avon), 2002. 17(9–10):p.650–659.

121. Pappas, A.M., R.M. Zawacki, and C.F. McCarthy, *Rehabilitation of the pitching shoulder.* Am J Sports Med, 1985. 13(4):p.223–235.

122. DiVeta, J., M.L. Walker, and B. Skibinski, *Relationship between performance of selected scapular muscles and scapular abduction in standing subjects.* Phys Ther, 1990. 70(8):p.470–476; discussion 476–479.

123. Neiers, L. and T.W. Worrel, *Assessment of scapular position.* J Sports Rehab, 1993. 2:p.20–25.

124. Kibler, W.B., *The role of the scapula in the overhead throwing motion.* Contemp Orthop, 1991. 22:p.525–532.

125. Kibler, W.B., *Normal shoulder mechanics and function.* Instr Course Lect, 1997. 46:p.39–42.

126. Kibler, W.B., T.J. Chandler, and B.K. Pace, *Principles of rehabilitation after chronic tendon injuries.* Clin Sports Med, 1992. 11(3): p.661–671.

127. Kibler, W.B., T.L. Uhl, J.W. Maddux, P.V. Brooks, B. Zeller, and J. McMullen, *Qualitative clinical evaluation of scapular dysfunction: a reliability study.* J Shoulder Elbow Surg, 2002. 11(6):p.550–556.

128. Odom, C.J., A.B. Taylor, C.E. Hurd, and C.R. Denegar, *Measurement of scapular asymetry and assessment of shoulder dysfunction using the Lateral Scapular Slide Test: a reliability and validity study.* Phys Ther, 2001. 81(2):p.799–809.

129. Daniels, T.P., R.A. Harter, and R.D. Wobig, *Evaluation of the lateral scapular test using radiographic imaging: A validity and reliability study.* J. Athletic training, 2002. 37:p.16.

130. Gibson, M.H., G.V. Goebel, T.M. Jordan, S. Kegerreis, and T.W. Worrell, *A reliability study of measurement techniques to determine static scapular position.* J Orthop Sports Phys Ther, 1995. 21(2):p.100–106.

131. Koslow, P.A., L.A. Prosser, G.A. Strony, S.L. Suchecki, and G.E. Mattingly, *Specificity of the lateral scapular slide test in asymptomatic competitive athletes.* J Orthop Sports Phys Ther, 2003. 33(6):p.331–336.

132. Crotty, N.M. and J. Smith, *Alterations in scapular position with fatigue: a study in swimmers.* Clin J Sport Med, 2000. 10(4):p.251–258.

133. Barnett, N.D., R.D. Duncan, and G.R. Johnson, *The measurement of three dimensional scapulohumeral kinematics—a study of reliability.* Clin Biomech (Bristol, Avon), 1999. 14(4):p.287–290.

134. Kelly, B.T., L.A. Roskin, D.T. Kirkendall, and K.P. Speer, *Shoulder muscle activation during aquatic and dry land exercises in nonimpaired subjects.* J Orthop Sports Phys Ther, 2000. 30(4):p.204–210.

135. Kelly, M.J. and S.K. Brenneman, *An examination sign to identify the presence of spinal accessory nerve palsy.* J Orthop Sports Phys Ther, 2000. 30:p.A–27.

136. McClure, P.W., A.R. Tate, M.C. Egner, E.M. Greenberg, R.M. Yops, and N.P. Neff, *Development and Interrater Reliability Testing of a System Of Classification For Scapular Dysfunction.* J Orthop Sports Phys Ther, 2002. 33:p.23–A.

137. Johnson, M.P., S. Adessi, and D.D. Ebaugh. *Development of a model to classify Scapular motion: A pilot study.* in *Pennsylvania physical therapy association.* 2001. Harrisburg.

138. Johnson, M.P., V.D. Heuvel, and S. E.L. *Reliability of a classification protocol for the Assessment of Scapular Motion in Patients with Shoulder Pathology.* in *1 st international congress of shoulder and elbow therapist.* 2004. Washington DC.

139. Ludewig, P.M. and T.M. Cook, *Alterations in shoulder kinematics and associated muscle activity in people with symptoms of shoulder impingement.* Phys Ther, 2000. 80(3):p.276–291.

140. Su, K.P., M.P. Johnson, E.J. Gracely, and A.R. Karduna, *Scapular rotation in swimmers with and without impingement syndrome: practice effects.* Med Sci Sports Exerc, 2004. 36(7):p.1117–1123.

141. MacWilliams, B.A., T. Choi, M.K. Perezous, E.Y. Chao, and E.G. McFarland, *Characteristic ground-reaction forces in baseball pitching.* Am J Sports Med, 1998. 26(1):p.66–71.

142. Magee, D.J., *Orthopaedic physical examination.* Vol. 1. 2002, Philadelphia: W.B. Saunders. 1020.

143. Sauers, E.L., M.P. Johnson, G. Keuter, S. M.F., and K.L. Koh, *The relationship between hip and shoulder range of motion in healthy professional baseball players.* J Athletic Training, 2004. 39(2):p.S–44.

144. Greenfield, B., P.A. Catlin, P.W. Coats, E. Green, J.J. McDonald, and C. North, *Posture in patients with shoulder overuse injuries and healthy individuals.* J Orthop Sports Phys Ther, 1995. 21(5): p.287–295.

145. Griegel-Morris, P., K. Larson, K. Mueller-Klaus, and C.A. Oatis, *Incidence of common postural abnormalities in the cervical, shoulder, and thoracic regions and their association with pain in two age groups of healthy subjects.* Phys Ther, 1992. 72(6):p.425–431.

146. Kebaetse, M., P. McClure, and N.A. Pratt, *Thoracic position effect on shoulder range of motion, strength, and three-dimensional scapular kinematics.* Arch Phys Med Rehabil, 1999. 80(8):p.945–950.

147. Paletta, G.A., Jr., J.J. Warner, R.F. Warren, A. Deutsch, and D.W. Altchek, *Shoulder kinematics with two-plane x-ray evaluation in patients with anterior instability or rotator cuff tearing.* J Shoulder Elbow Surg, 1997. 6(6):p.516–527.

148. Kibler, W.B., *Biomechanical analysis of the shoulder during tennis activities.* Clin Sports Med, 1995. 14(1):p.79–85.

149. Bhargav, D. and G.A. Murrell, *Shoulder stiffness: diagnosis.* Aust Fam Physician, 2004. 33(3):p.143–147.

150. Rundquist, P.J., D.D. Anderson, C.A. Guanche, and P.M. Ludewig, *Shoulder kinematics in subjects with frozen shoulder.* Arch Phys Med Rehabil, 2003. 84(10):p.1473–1479.

151. Chambler, A.F. and A.J. Carr, *The role of surgery in frozen shoulder.* J Bone Joint Surg Br, 2003. 85(6):p.789–795.

152. Cutts, S. and D. Clarke, *The patient with frozen shoulder.* Practitioner, 2002. 246(1640):p.730, 734–736, 738–739.

153. Gerber, C., N. Espinosa, and T.G. Perren, *Arthroscopic treatment of shoulder stiffness.* Clin Orthop, 2001(390):p.119–128.

154. Hertel, R., *[The frozen shoulder].* Orthopade, 2000. 29(9): p. 845–851.

155. Goldberg, B.A., M.M. Scarlat, and D.T. Harryman, 2nd, *Management of the stiff shoulder.* J Orthop Sci, 1999. 4(6):p.462–471.

156. Simotas, A.C. and P. Tsairis, *Adhesive capsulitis of the glenohumeral joint with an unusual neuropathic presentation: a case report.* Am J Phys Med Rehabil, 1999. 78(6):p.577–581.

157. Noel, E., T. Thomas, T. Schaeverbeke, P. Thomas, M. Bonjean, and M. Revel, *Frozen shoulder.* Joint Bone Spine, 2000. 67(5):p.393–400.

158. Warner, J.J., *Frozen Shoulder: Diagnosis and Management.* J Am Acad Orthop Surg, 1997. 5(3):p.130–140.

159. Muller, L.P., M. Rittmeister, J. John, J. Happ, and F. Kerschbaumer, *Frozen shoulder—an algoneurodystrophic process?* Acta Orthop Belg, 1998. 64(4):p.434–440.

160. Herold, H.Z., *[Frozen shoulder].* Harefuah, 1982. 103(1–2): p. 26–27.

161. Rydell, N., *[The frozen shoulder—a mysterious pain].* Lakartidningen, 1982. 79(19):p.1882–1883.

162. Rizk, T.E. and R.S. Pinals, *Frozen shoulder.* Semin Arthritis Rheum, 1982. 11(4):p.440–452.

163. Bruckner, F.E., *Frozen shoulder (adhesive capsulitis).* J R Soc Med, 1982. 75(9): p. 688–689.

164. Bunker, T.D. and P.P. Anthony, *The pathology of frozen shoulder. A Dupuytren-like disease.* J Bone Joint Surg Br, 1995. 77(5): p.677–683.

165. Ha'eri, G.B. and A. Maitland, *Arthroscopic findings in the frozen shoulder.* J Rheumatol, 1981. 8(1):p.149–152.

166. Bunker, T.D., J. Reilly, K.S. Baird, and D.L. Hamblen, *Expression of growth factors, cytokines and matrix metalloproteinases in frozen shoulder.* J Bone Joint Surg Br, 2000. 82(5):p.768–773.

167. Kilian, O., J. Kriegsmann, K. Berghauser, J.P. Stahl, U. Horas, and R. Heerdegen, *[The frozen shoulder. Arthroscopy, histological findings and transmission electron microscopy imaging].* Chirurg, 2001. 72(11):p.1303–1308.

168. Bhargav, D. and G.A. Murrell, *Shoulder stiffness: management.* Aust Fam Physician, 2004. 33(3):p.149–152.

169. Kordella, T., *Frozen shoulder & diabetes. Frozen shoulder affects 20 percent of people with diabetes. Proper treatment can help you work through it.* Diabetes Forecast, 2002. 55(8):p.60–64.

170. Xu, H.Z., B. Yu, Q.G. Zhang, and X.R. Chen, *[Treatment of 48 cases of frozen shoulder with manual therapy under brachial plexus anesthesia through a retained tube].* Di Yi Jun Yi Da Xue Xue Bao, 2003. 23(1):p.87–88.

171. Chen, S.K., S.H. Chien, Y.C. Fu, P.J. Huang, and P.H. Chou, *Idiopathic frozen shoulder treated by arthroscopic brisement.* Kaohsiung J Med Sci, 2002. 18(6):p.289–294.

172. Gam, A.N., P. Schydlowsky, I. Rossel, L. Remvig, and E.M. Jensen, *Treatment of "frozen shoulder" with distension and glucorticoid compared with glucorticoid alone. A randomised controlled trial.* Scand J Rheumatol, 1998. 27(6):p.425–430.

173. Donatelli, R., *Physical therapy of the shoulder.* Vol. 1. 2004, St.Louis, Missouri: Elsevier. 574.

174. Kendall, S.A., F.P. Kendall, and G.E. Wadsworth, *Muscles: testing and function.* Vol. 1. 1971, Baltimore: Williams and Wilkins.

175. Tyler, T.F., T. Roy, S.J. Nicholas, and G.W. Gleim, *Reliability and validity of a new method of measuring posterior shoulder tightness.* J Orthop Sports Phys Ther, 1999. 29(5):p.262–269; discussion 270–264.

176. Tyler, T.F., S.J. Nicholas, T. Roy, and G.W. Gleim, *Quantification of posterior capsule tightness and motion loss in patients with shoulder impingement.* Am J Sports Med, 2000. 28(5):p.668–673.

177. Tyler, T.F., S.J. Nicholas, R.J. Campbell, and M.P. McHugh, *The association of hip strength and flexibility with the incidence of adductor muscle strains in professional ice hockey players.* Am J Sports Med, 2001. 29(2):p.124–128.

178. Mourtacos, S., J. Downar, and E.L. Sauers, *Clinical measures of shoulder mobility in the adolescent baseball player.* J. Athletic training, 2003. 38(2):p.S–72.

179. Turkel, S.J., M.W. Panio, J.L. Marshall, and F.G. Girgis, *Stabilizing mechanisms preventing anterior dislocation of the glenohumeral joint.* J Bone Joint Surg Am, 1981. 63(8):p.1208–1217.

180. Mullen, F., S. Slade, and C. Briggs, *Bony and capsular determinants of glenohumeral 'locking' and 'quadrant' positions.* Austral J Physiother, 1989. 35:p.202–208.

181. Browne, A.O., P. Hoffmeyer, S. Tanaka, K.N. An, and B.F. Morrey, *Glenohumeral elevation studied in three dimensions.* J Bone Joint Surg Br, 1990. 72(5):p.843–845.

182. Codman, E.A., *The shoulder.* 1934, Boston: Thomas Todd.

183. Nobuhara, K., *The Shoulder: It's function and clinical aspects.* Vol. 1. 2003, Singapore: World Scientific Publishing.

184. Beetham, W.P., H.F. Polley, and C.H. Slocum, *Physical examination of the joints.* 1965, Philadelphia: W.B. Sauders.

185. Hoppenfeld, S., *Physical Examination of the Spine and Extremities.* 1976, New York: Appleton-Century-Crofts. 276.

186. Riddle, D.L., J.M. Rothstein, and R.L. Lamb, *Goniometric reliability in a clinical setting. Shoulder measurements.* Phys Ther, 1987. 67(5): p.668–673.

187. Fiebert, I.M., P.A. Downey, and J.S. Brown, *Active shoulder range of motion in persons aged 60 years and older.* Phys Occupat Ther Geriatr, 1995. 13(1/2):p.115–128.

188. Andrews, A.W. and R.W. Bohannon, *Decreased shoulder range of motion on paretic side after stroke.* Phys Ther, 1989. 69(9):p.768–772.

189. Green, S., R. Buchbinder, A. Forbes, and N. Bellamy, *A standardized protocol for measurement of range of movement of the shoulder using the Plurimeter-V inclinometer and assessment of its intrarater and interrater reliability.* Arthritis Care Res, 1998. 11(1):p.43–52.

190. Clarke, G., Willis, L., Fish, W., Nichols, P., *Assessment of movement at the glenohumeral joint.* Orthopaedics, 1974. 7:p.55–71.

191. Doody, S.G., L. Freedman, and J.C. Waterland, *Shoulder movements during abduction in the scapular plane.* Arch Phys Med Rehabil, 1970. 51(10):p.595–604.

192. Poppen, N.K. and P.S. Walker, *Normal and abnormal motion of the shoulder.* J Bone Joint Surg Am, 1976. 58(2):p.195–201.

193. Bagg, S.D. and W.J. Forrest, *A biomechanical analysis of scapular rotation during arm abduction in the scapular plane.* Am J Phys Med Rehabil, 1988. 67(6):p.238–245.

194. Downar, J.M., E.L. Sauers, and S.L. Mourtacos, *Chronic adaptations in the throwing shoulder of professional baseball players.* J of Athletic Training, 2002. 36(2):p.S–17.

195. Baltaci, G., R. Johnson, and H. Kohl, 3rd, *Shoulder range of motion characteristics in collegiate baseball players.* J Sports Med Phys Fitness, 2001. 41(2):p.236–242.

196. Johnson, L., *Patterns of shoulder flexibility among college baseball players.* J Athl Train, 1992. 27:p.44–49.

197. Ellenbecker, T.S., E.P. Roetert, D.S. Bailie, G.J. Davies, and S.W. Brown, *Glenohumeral joint total rotation range of motion in elite tennis players and baseball pitchers.* Med Sci Sports Exerc, 2002. 34(12): p.2052–2056.

198. Ellenbecker, T.S. and E.P. Roetert, *Effects of a 4-month season on glenohumeral joint rotational strength and range of motion in female collegiate tennis players.* J Strength Cond Res, 2002. 16(1):p.92–96.

199. Roetert, E.P., T.S. Ellenbecker, and S.W. Brown, *Shoulder internal and external rotation range of motion in nationally ranked junior tennis players: a longitudinal analysis.* J Strength Conditioning Res, 2000. 14(2):p.140–143.

200. Kondo, M., S. Tazoe, and M. Yamada, *Changes of the tilting angle of the scapula following elevation of the arm,* in *Surgery of the Shoulder,* J.E. Bateman, Welsh, R.P., Editor. 1984, BC Decker, Inc.: Philadelphia.p.12–16.

201. Johnson, G.R., P.R. Stuart, and S. Mitchell, *A method for the measurement of three-dimensional scapular movement.* Clin Biomech, 1993. 8:p.269–273.

202. van der Helm, F.C. and G.M. Pronk, *Three-dimensional recording and description of motions of the shoulder mechanism.* J Biomech Eng, 1995. 117(1):p.27–40.

203. Ludewig, P.M., T.M. Cook, and D.A. Nawoczenski, *Three-dimensional scapular orientation and muscle activity at selected positions of humeral elevation.* J Orthop Sports Phys Ther, 1996. 24(2):p.57–65.

204. Meskers, C.G., F.C. van der Helm, L.A. Rozendaal, and P.M. Rozing, *In vivo estimation of the glenohumeral joint rotation center from scapular bony landmarks by linear regression.* J Biomech, 1998. 31(1):p.93–96.

3

Strength Testing

An important component of the physical examination of the shoulder is strength testing of both the shoulder and of the whole upper extremity (**Figs. 3–1, 3–2**). Weakness, particularly painless weakness, can have a variety of etiologies. These should be ruled out with a careful history and thorough examination. In our clinic we have had patients referred to us diagnosed with rotator cuff disease who had tumors of the cervical spine, myasthenia gravis, amyotrophic lateral sclerosis, Parkinson's disease, and a myriad of other conditions. Although these conditions are rare, a careful assessment that includes strength testing may be needed before the diagnosis can be made accurately.

The term *muscular strength* refers to a measure describing an individual's ability to exert maximum muscular force statically or dynamically.[1] Objective measurement of shoulder strength is an important part in the comprehensive evaluation and rehabilitation of an injured shoulder. There are several applications of strength testing in the shoulder:

1. Neurologic impairment[2–8]
2. Rotator cuff tears diagnosis and evaluation after surgery[9–14]
3. Return to sports after injury[15,16]
4. Weakness as risk factor for an injury in an athlete[17]
5. Evaluation of postsurgical rehabilitation[18,19]
6. Testing of normal individuals before sports participation[15,20–23]
7. Personal injury litigation and worker's compensation[24]

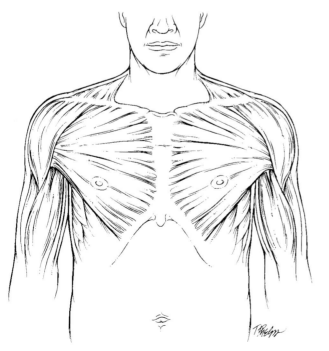

FIGURE 3–1 Anterior view of the shoulder musculature.

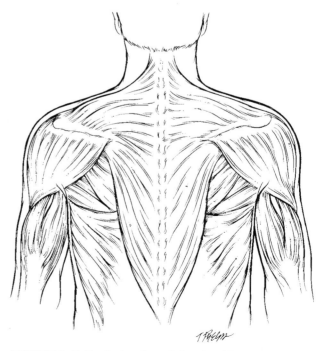

FIGURE 3–2 Posterior view of the shoulder musculature.

■ Basic Principles

Muscle physiology can be a difficult subject for the clinician. Only a minimal knowledge of muscle physiology is fortunately necessary to conduct a thorough examination of muscle strength. Several texts[25–27] describe a few basic principles necessary for understanding muscle testing. These principles and the relationship between manual muscle testing and more objective measures of muscular strength will be discussed throughout this chapter.

Correctly positioning the extremity to perform manual muscle testing is important. Each muscle has an optimum length for creating force. This relationship between force and length is known as Blix's curve (**Fig. 3–3**). If the muscle is tested at any other length other than the optimum, the muscle may be at a mechanical disadvantage to perform efficiently. This principle is also the basis of lag signs, which have been described for use in the examination of the shoulder by Hertel et al.[28] In these signs the weakened muscle is placed in a position of maximum shortening, and the patient is asked to hold the position. If the muscle is weak for any reason, then the patient will not be able to hold the arm in this position, and the arm will fall back into a position where the muscle force is not needed

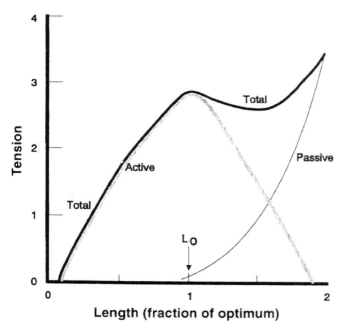

FIGURE 3–3 Blix's curve describes the optimum length of a muscle to generate force and the effects of the muscle being too long or too short on generating force. (Adapted with permission from Garret W, Best TM. Anatomy, physiology, and mechanics of skeletal muscle. In: Buckwalter J, Einhorn TA, Simon SR, eds. Orthopaedic Basic Science: Biology and Biomechanics of the Musculoskeletal System. Rosemont, IL: American Academy of Orthopaedic Surgeons;2000: 683–717.)

and the joint position is maintained by other factors (e.g., the functioning muscle–tendon units, the ligaments, and the bony confirmation). These lags signs have been used to test the infraspinatus and subscapularis muscle–tendon units[28,29] and will be described in more detail in Chapter 4.

Isolation of One Muscle

Because many muscles can perform similar functions at a given joint, it is important to position the extremity so as to isolate and differentiate the contraction of the tested muscle as much as possible. Although this concept has been advocated as a way to isolate a muscle for strength testing, it is rarely possible to completely isolate only one muscle in the shoulder when performing manual muscle testing of the upper extremity. This is particularly true in the shoulder, where so many muscles are capable of functioning for more than one purpose and where muscle substitution may hide isolated weakness in one muscle out of a muscle group.

In some settings it may be more important to test groups of muscles that make up a given myotome rather than individual muscles. Functional assessments and grading systems of muscle strength are notoriously inexact, so it is important to have a consistent system of measurement and grading to be able to communicate with other health practitioners. We favor a system that relates the upper extremity motion to strength, such as motion against gravity or motion only with gravity eliminated.

Electromyography Muscle Strength Testing

Many studies have used quantitative electromyography (EMG) techniques to delineate and evaluate the optimum position for muscle testing. These techniques have certain limitations that impact the interpretation of manual muscle testing of specific muscles. The studies are performed by placing an electrode on the skin over the muscle (surface EMG), or a fine wire is placed into the muscle itself (intramuscular fine-wire EMG). The electrode records the electrical activity of the muscle, which can then be interpreted as seen on oscilloscope.

The amount of electrical activity that is recorded is influenced by several factors, including the type of muscle fiber type, diameter, depth, and location compared with the electrode. Other factors include the electrode type and shape or amount of tissue between the electrode and muscle.[30] Fine-wire EMG evaluates the voluntary recruitment of the motor units within an activated muscle; however, it is limited by the small sample area of muscle fibers and high variability with physical activity. The surface EMG is easier to implement with a wider range of activities and samples a greater number of muscle fibers, but it is less accurate in assessing motor unit recruitment.[31]

The electrical activity detected by EMG is converted into a number that quantifies the amount of muscle activity. Most studies now attempt to standardize the method assessing muscle activity through a normalization technique. Specifically, EMG muscle activity is recorded while the subject is performing a muscle contraction. That recorded value is then compared with a reference value of EMG generated from a maximal voluntary contraction (MVC) of the same muscle. The comparison of the two values is recorded as a percentage that theoretically allows a reliable comparison of activity between subjects.[32,33]

The best method for assessing motor unit activity is unclear. Early studies suggested that EMG from an isometric MVC is less reliable than a signal obtained from an isometric submaximal contraction,[34] yet this method may yield higher intraclass correlation coefficients between trials.[35] To be specific, EMG activity for the biceps brachii is unaffected by joint angle, or concentric/eccentric muscle, action. As a result, the isometric and isokinetic MVC should be used to normalize the EMG.[30] In contrast, EMG activity during the isokinetic MVCs of the knee extensor muscles is greatest during concentric activity between 60 and 65 degrees.[36]

It is important to note that higher EMG activity does not necessarily mean that the muscle is creating more force to its tendon or upon the joint it crosses. For example, a muscle firing concentrically may generate less force than a muscle firing eccentrically with the same EMG activity.[37] An EMG is only a measure of electrical activity. It is important to realize that there is generally not a linear relationship between EMG activity and the generation of force. Other factors, such as the position of the muscle and its bipennate or unipennate configuration, influence whether this electrical activity is actually transmitted into force.[37]

Muscles as Functional Groups

Many attempts have been made to divide the muscles of the shoulder and upper extremity into functional groups specific to a particular joint motion or neurologic level. The muscles around the shoulder can also be divided anatomically into the thoracohumeral muscles, the scapulohumeral muscles, and the scapulothoracic muscles. When performing neurologic testing, it is important to test both individual muscles innervated by common peripheral nerves and groups of muscles innervated by a particular cervical level or myotome. Still others have suggested testing particular combinations of muscles that have complementary functions and create "force couples" about the shoulder.

Pink et al[38] proposed a system for conceptualizing the muscle groups around the shoulder so that their function

was emphasized. These functional groups serve as a way to remember the concepts of strengthening of shoulder muscles for what they called an E[3] (Effective and Efficient Exercise) program. An E[3] program is focused on the four *P*s, or muscles grouped according to function: the glenohumeral protectors (rotator cuff muscles), the scapulohumeral pivotors (scapular rotator muscles), the humeral positioners (three heads of the deltoid), and the power drivers (pectoralis major and latissimus dorsi). Although this classification system is a convenient way to think about the muscles around the shoulder and their functions, it has not yet been used on a widespread basis to guide treatment.

■ Examination for Muscle Strength

The examination of muscle strength varies depending on the purpose of the examination. The physician who is examining the patient for gross neurologic deficits may do an examination that differs in detail from an examination by a physical therapist or athletic trainer who is preparing an individual to return to his or her sport or activities. Strength testing also can be employed to provide normative values in a particular sport or discipline, also called athletic profiling.[20–23,39–41] This has been performed to evaluate young athletes to determine their candidacy for further training,[22,42] to distinguish among the different performance levels,[22,42,43] and to evaluate the effects of physical exercise or athletic training procedures.[44–47]

There are several factors that influence strength testing; these can be divided roughly into two broad groups. The first group comprises those related to the differences between tested participants.[18,19,41,48] These include differences in age, gender, physical activity, side, weight or body size,[21] pain,[48] motivational factors,[18] and body composition.[19] The second group of factors is related to the methods of testing. Differences in testing instruments, protocols, the position of the extremity/shoulder or the plane of motion, gravitational forces,[49] stabilization of the body,[50] and test sequences[49–53] all give different results. For example, some authors suggest that a prone examination is better than a supine examination.[27] The most important factor for an individual clinician is probably to perform the examination consistently and in a fashion that is reproducible and accurate.

Factors Affecting Muscle Strength

The variables that influence accurate strength testing are important to consider when examining a patient and when reading and comparing the literature regarding strength as a variable in the mechanism of injury,

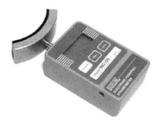

FIGURE 3–4 An example of a commercially available handheld spring scale–type of dynamometer. (Courtesy of Fabrication Enterprises, Inc.)

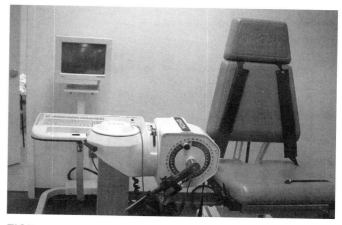

FIGURE 3–6 An example of a commercially available isokinetic dynamometer. (Kin-Com dynamometer, Chattecx Co., Chattanooga, TN)

the force measurements by the perpendicular distance measured between the joint's axis of rotation and the point of application of the dynamometer.[70] The dynamometers typically are marked with some predetermined increments in either newtons or kilograms. The strain gauge handheld dynamometers provide digital readouts of force in newtons, and the spring-scale dynamometers provide the values of strength in kilograms or pounds.

Advantages of handheld dynamometers are that they are portable, simple to use, and have a satisfactory degree of accuracy, good intrarater reproducibility, and fair to good interrater reliability. The reliability of these devices depends on their type of construction and other factors that are discussed later.

Different types of dynamometers are available (**Figs. 3–4, 3–5, 3–6**). Dynamometers can be handheld or mounted to a table or other device. There are three types of handheld dynamometers based on the mechanism inside; these include strain gauge, spring-scale, and isokinetic dynamometers. Several devices have been produced that purport to measure muscle strength[3,16,81,82] in a standardized and reproducible fashion.

Since the development of the earliest dynamometers in 1763 by Graham and Desaguliers,[83] and the earliest spring-scale device by Lovett and Martin[76] in 1916, investigators have attempted to examine the variables that affect the reliability of strength assessment using these devices. Bohannon and Andrews[84] compared the

accuracy of two spring gauge and two strain gauge dynamometers and concluded that initially the two were comparable in accuracy, but over a period of time the strain gauge dynamometer was more accurate. They advised the clinicians to check the accuracy of their dynamometers on a timely basis as the springs become fatigued in the spring dynamometer.

Hayes et al[11] studied subjects with shoulder dysfunction and compared the reliability of manual muscle tests, handheld dynamometers, and a spring-scale dynamometer for assessing shoulder strength (**Table 3–3**). They found that the reliability of manual muscle tests was less consistent than that of handheld dynamometers and

TABLE 3–3 Interrater Reliability of Three Methods of Assessing Shoulder Strength

Test*	Intraclass Correlation Coefficient (p)†	95% CI
Manual muscle test		
Elevation	.72	.38–.93
External rotation	.55	.17–.88
Internal rotation	.61	.26–.89
Liftoff	.38	.02–.81
Dynamometry		
Elevation	.92	.75–.99
External rotation	.82	.55–.96
Internal rotation	.85	.62–.97
Liftoff	.79	.50–.95
Spring-scale dynamometer		
Elevation	.96	.84–1.00
External rotation	.75	.40–.95
Internal rotation	.88	.68–.98
Adduction	.90	.72–.98

Source: Adapted with permission from Hayes K, et al. Reliability of 3 methods for assessing shoulder strength. J Shoulder Elbow Surg 2002;11(1):33–39.

*Each test was performed on eight subjects by four raters.

†Intraclass correlation coefficients (p) were calculated with use of a two-way random effects model.

CI, Confidence interval.

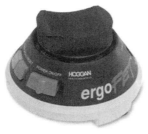

FIGURE 3–5 An example of a commercially available handheld strain gauge–type of dynamometer. (Courtesy of Hoggan Healthcare.)

TABLE 3–4 Details of Test Positions and Dynamometer Placements during the Testing of Shoulder Muscles

Muscle Action	Extremity/Joint Position	Dynamometer Placement
Shoulder Flexion	Shoulder flexed 90 degrees; elbow extended	Just proximal to epicondyles of humerus
Shoulder extension	Shoulder flexed 90 degrees; elbow flexed	Just proximal to epicondyles of humerus
Shoulder abduction	Shoulder abducted 45 degrees; elbow extended	Just proximal to lateral epicondyle of humerus
Shoulder lateral rotation	Shoulder abducted 45 degrees; elbow at 90 degrees	Just proximal to styloid processes
Shoulder medial rotation	Shoulder abducted 45 degrees; elbow at 90 degrees	Just proximal to styloid processes

Source: Adapted with permission from Andrews AW, Thomas MW, Bohannon RW. Normative values for isometric muscle force measurements obtained with handheld dynamometers. Phys Ther, 1996;76(3):248–259.

the spring-scale dynamometer. The results supported the observation of the presence of examiner bias in the use of manual muscle tests using these devices.

There have been several studies examining the reliability of dynamometers. Hosking et al[85] studied the test–retest reliability of handheld dynamometers and reported that variation in the recorded strength measurements after repeated testing did not exceed ± 15% of the initial values. Bohannon,[4] in his study on the test–retest reliability of handheld dynamometer strength testing for 18 extremity muscle groups, found that it was highly reliable, with a mean correlation coefficient of .97. He further speculated that the test–retest reliability is higher for tests performed on adult patients who are weak and have a greater distribution of strength values than the test results of healthy adults.

Some researchers have advocated that more accuracy can be obtained by testing the muscle on more that one occasion.[19,67] Others have argued, however, that a single test of muscle strength may be adequate, and that testing only once could save time and prevent fatigue of the tested person.[64–66]

Intra- and interater reliability of handheld dynamometers has been demonstrated with able-bodied subjects[86,87] and subjects with neuromuscular or orthopedic disorders.[8,88–90] Bohannon[91] summarized 18 studies on intertester reliability coefficients and found that reliability coefficients for the upper extremity actions were generally high. He further cautioned that such reliability should not be taken for granted, particularly if, relative to the testers, the muscle actions of tested subjects are strong. He advocated the training of personnel taking such readings and the standardization of their methods (**Table 3–4**).

Another issue with the use of handheld dynamometers is of the duration of the force applied, because fatigue could become a factor. Nicholas et al[92] studied the influence of the amount or duration of force applied manually by the tester, or both, on 65 patients. They evaluated the strength of hip flexors and abductor muscles with an electromechanical device. Nicholas et al concluded that the product of force with which the patient resists the tester and the time required in moving the limb through a certain range of motion were significant factors. These factors could influence the tester's perceptions of deficits in strength. These findings were consistent with the study of Ryan and Agnew[93] in 1917, who had proposed that the product of force and time was a significant factor in assessing muscle power and fatigability.

Murray et al[58] tested 40 healthy subjects with a dynamometer and presented reference values for shoulder flexors, extensors, adductors, abductors, and medial and lateral rotators (**Table 3–5**). They proposed that the data could serve as the basis of comparison in the evaluation of patients with shoulder dysfunction. In a study of 231 healthy volunteers ages 20 to 79 using handheld dynamometers, Bohannon[55] also provided reference values for shoulder abduction, extension, and lateral rotation muscle strength.

TABLE 3–5 Average Shoulder Muscle Torque (kg/cm) during Maximum Isometric Contraction*

	Men		Women	
Muscles/Joint Position	Younger	Older	Younger	Older
Number	20	20	20	20
Extensors/0 degree of flexion	812 ± 40	755 ± 30	536 ± 30	359 ± 23
Flexors/0 degree of flexion	1058 ± 47	852 ± 42	514 ± 17	384 ± 29
Flexors/45 degrees of flexion	566 ± 24	478 ± 23	338 ± 16	224 ± 18
Abductors/45 degrees of abduction	562 ± 23	426 ± 21	275 ± 15	222 ± 16
Adductors/45 degrees of abduction	1051 ± 59	833 ± 49	561 ± 33	387 ± 25
Inward rotators/0 degree of rotation	592 ± 27	444 ± 17	289 ± 12	229 ± 15
Outward rotators/0 degree of rotation	335 ± 15	280 ± 10	186 ± 8	152 ± 11

Source: Adapted with permission from Murray MP, et al. Shoulder motion and muscle strength of normal men and women in two age groups. Clin Orthop; 1985(192):268–273.

*The higher torque value from the two consecutive attempts at a maximum contraction was used to calculate average values (mean ± 1 standard error).

Donatelli et al[17] studied 39 professional baseball pitchers to compare the passive range of motion and muscle strength of the glenohumeral and scapular rotators in the pitching and nonpitching arms with the help of a handheld dynamometer. They found that the internal rotators of the pitching arm when tested in abduction were significantly stronger than those in the nonpitching arm; however, the external rotator strength of the nondominant arm in the plane of the scapula and in abduction was significantly greater than that of the pitching arm. The researchers proposed a baseline for assessment of strength in overhead throwing athletes at the beginning of the season to monitor this weakness in external rotation observed in some players.

The relative weakness of the external rotators of the dominant arm of athletes involved in throwing or overhead sports has been noticed by many researchers.[17,94–96] The exact etiology of this weakness is unknown, but there are several competing theories. The first is that the external rotators fatigue due to their function to decelerate the arm in the follow-through portion of the throw or swing.[97,98] The second is that the nerve to the infraspinatus may be damaged due to traction produced in the extremely protracted position seen in the follow-through of the throw or swing. The third is that pain and scapular dyskinesia can produce weakness due to inhibition produced by the pain of rotator cuff tendinitis or labrum lesions.[99]

> Higher internal rotation strength in the shoulder of athletes is common, and the etiology currently is unknown.

The main disadvantages of handheld dynamometers are (1) the concern of stabilization of the dynamometer and subject during the test and (2) the sufficient examiner strength needed to resist the subject's muscle contraction, particularly in muscle groups capable of high-force output.[4,86,87,100,101] This is more for lower limb muscle groups than for the upper limb muscle groups. Bohannon[4] commented that handheld dynamometers may not be good for measuring higher muscle force because the clinician's physical strength may be a factor. Because the physician is measuring the muscle strength with a handheld dynamometer, which is placed on the wrist of the patient, when the patient is asked to push against the device (which is being held by the physician), there may be error in recording the force if the physician is not able to counter the force of the patient. The maximum force may not be recorded if the patient has pushed away the device despite the countering force from the physician. Clinicians who are strong enough may consider using dynamometers with higher muscle force for measuring capacities.

Another disadvantage is that calculation of torque is not practical in the office setting as it takes additional time to calculate the torque from the force readings given by the dynamometers and the distance measurement between the joint axis and the point of application of the dynamometer. Such distance measurements are sources of error for the measurement of strength. The previously mentioned disadvantages are not a problem with isokinetic dynamometers; however, the advantages of handheld dynamometers, which include the portability, limited expense, ease, and speed with which the patient can be tested, still make them clinically more practical.[102,103]

> Handheld dynamometers are helpful but not necessary for routine evaluations; additionally, they are most useful for specific purposes, such as research and disability evaluations.

Isokinetic Testing of Muscle Strength

For isokinetic measurement of shoulder strength, equipment such as Cybex II[68] and Biodex (Biodex Corp., Shirley, NY) is commonly used (**Fig. 3–6**). These machines can test strength in isometric, concentric, and eccentric modes. They measure peak torque using a force transducer and joint angle using an electrogoniometer. The evaluation of the strength in multiaxial component motions is an advantage with isokinetic dynamometers.

Studies have shown that reliable and reproducible objective measurements of shoulder strength can be made with devices as the Cybex II[86,104] and Kincom (Chattanooga Group, Hixson, TN) isokinetic dynamometers.[105] With the addition of the Upper Body Exercise Table (UBXT) (Cybex, CSMI Norwood, MA), the Cybex II affords several multiaxial modes of testing shoulder rotational strength over a wide range of shoulder positions. Ivey et al[15] measured the strength of shoulder flexion, extension, abduction, adduction, and internal and external rotation in 31 normal volunteers with a Cybex II isokinetic dynamometer and presented the normal values for the same. They found that internal rotation strength was greater than external rotation by a ratio of 3:2, adduction strength was greater than abduction by a ratio of 2:1, and extension strength was greater than flexion strength by a ratio of 5:4. They also found that male strength was greater than female, but the advantage decreased when normalized for lean body mass and exercise habits. The researchers also found that strength was directly proportional to exercise patterns; that is, the subjects who exercised a particular group of muscles more than others had more strength in that muscle group.

Despite its good reliability and objective measurements, isokinetic equipment is usually impractical in the clinical setting, due to expenses, space requirements, specialized training, and time constraints. The use of isokinetic devices to determine the ability to perform job or sports tasks may not replicate the activity enough to be helpful for return to work or play decisions.

> Isokinetic strength testing has uses primarily for returning athletes to competition and is not a necessary part of a routine clinical evaluation.

■ Relationship of Muscle Strength to Function

One controversial area regarding muscle testing is the relationship between muscle strength testing and the activity of the muscle needed to fulfill its functions. For example, a patient may be weak with resisted abduction but have normal range of motion and nearly normal function for activities of daily living. Some authors have suggested that the function of a muscle in terms of the movements it creates can be determined by examining its origin and insertion.[106,107] Others suggest that one can only speculate on muscle function by examining the origin and insertions.[108]

When testing muscles of the shoulder used in activities of daily living or for sports activity, it is important to try to determine the function of the muscle whenever possible. This is not as easy as it sounds when considering muscles around the shoulder and scapula, as particular muscle alignments and lengths change with different positions of the shoulder. Also, the muscle may be contracting concentrically or eccentrically with a certain motion. If the muscle is not firing at a maximal level, it is not clear whether its function is to stabilize the joint or to fine-tune the motion that is being performed. For example, the serratus anterior muscle has been implicated in the development of shoulder pain in athletes.[109,110] EMG studies of athletes throwing a baseball demonstrate that the serratus anterior fires at low levels during the throwing motion,[111] and it has been postulated that abnormalities in the muscle firing pattern contributes to injury.

Variations in muscle function are important when considering strength testing of the muscles. Moseley et al[107] examined exercises that produced the most manual muscle testing in the serratus anterior muscle. They found that the highest MMT in the middle portion of this muscle was produced by arm flexion and with a military press. The lower portion of the muscle had the highest MMT in a push-up, with a plus where the scapula is retracted or "pinched" in the back once full elbow extension is reached. So are these the best positions to strengthen the serratus for a baseball player or swimmer whose sport does not typically include these motions?

The relationship between strength and function has been the subject of a long-standing debate. Most agree that the best way to train and strengthen the muscles used in a particular sport is to play that sport. A logical conclusion would be that the role of isolated strength testing of muscles in positions or motions used in a particular sport may or may not be predictive of function or ability to return to the sport after training or after medical or surgical treatment.

One goal of strength testing is to predict the function of the extremity for the tasks being asked of it by the individual being tested. It can be used as a rough measure of whether a muscle is capable of beginning more functional activities. It is generally accepted, however, that manual muscle testing can give only rough measures of the function of the extremity.

Muscle strength has been of some use in examining weakness in athletes who participate in throwing or overhead sports. Using dynamometers in athletes, several authors[17,112–114] have studied antagonistic strength ratios in baseball players and concluded that there is significant decrease in the shoulder strength ratio of external/internal rotation in a pitcher's throwing arm as compared with the nonthrowing arm, and there is significant difference between a pitcher's and a nonpitcher's dominant arm for both shoulder flexion/extension and internal/external rotation. Hence, several authors have suggested that particular attention should be paid to the maintenance of external rotation strength to prevent shoulder injuries in overhead athletes.

Shoulder muscle weakness has been proposed as a possible risk factor for developing injury in an athlete. This relationship between weakness and injury has been used as an argument for the importance of accurate strength testing in this group. More accurate methods for testing strength can be used to monitor a therapy program, to improve performance, and to prevent injury. Mayer et al[115] and others[17] are of the opinion that muscular imbalances (i.e., change in strength ratios between internal and external rotation) are more important for the onset of shoulder complaints than their influence on athletic performance capacity.

■ Testing Specific Shoulder Muscles

Thorax Muscles

Trapezius

The trapezius is the largest and most superficial of the scapulothoracic muscles (**Fig. 3–7**). It takes origin from the spinous processes of the C7 through T12 vertebrae. The upper fibers are inserted over the distal third of the clavicle, the middle fibers over the acromion and spine of the scapula, and the lower fibers at the base of the scapular spine.

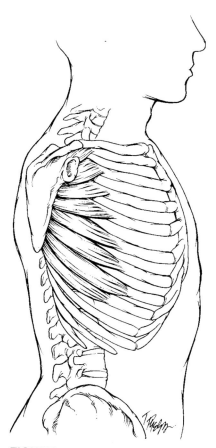

FIGURE 3–19 The serratus anterior muscle stabilizes the medial border of the scapula.

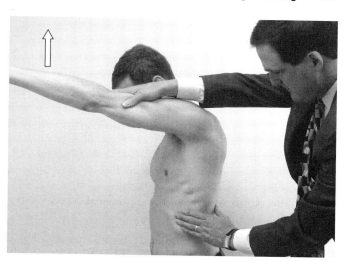

FIGURE 3–21 Strength testing of the serratus anterior muscle can be performed as shown.

(**Fig. 3–22**). A wall push-up is done by placing the arms against the wall, leaning into the wall, then pushing away from the wall, like a prone push-up.

Scapular winging can be graded as mild, moderate, or severe. In severe cases, there is prominent winging, even with the arms at the side. In severe cases, the ability to elevate the arm over 120 degrees may be limited. Moderate cases can be seen with forward elevation of the arms alone. Mild cases can be detected only with a wall push-up or if there is only minimal winging.

> The best way to test the serratus anterior is to have the subject flex the arm forward; more stress can be added if more subtle injury is suspected.

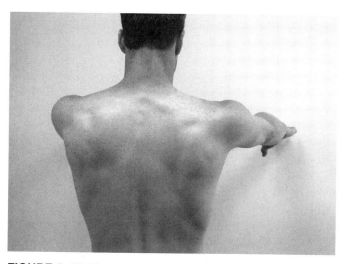

FIGURE 3–20 The serratus anterior muscle can be tested by merely having the subject flex the arms forward.

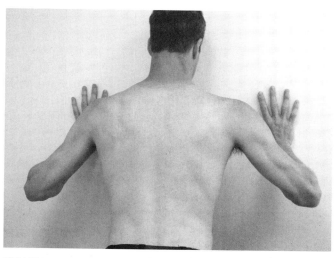

FIGURE 3–22 Subtle scapular winging due to weakness of the serratus anterior muscle may be detected by having the subject perform a push-up off the wall.

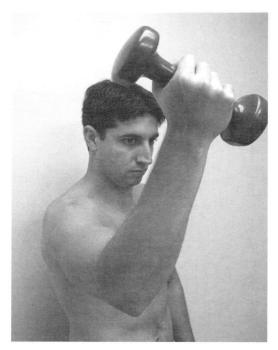

FIGURE 3–23 Elkstrom et al found the optimum position for creating electromyographic activity in the serratus anterior muscle. (Adapted with permission from Ekstrom RA, Donatelli RA, Soderberg GL. Surface electromyographic analysis of exercises for the trapezius and serratus anterior muscles. J Orthop Sports Phys Ther; 2003;33(5):247–258.

Ekstrom et al[121] found that the exercises that produced the most muscle activity in the serratus anterior muscle were diagonal exercises that had a combination of flexion, horizontal flexion, and external rotation (**Fig. 3–23**). The second position that produced the most muscle activation was with shoulder abduction above 120 degrees in the plane of the scapular. The serratus anterior muscle activity was very low with arm elevation below 80 degrees of abduction.[127]

Some scapular movement abnormalities in athletes may be due to fatigue in the serratus anterior.[110,128] This conclusion is based on EMG studies that show a low-grade contraction of the serratus anterior during the overhead motion or during the swimming stroke. Glousman et al[111] found that in overhead throwers with painful occult anterior instability serratus activity was lower than in throwers who did not have pain. Although the pattern of firing was similar between the two groups, the researchers speculated that decreased activity of the serratus anterior may alter scapular horizontal protraction and contribute to injury.

Rhomboids

The rhomboids take origin from the lower ligamentum nuchae at C7 and T1 for the rhomboid minor and T2 through T5 for the rhomboid major (**Fig. 3–24**).

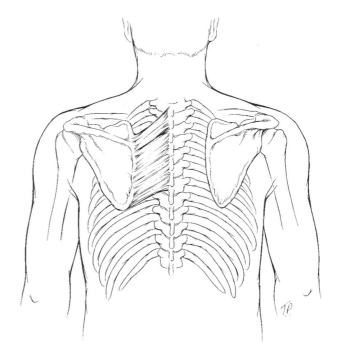

FIGURE 3–24 The rhomboid muscles.

The rhomboid minor inserts on the posterior portion of the medial base of the spine of the scapula. The rhomboid major inserts into the posterior surface of the medial border from the point at which the minor leaves off down to the inferior angle of the scapula. Innervation to the rhomboid muscle is the dorsal scapular nerve (C5).

The action of the rhomboids is adduction, elevation, and rotation of the scapula, so that the glenoid faces inferiorly. The muscle is tested with hands on the hips and pushing the elbows backward against resistance (**Fig. 3–25**). Kendall et al[27] described testing this muscle

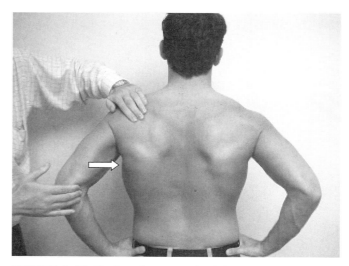

FIGURE 3–25 Testing the strength of the rhomboid muscles can be performed as shown.

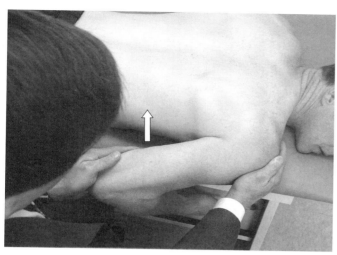

FIGURE 3–26 Kendall et al described testing the rhomboid muscles in the position shown. (Adapted with permission from Kendall H, Kendall FO, Wadsworth GE. Muscles; Testing and Function. Baltimore: Williams & Wilkins;1971:283.)

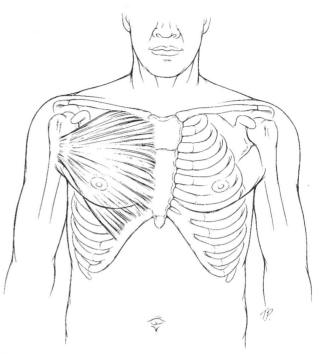

FIGURE 3–27 The pectoralis major muscle has two major portions: an upper or clavicular portion and a lower or sternal portion.

with the subject prone and with the arm adducted in slight external rotation and extension (**Fig. 3–26**). It is difficult to assess the rhomboids independently of the trapezius, which covers the rhomboids. We know of no study that has demonstrated that this position is the best test for rhomboid strength.

The exact clinical implications of weak rhomboids have not been fully elucidated; however, it has been postulated that the rhomboids act in conjunction with the trapezius and serratus to form a "force couple" controlling scapular movement.

> Isolated strength testing of the rhomboids is typically not clinically necessary, as this muscle is seldom weak.

Pectoralis Major

The pectoralis major comprises two heads of origin from the thorax (**Fig. 3–27**). The clavicular head originates from the clavicle and upper ribs, whereas the sternal head arises from the ribs and lateral border of the sternum. The two tendons rotate around each other to insert on the proximal humerus just lateral to the biceps tendon. The pectoralis major is innervated by the medial and lateral pectoral nerves, which originate from the medial and lateral cords of the brachial plexus, respectively.

The pectoralis major functions primarily as an adductor and internal rotator of the shoulder, in addition to it being a weak shoulder flexor. Pearl et al[124] found that when performing circular motions the clavicular portion of the pectoralis major functions primarily to adduct the arm medially along the horizontal plane.

There are no known isolated nerve lesions of the pectoralis that affect its function. Isolated atrophy of this muscle has not been reported to our knowledge, but deformity can be present in cases of congenital absence of the pectoralis major. This congenital absence of the pectoralis muscle may not be detected until an individual gets older, when the muscle size typically increases. Congenital deficiency of the pectoralis muscle rarely leads to any deficiencies in shoulder function, but the cosmetic deformity sometimes is a concern of patients.[128,129] Because there are so many other muscles around the shoulder that can substitute for the absent muscle, functional deficits are rarely noticed.

To test the strength of the pectoralis major muscle, the patient can be standing or supine. The arm is forward flexed to 90 degrees and slight internal rotation. The examiner resists adduction of the arm by applying pressure to the distal forearm in line with the muscle fibers. If necessary, the tendon can be palpated during testing.[27] The upper portion of the pectoralis major can be tested with the arm in 90 degrees of elevation (**Fig. 3–28**), whereas the lower portion can be tested in less forward flexion (**Fig. 3–29**).

Ruptures of the pectoralis major muscle are common and typically are seen in weight lifters, particularly when performing a bench press.[130] These acute ruptures are accompanied by pain, swelling, and ecchymosis into the arm and chest. There may be some limited motion early on, but most patients recover rapidly after this injury. Once the swelling diminishes, there is frequently an

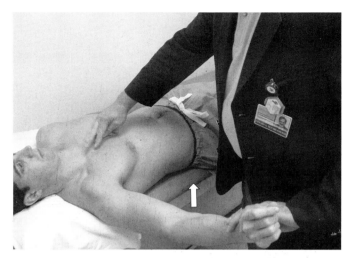

FIGURE 3–28 Testing of the strength of the upper portion of the pectoralis major can be performed as shown.

obvious defect in the tendon (**Fig. 3–30**). The deformity can be accentuated by having the patient press his or her hands together in front of the body (**Fig. 3–31**).

> To accentuate the deformity of a pectoralis tendon rupture, have the patient press his or her hands together in front of the body.

Pectoralis Minor

The pectoralis minor muscle has a fleshy origin from the second through the fifth ribs, anteriorly on the chest wall, and inserts into the base of the medial side of the coracoid. Innervation of the muscle is from the medial

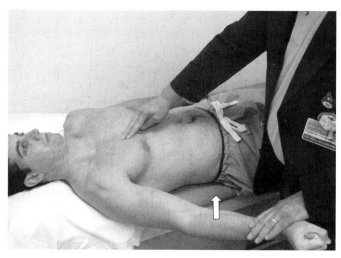

FIGURE 3–29 Testing of the strength of the lower portion of the pectoralis major can be performed as shown.

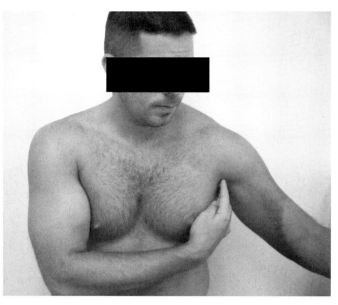

FIGURE 3–30 Rupture of the pectoralis major tendon typically produces swelling and ecchymosis on the chest and arm.

pectoral nerve (C8, T1) (**Fig. 3–32**). The pectoralis minor covers the brachial plexus as it exits the thoracic outlet, and the divisions of the brachial artery are named in relationship to this muscle.

Based on its orientation and position, the postulated function of the pectoralis minor is protraction of the scapula.[131] It has also been postulated that spasm of the muscle or contracture of this muscle can result in

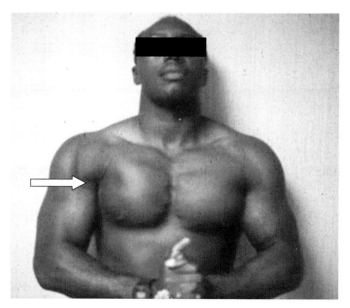

FIGURE 3–31 A rupture of the pectoralis major tendon can be accentuated by having the subject push his or her hands together with the arms elevated, as shown.

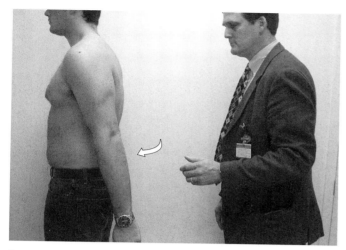

FIGURE 3–42 The deltoid lag sign is performed by having the patient extend the arm and then hold the arm in that position. If the arm falls, it is a positive test (See Chapter 4).

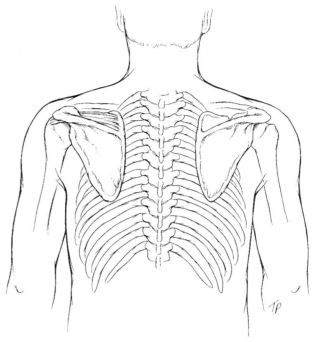

FIGURE 3–44 The supraspinatus muscle fills the supraspinatus fossa of the scapula.

tendon near the bicipital groove (**Fig. 3–43**). As the tendon of the teres minor approaches its attachment to the humerus, its tendon becomes intimately in contact with the tendon of the latissimus dorsi tendon. It is innervated by the lower subscapular nerve.

The teres major muscle functions like the latissimus dorsi muscle as an internal rotator, adductor, and extender of the shoulder.[131] Pearl et al[124] found that it fires with the latissimus dorsi muscle in motions that move the arm obliquely downward away from the midline. There are no known isolated tests of the teres major

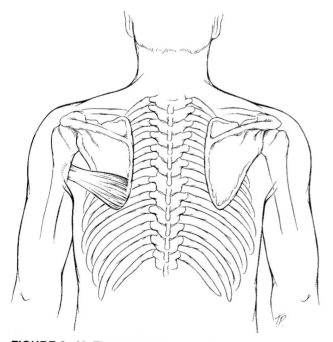

FIGURE 3–43 The teres major muscle.

muscle because it essentially has the same function as the latissimus dorsi. The teres major has been recommended as a muscle transfer for massive rotator cuff tears.[139]

Supraspinatus

The supraspinatus muscle originates in the suprascapular fossa and transitions into a thick tendon approximately at the level of the glenohumeral joint (**Fig. 3–44**). It is innervated by the suprascapular nerve, which enters the muscle after passing through the scapular notch. The supraspinatus tendon is more tendinous anteriorly than posteriorly, and the tendon inserts on the greater tuberosity.[140]

This region of attachment of the supraspinatus tendon on the greater tuberosity is called the "footprint" of the tendon insertion (**Fig. 3–45**). It should be noted that the footprint is about 1 cm in medial–lateral distance and 3 cm in width. A cadaveric study by Ruotolo et al[141] found that the mean anteroposterior dimension of the supraspinatus insertion was 25 mm. The mean superior to inferior tendon thickness at the rotator interval was 11.6 mm, 12.1 mm at the midtendon, and 12 mm at the posterior edge. The distance from the articular cartilage margin to the bony tendon insertion was 1.5 to 1.9 mm, with a mean of 1.7 mm.

The extent of this attachment of the supraspinatus tendon to the greater tuberosity of the humerus has important implications for interpreting the results of strength testing of the supraspinatus. Biomechanically, studies have shown that up to two thirds of the

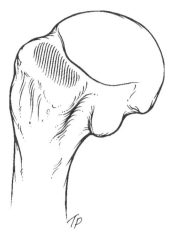

FIGURE 3–45 The supraspinatus inserts on an area of the greater tuberosity called the "footprint" of the supraspinatus tendon.

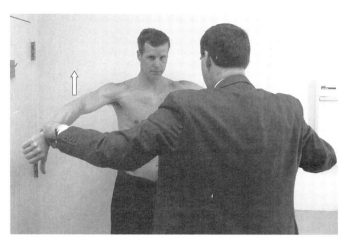

FIGURE 3–46 The strength of the supraspinatus muscle can be tested with the arm abducted in the plane of the scapula with the thumb down, known as the "empty can" position.

supraspinatus tendon must be detached before there is a large increase in the stress on the muscle unit.[142]

> In an asymptomatic supraspinatus tendon tear where the patient does not have pain, strength in the supraspinatus muscle may not be diminished until over two thirds of the tendon is torn.

There have been several studies examining the optimum position for testing the supraspinatus muscle. Jobe[143] recommended testing the supraspinatus with the arm at 90 degrees of elevation in the scapular plane, with maximum internal rotation of the shoulder, so that the thumb is pointing toward the floor and the elbow is fully extended (**Fig. 3–46**). This has been called the "empty can" position. The rationale for testing the supraspinatus in this arm position is based this on EMG testing that

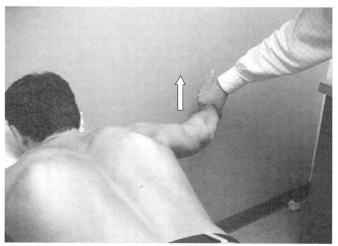

FIGURE 3–47 The strength of the supraspinatus muscle can be tested with the subject prone and the arm elevated with the arm in external rotation, a position described by Blackburn et al.[144]

showed most muscle activity occurs in this position compared with other arm positions.[107]

Blackburn et al[144] conducted an extensive EMG study of various arm positions and the effect of resistance on EMG activity in the supraspinatus. Their study confirmed that the position that seemed to isolate the supraspinatus tendon the most was abduction of the arm elevated 90 degrees and the hand in neutral rotation; however, they found that the position that created the most electrical activity in the muscle was with the subject prone with the arm elevated 100 degrees and in maximum external rotation (**Fig. 3–47**). Furthermore, they found that, although this position created the greatest EMG activity in the supraspinatus, there was also EMG activity in the infraspinatus and teres minor muscles. Worrell et al[145] found that the Blackburn position created more EMG activity in the supraspinatus, but they suggested that the Jobe position may generate more torque because of activation of the anterior and middle deltoids.

Malanga et al[146] evaluated the EMG activity of the supraspinatus and 16 other muscles around the shoulder with the arm in both the Jobe "empty can" position and the Blackburn position. They found that there were no significant differences in the EMG activation of the supraspinatus between the two positions; however, they noted that neither position isolated the supraspinatus and that other muscles influenced the strength of the arm in this position. They also noted that exercises designed to strengthen the supraspinatus in either of these positions would not isolate the supraspinatus.

> The Jobe "empty can" position does not isolate the supraspinatus and tests that muscle and the anterior and middle deltoid muscles.

Injection studies into the suprascapular and axillary nerves substantiate that both the supraspinatus and deltoid muscle function in elevation of the arm.[147] After injecting local anesthetic into the suprascapular nerve, which paralyzes the supraspinatus and infraspinatus muscles, Colachis et al[137] found that the subjects had full elevation but that the arm was slightly weak in abduction. This finding is confirmed in clinical practice, where some patients with complete tears of the supraspinatus have relatively normal shoulder function and very good shoulder strength to resisted abduction. Likewise, injecting local anesthetic into the axillary nerve (which paralyzes the deltoid muscle) left the subjects weak but still able to obtain full elevation. These studies substantiate that one can still elevate the arm without either the deltoid or the supraspinatus muscle, but if both are affected, then the patient will have significant weakness in elevation.

> The supraspinatus tendon can be completely torn, and the shoulder can have full range of motion; the only deficit will be weakness using the arm for lifting above shoulder level and with the arm away from the body.

One of the disadvantages of the Jobe "empty can" position is that this arm position can be painful in a patient with rotator cuff disease or with other shoulder pathologies.[146] Kelly et al[148] evaluated the EMG activity in the supraspinatus with the arm in three variations of the Jobe position of 90 degrees of elevation in the plane of the scapula: with the arm in maximum external rotation so that the thumb was up; with the arm in neutral rotation, with the thumb parallel to the floor (**Fig. 3–48**); and with the arm in full internal rotation so that the thumb faced the floor. The latter has become known as

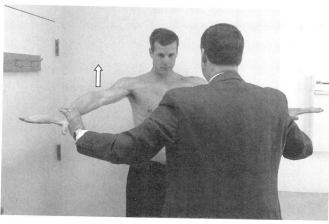

FIGURE 3–48 The strength of the supraspinatus muscle can be tested with the arm abducted in the plane of the scapula with the thumb in a neutral position parallel to the floor.

the "full can" position (**Fig. 3–49**). The researchers found no difference in the EMG activity, and they concluded that there is no advantage to testing the arm in the classic Jobe position with the thumb down.

> When testing abduction strength, the arm does not have to be in internal rotation (classic Jobe "empty can" position), but the arm can be tested in neutral rotation.

As a result of these studies, we no longer test abduction strength in the classic Jobe "empty can" position. Instead, we test the supraspinatus with the arm elevated 90 degrees and with the arm placed in the neutral position of rotation because it is less painful for patients. We recommend first testing resisted elevation of the shoulder with the arm elevated 90 degrees in the scapular plane with the elbow bent (**Fig. 3–50**). Downward pressure to the elbow

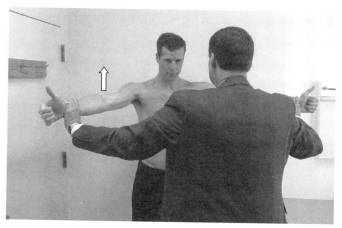

FIGURE 3–49 The strength of the supraspinatus muscle can be tested with the arm abducted in the plane of the scapula with the thumb up, known as the "full can" position.

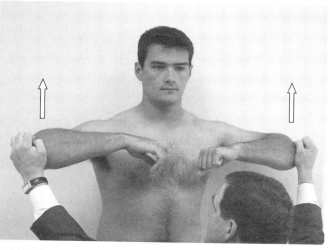

FIGURE 3–50 The strength of the supraspinatus muscle can be tested with the elbows flexed rather than extended to decrease the stress.

is then applied by the examiner, and both arms are compared. It is important to apply pressure gently at first and increase the pressure if the patient does not have pain. If the patient is not weak and does not have pain with resistance to elevation in this position, then the arm can be extended and pressure applied to the wrist. This increases the lever arm that is being tested and can be helpful in detecting more subtle weakness or pain in the shoulder.

> When evaluating elevation of the arm, testing first with the elbow bent can be followed by testing with the arm extended to detect more subtle weakness in the shoulder muscles.

EMG studies confirm that the supraspinatus muscle also functions as an external rotator of the shoulder. Jenp et al[149] studied supraspinatus muscle activity using EMGs and an isokinetic device with arm movements in several positions. They did not test the supraspinatus in abduction, nor did they try to find a test that isolated the supraspinatus; however, they found that most supraspinatus muscle activation occurred with resisted external rotation when the arm was at the side and in external rotation of ~30 degrees. In this position the other muscles that fired with resisted external rotation included the posterior deltoid, the infraspinatus, and the teres minor. Their findings suggest that strength testing of the infraspinatus with the arm at the side can be influenced by the supraspinatus if the testing position is in external rotation.

Another important aspect of testing shoulder abduction strength is to ascertain whether the patient has pain with resisted abduction. When testing for rotator cuff disease, this test typically should produce pain into the deltoid, proximal shoulder, or biceps region. This pain may radiate down the arm to the hand; however, it should be noted that many patients with large rotator cuff tears may have weakness yet no pain with resisted abduction. Also, pain with abduction is not specific for tears of the rotator cuff and can be caused by any cause of pain or inflammation in the shoulder.

> Shoulder pain with resisted abduction of the arm should raise suspicion for supraspinatus tendon pathology, but pain in this position can be due to a variety of shoulder pathologies.

Infraspinatus

The infraspinatus fills the infraspinatus fossa of the scapula. It becomes tendinous more distally in relation to the shoulder joint than the supraspinatus (**Fig. 3–51**). Its attachment to the greater tuberoses is posterior and inferior, and its tendon attachment is nearly indistinguishable from the teres minor tendon. In some patients

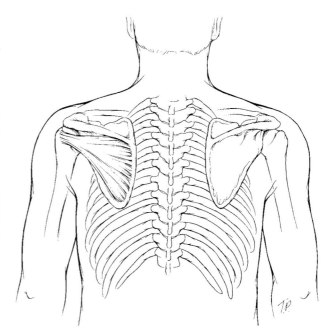

FIGURE 3–51 The infraspinatus muscle.

there is a cleft between the infraspinatus tendon and the supraspinatus tendon, but a true rotator cuff interval as seen anteriorly between the supraspinatus and subscapularis tendons is not common.

The infraspinatus is innervated by the infraspinatus branches of the suprascapular nerve. These branches are the continuation of the nerve after it has given off its motor branches to the supraspinatus muscle, and the nerve courses through the spinoglenoid notch at the base of the scapular spine. The infraspinatus branch makes a turn medially around the scapular spin and then courses for several centimeters before splitting into several branches to the infraspinatus muscle.

Atrophy of the infraspinatus can be due to several etiologies, but the most common are infraspinatus tendon tears or damage to the infraspinatus branch of the suprascapular nerve by compressive lesions (usually synovial cysts) or by traction injuries. The exact cause of traction injuries to the infraspinatus branches is unknown, but such injuries are seen in overhead athletes such as baseball pitchers and volleyball players.[150] These lesions are often asymptomatic, but they also can produce pain, a nonspecific dull ache.[151] In a study conducted by Ferretti et al[152] on 96 top-level volleyball players who competed during the European championships, 12 players were found to have asymptomatic isolated paralysis of the infraspinatus of the dominant side.

> Isolated infraspinatus weakness and atrophy can be tolerated enough by the shoulder to allow athletes to participate in overhead sports with few limitations.

44. Bell, G.J. and H.A. Wenger, *Physiological adaptations to velocity-controlled resistance training.* Sports Med, 1992. **13**(4):p.234–44.

45. Bemben, M.G. and R.E. Murphy, *Age related neural adaptation following short term resistance training in women.* J Sports Med Phys Fitness, 2001. **41**(3):p.291–9.

46. Kanehisa, H. and M. Miyashita, *Specificity of velocity in strength training.* Eur J Appl Physiol Occup Physiol, 1983. **52**(1):p.104–6.

47. Kraemer, W.J., S.A. Mazzetti, B.C. Nindl, L.A. Gotshalk, J.S. Volek, J.A. Bush, J.O. Marx, K. Dohi, A.L. Gomez, M. Miles, S.J. Fleck, R.U. Newton, and K. Hakkinen, *Effect of resistance training on women's strength/power and occupational performances.* Med Sci Sports Exerc, 2001. **33**(6):p.1011–25.

48. Ben-Yishay, A., J.D. Zuckerman, M. Gallagher, and F. Cuomo, *Pain inhibition of shoulder strength in patients with impingement syndrome.* Orthopedics, 1994. **17**(8):p.685–8.

49. Winter, D.A., R.P. Wells, and G.W. Orr, *Errors in the use of isokinetic dynamometers.* Eur J Appl Physiol Occup Physiol, 1981. **46**(4):p.397–408.

50. Mendler, H.M., *Effect of stabilization on maximum isometric knee extensor force.* Phys Ther, 1967. **47**(5): p.375–9.

51. Cahalan, T.D., M.E. Johnson, and E.Y. Chao, *Shoulder strength analysis using the Cybex II isokinetic dynamometer.* Clin Orthop, 1991(271): p.249–57.

52. Ellenbecker, T.S., G.J. Davies, and M.J. Rowinski, *Concentric versus eccentric isokinetic strengthening of the rotator cuff. Objective data versus functional test.* Am J Sports Med, 1988. **16**(1):p. 64–9.

53. Kuhlman, J.R., J.P. Iannotti, M.J. Kelly, F.X. Riegler, M.L. Gevaert, and T.M. Ergin, *Isokinetic and isometric measurement of strength of external rotation and abduction of the shoulder.* J Bone Joint Surg Am, 1992. **74**(9):p.1320–33.

54. Andrews, A.W., M.W. Thomas, and R.W. Bohannon, *Normative values for isometric muscle force measurements obtained with hand-held dynamometers.* Phys Ther, 1996. **76**(3): p. 248–59.

55. Bohannon, R.W., *Reference values for extremity muscle strength obtained by hand-held dynamometry from adults aged 20 to 79 years.* Arch Phys Med Rehabil, 1997. **78**(1):p.26–32.

56. Connelly Maddux, R.E.C., W.B. Kibler, and T. Uhl, *Isokinetic peak torque and work values for the shoulder.* J Orthop Sports Phys Ther, 1989. **10**:p.264–69.

57. Davies, G.J., *A compendium of isokinetics in clinical usage.* Vol. 4. 1984, Lacrosse,WI: S&S Publishers. p.261–91.

58. Murray, M.P., D.R. Gore, G.M. Gardner, and L.A. Mollinger, *Shoulder motion and muscle strength of normal men and women in two age groups.* Clin Orthop, 1985(192):p.268–73.

59. Warner, J.J., L.J. Micheli, L.E. Arslanian, J. Kennedy, and R. Kennedy, *Patterns of flexibility, laxity, and strength in normal shoulders and shoulders with instability and impingement.* Am J Sports Med, 1990. **18**(4):p.366–75.

60. Edwards, R.H. and M. McDonnell, *Hand-held dynamometer for evaluating voluntary-muscle function.* Lancet, 1974. **2**(7883): p.757–8.

61. Hyde, S.A., C.M. Goddard, and O.M. Scott, *The myometer: the development of a clinical tool.* Physiotherapy, 1983. **69**(12):p.424–7.

62. Figoni, S.F. and A.F. Morris, *Effects of knowledge of results on reciprocal, isokinetic strength and fatigue.* J Orthop Sports Phys Ther, 1984. **6**:p.190–97.

63. McGarvey, S.R., B.F. Morrey, L.J. Askew, and K.N. An, *Reliability of isometric strength testing. Temporal factors and strength variation.* Clin Orthop, 1984(185):p.301–5.

64. Bohannon, R., *Hand-held dynamometry; stability of muscle strength over multiple measurements.* Clin Biomech (Bristol, Avon), 1987. **2**:p.74–77.

65. Bohannon, R. and N. Saunders, *Hand-held dynamometry: A single trial may be adequate for measuring muscle strength in healthy individuals.* Physiotherapy Canada, 1990. **42**:p.6–9.

66. Schenck, J.M. and E.M. Forward, *Quantitative strength changes with test repetitions.* Phys Ther, 1965. **45**:p.562–69.

67. Whitley, J.D. and L.E. Smith, *Larger correlations obtained by using average rather than "best" strength scores.* Res Quart, 1963. **34**:p.248–49.

68. Cybex, *Isolated joint testing and exercise: A handbook for using the Cybex II and U.B.X.T.* 1984, New York: Ronkonkoma.

69. Saha, A.K., *The classic. Mechanism of shoulder movements and a plea for the recognition of "zero position" of glenohumeral joint.* Clin Orthop, 1983(173):p.3–10.

70. Bohannon, R., *Testing isometric limb muscle strength with dynamometers.* Phys Rehab Med, 1990. **2**(2):p.75–86.

71. Kelly, B.T., W.R. Kadrmas, D.T. Kirkendall, and K.P. Speer, *Optimal normalization tests for shoulder muscle activation: an electromyographic study.* J Orthop Res, 1996. **14**(4):p.647–53.

72. Soderberg, G.J. and M.J. Blaschak, *Shoulder internal and external rotation peak torque production through a velocity spectrum in differing positions.* J Orthop Sports Phys Ther, 1987. **8**:p.518–23.

73. Neer, C.S., 2nd, *Anterior acromioplasty for the chronic impingement syndrome in the shoulder: a preliminary report.* J Bone Joint Surg Am, 1972. **54**(1):p.41–50.

74. Neer, C.S., 2nd and R.P. Welsh, *The shoulder in sports.* Orthop Clin North Am, 1977. **8**(3):p.583–91.

75. Daniels, L. and C. Worthingham, *Muscle testing techniques of manual examination.* 5th ed. 1986, Philadelphia: W.B. Saunders.

76. Lovett, P.W. and E.G. Martin, *Certain aspects of infantile paralysis with a description of a method of muscle testing.* JAMA, 1916. **66**: p.729–33.

77. Hoppenfeld, S., *Physical examination of the spine and extremities.* 1976, New York: Appleton-Century-Crofts. 26.

78. Council, M.R., *Aids to the evaluation of peripheral nerve injuries,* in *Her Majesty's stationary office.* 1943: London.

79. Gonnella, C., G. Harmon, and M. Jacobs, *The role of the physical therapist in the gamma globulin poliomyelitis prevention study.* Phys Ther Rev, 1953. **33**(7):p.337–45.

80. Brooke, M.H., R.C. Griggs, J.R. Mendell, G.M. Fenichel, J.B. Shumate, and R.J. Pellegrino, *Clinical trial in Duchenne dystrophy. I. The design of the protocol.* Muscle Nerve, 1981. **4**(3):p.186–97.

81. Clarke, H., *Improvemnet of objective strength tests of muscle groups by cable-tension methods.* Res Q, 1951. **22**:p.399–419.

82. Hunsicker, P.A. and R. Donnelly, *Instruments to measure strength.* Res Q, 1955. **26**:p.408–420.

83. Pearn, J., *Two early dynamometers. An historical account of the earliest measurements to study human muscular strength.* J Neurol Sci, 1978. **37**(1–2):p.127–34.

84. Bohannon, R. and A.W. Andrews, *Accuracy of spring and strain gauge hand-held dynamometers.* J Orthop Sports Phys Ther, 1989. **10**:p.323–325.

85. Hosking, J.P., U.S. Bhat, V. Dubowitz, and R.H. Edwards, *Measurements of muscle strength and performance in children with normal and diseased muscle.* Arch Dis Child, 1976. **51**(12):p.957–63.

86. Agre, J.C., J.L. Magness, S.Z. Hull, K.C. Wright, T.L. Baxter, R. Patterson, and L. Stradel, *Strength testing with a portable dynamometer: reliability for upper and lower extremities.* Arch Phys Med Rehabil, 1987. **68**(7):p.454–8.

87. Byl, N.N., S. Richards, and J. Asturias, *Intrarater and interrater reliability of strength measurements of the biceps and deltoid using a hand held dynamometer.* J Orthop Sports Phys Ther, 1988. **9**:p.399–405.

88. Bohannon, R.W. and A.W. Andrews, *Interrater reliability of hand-held dynamometry.* Phys Ther, 1987. **67**(6):p.931–3.

89. Hayes, K.W. and J. Falconer, *Differential muscle strength decline in osteoarthritis of the knee. A developing hypothesis.* Arthritis Care Res, 1992. **5**(1):p.24–8.

90. Stuberg, W.A. and W.K. Metcalf, *Reliability of quantitative muscle testing in healthy children and in children with Duchenne muscular dystrophy using a hand-held dynamometer.* Phys Ther, 1988. **68**(6): p.977–82.

91. Bohannon, R.W., *Intertester reliability of hand-held dynamometry: a concise summary of published research.* Percept Mot Skills, 1999. **88**(3 Pt 1):p.899–902.

92. Nicholas, J.A., A. Sapega, H. Kraus, and J.N. Webb, *Factors influencing manual muscle tests in physical therapy.* J Bone Joint Surg Am, 1978. **60**(2):p.186–90.

93. Ryan, A.H. and J.H. Agnew, *Studies in muscular power and fatigue.* Am J Physiol, 1917. **42**:p.599–600.

94. Chandler, T.J., W.B. Kibler, E.C. Stracener, A.K. Ziegler, and B. Pace, *Shoulder strength, power, and endurance in college tennis players.* Am J Sports Med, 1992. **20**(4):p.455–8.

95. Ellenbecker, T. and E.P. Roetert, *Age specific isokinetic glenohumeral internal and external rotation strength in elite junior tennis players.* J Sci Med Sport, 2003. **6**(1):p.63–70.

96. Ellenbecker, T.S. and A.J. Mattalino, *Concentric isokinetic shoulder internal and external rotation strength in professional baseball pitchers.* J Orthop Sports Phys Ther, 1997. **25**(5):p.323–8.

97. Glousman, R., *Electromyographic analysis and its role in the athletic shoulder.* Clin Orthop, 1993(288):p.27–34.

98. Jobe, F.W., D.R. Moynes, J.E. Tibone, and J. Perry, *An EMG analysis of the shoulder in pitching. A second report.* Am J Sports Med, 1984. **12**(3):p.218–20.

99. Kibler, W.B., *The role of the scapula in athletic shoulder function.* Am J Sports Med, 1998. **26**(2):p.325–37.

100. Brinkmann, J.R., *Comparison of a hand-held and fixed dynamometer in measuring strength of patients with neuromuscular disease.* J Orthop Sports Phys Ther, 1994. **19**(2):p.100–4.

101. Wikhom, J.B. and R. Bohannon, *Hand-held dynamometer measurements: tester strength makes a difference.* J Orthop Sports Phys Ther, 1991. **13**:p.191–98.

102. Bohannon, R.W., *Manual muscle test scores and dynamometer test scores of knee extension strength.* Arch Phys Med Rehabil, 1986. **67**(6):p.390–2.

103. Bohannon, R.W., *Research incorporating hand-held dynamometry: publication trends since 1948.* Percept Mot Skills, 1998. **86**(3 Pt 2): p.1177–8.

104. Noreau, L. and J. Vachon, *Comparison of three methods to assess muscular strength in individuals with spinal cord injury.* Spinal Cord, 1998. **36**(10):p.716–23.

105. Plotnikoff, N.A. and D.L. MacIntyre, *Test-retest reliability of glenohumeral internal and external rotator strength.* Clin J Sport Med, 2002. **12**(6):p.367–72.

106. Mackenzie, W.C., Sir, *The action of muscles, including muscle rest and muscle re-education.* 2nd ed. 1930, New York: Paul B. Hoeber. 44,45.

107. Moseley, J.B., Jr., F.W. Jobe, M. Pink, J. Perry, and J. Tibone, *EMG analysis of the scapular muscles during a shoulder rehabilitation program.* Am J Sports Med, 1992. **20**(2):p.128–34.

108. Brunnstrom, S., *Muscle testing around the shoulder girdle.* J Bone Joint Surg Am, 1941. **23**:p.263–272.

109. Patel, D.R. and T.L. Nelson, *Winging of the Scapula in a Young Athlete.* Adolesc Med, 1996. **7**(3):p.433–438.

110. Pink, M., F.W. Jobe, J. Perry, A. Browne, M.L. Scovazzo, and J. Kerrigan, *The painful shoulder during the butterfly stroke. An electromyographic and cinematographic analysis of twelve muscles.* Clin Orthop Relat Res, 1993(288):p.60–72.

111. Glousman, R., F. Jobe, J. Tibone, D. Moynes, D. Antonelli, and J. Perry, *Dynamic electromyographic analysis of the throwing shoulder with glenohumeral instability.* J Bone Joint Surg Am, 1988. **70**(2): p.220–6.

112. Cook, E.E., V.L. Gray, E.S. Nogue, and J. Medeiros, *Shoulder antaganostic strength ratios: A comparison between college-level baseball pitchers and nonpitchers.* J Orthop Sports Phys Ther, 1987. **8**:p.451–61.

113. Hinton, R.Y., *Isokinetic evaluation of shoulder rotational strength in high school baseball pitchers.* Am J Sports Med, 1988. **16**(3):p.274–9.

114. Mackinnon, S.E., S. McCabe, J.F. Murray, J.P. Szalai, L. Kelly, C. Novak, B. Kin, and G.M. Burke, *Internal neurolysis fails to improve the results of primary carpal tunnel decompression.* J Hand Surg [Am], 1991. **16**(2):p.211–8.

115. Mayer, F., D. Axmann, T. Horstmann, F. Martini, J. Fritz, and H.H. Dickhuth, *Reciprocal strength ratio in shoulder abduction/adduction in sports and daily living.* Med Sci Sports Exerc, 2001. **33**(10): p.1765–9.

116. Lindman, R., A. Eriksson, and L.E. Thornell, *Fiber type composition of the human male trapezius muscle: enzyme-histochemical characteristics.* Am J Anat, 1990. **189**(3):p.236–44.

117. Lindman, R., A. Eriksson, and L.E. Thornell, *Fiber type composition of the human female trapezius muscle: enzyme-histochemical characteristics.* Am J Anat, 1991. **190**(4):p.385–92.

118. Inman, V.T., J.B. Saunders, and L.C. Abbott, *Observations of the function of the shoulder joint. 1944.* Clin Orthop Relat Res, 1996(330):p.3–12.

119. Inman, V.T., M. Saundersm, and L.C. Abbott, *Observations of the function of the shoulder joint.* J Bone Joint Surg, 1944. **26A**:p.1–31.

120. Silliman, J.F. and M.T. Dean, *Neurovascular injuries to the shoulder complex.* J Orthop Sports Phys Ther, 1993. **18**(2):p.442–8.

121. Ekstrom, R.A., R.A. Donatelli, and G.L. Soderberg, *Surface electromyographic analysis of exercises for the trapezius and serratus anterior muscles.* J Orthop Sports Phys Ther, 2003. **33**(5):p.247–58.

122. Townsend, H., F.W. Jobe, M. Pink, and J. Perry, *Electromyographic analysis of the glenohumeral muscles during a baseball rehabilitation program.* Am J Sports Med, 1991. **19**(3):p.264–72.

123. Scheving, L.E. and J.E. Pauly, *An electromyographic study of some muscles acting on the upper extremity of man.* Anat Rec, 1959. **135**:p.239–45.

124. Pearl, M.L., J. Perry, L. Torburn, and L.H. Gordon, *An electromyographic analysis of the shoulder during cones and planes of arm motion.* Clin Orthop Relat Res, 1992(284):p.116–27.

125. Schickendantz, M.S., C.P. Ho, L. Keppler, and B.D. Shaw, *MR imaging of the thrower's shoulder. Internal impingement, latissimus dorsi/subscapularis strains, and related injuries.* Magn Reson Imaging Clin N Am, 1999. **7**(1):p.39–49.

126. Nobuhara, K., *The Shoulder: Its Function and Clinical Aspects.* Vol. 1. 2001, Singapore: World Scientific Publishing. p.515.

127. Decker, M.J., R.A. Hintermeister, K.J. Faber, and R.J. Hawkins, *Serratus anterior muscle activity during selected rehabilitation exercises.* Am J Sports Med, 1999. **27**(6):p.784–91.

128. Pink, M., J. Perry, A. Browne, M.L. Scovazzo, and J. Kerrigan, *The normal shoulder during freestyle swimming. An electromyographic and cinematographic analysis of twelve muscles.* Am J Sports Med, 1991. **19**(6):p.569–76.

129. Ireland, D.C., N. Takayama, and A.E. Flatt, *Poland's syndrome.* J Bone Joint Surg Am, 1976. **58**(1):p.52–8.

130. Jones, M.W. and J.P. Matthews, *Rupture of pectoralis major in weight lifters: a case report and review of the literature.* Injury, 1988. **19**(3):p.219.

131. Jobe, C.M. and M.J. Coen, *Gross anatomy of the shoulder,* in *The Shoulder,* C.A. Rockwood, et al., Editors. 2004, Elsevier: Philadelphia. p.33–96.

132. Jobe, C.M., *Gross anatomy of the shoulder,* in *The Shoulder, 3rd ed.,* F.A. Matsen, 3rd, Editor. 1998, WB Saunders: Philadelphia. p.1–33.

133. Mehallo, C.J., *Isolated tear of the pectoralis minor.* Clin J Sport Med, 2004. **14**(4):p.245–6.

134. DiVeta, J., M.L. Walker, and B. Skibinski, *Relationship between performance of selected scapular muscles and scapular abduction in standing subjects.* Phys Ther, 1990. **70**(8):p.470–6.

135. Saha, A.K., *Dynamic stability of the glenohumeral joint.* Acta Orthop Scand, 1971. **42**(6):p.491–505.

136. Lee, S.B. and K.N. An, *Dynamic glenohumeral stability provided by three heads of the deltoid muscle.* Clin Orthop Relat Res, 2002(400): p.40–7.

137. Colachis, S.C.J., B.R. Strohm, and V.L. Brechner, *Effects of axillary nerve block on muscle force in the upper extremity.* Arch Phys Med Rehabil, 1969. **50**(11):p.647–54.

138. Hertel, R., S.M. Lambert, and F.T. Ballmer, *The deltoid extension lag sign for diagnosis and grading of axillary nerve palsy.* J Shoulder Elbow Surg, 1998. **7**(2):p.97–9.

139. Magermans, D.J., E.K. Chadwick, H.E. Veeger, F.C. van der Helm, and P.M. Rozing, *Biomechanical analysis of tendon transfers for massive rotator cuff tears.* Clin Biomech (Bristol, Avon), 2004. **19**(4): p.350–7.

140. Volk, A.G. and C.T.J. Vangsness, *An anatomic study of the supraspinatus muscle and tendon.* Clin Orthop Relat Res, 2001(384):p.280–5.

141. Ruotolo, C., J.E. Fow, and W.M. Nottage, *The supraspinatus footprint: an anatomic study of the supraspinatus insertion.* Arthroscopy, 2004. **20**(3):p.246–9.

142. Halder, A.M., S.W. O'Driscoll, G. Heers, N. Mura, M.E. Zobitz, K.N. An, and R. Kreusch-Brinker, *Biomechanical comparison of effects of supraspinatus tendon detachments, tendon defects, and muscle retractions.* J Bone Joint Surg Am, 2002. **84-A**(5):p.780–5.

143. Jobe, F.W., *Operative Techniques in Upper Extremity Sports Injury.* Vol. 1996. 1996, St. Louis: Mosby.

144. Blackburn, T.A., W.D. McLeod, B. White, and L. Wofford, *EMG analysis of posterior rotator cuff exercise.* Athl Train, 1990. **25**:p.40–45.

145. Worrell, T.W., B.J. Corey, S.L. York, and J. Santiestaban, *An analysis of supraspinatus EMG activity and shoulder isometric force development.* Med Sci Sports Exerc, 1992. **24**(7):p.744–8.

146. Malanga, G.A., Y.N. Jenp, E.S. Growney, and K.N. An, *EMG analysis of shoulder positioning in testing and strengthening the supraspinatus.* Med Sci Sports Exerc, 1996. **28**(6):p.661–4.

147. Colachis, S.C., Jr. and B.R. Strohm, *Effect of suprascauular and axillary nerve blocks on muscle force in upper extremity.* Arch Phys Med Rehabil, 1971. **52**(1):p.22–9.

148. Kelly, B.T., W.R. Kadrmas, and K.P. Speer, *The manual muscle examination for rotator cuff strength. An electromyographic investigation.* Am J Sports Med, 1996. **24**(5):p.581–8.

149. Jenp, Y.N., G.A. Malanga, E.S. Growney, and K.N. An, *Activation of the rotator cuff in generating isometric shoulder rotation torque.* Am J Sports Med, 1996. **24**(4):p.477–85.

150. Cummins, C.A., T.M. Messer, and M.F. Schafer, *Infraspinatus muscle atrophy in professional baseball players.* Am J Sports Med, 2004. **32**(1):p.116–20.

151. Ferretti, A., A. De Carli, and M. Fontana, *Injury of the suprascapular nerve at the spinoglenoid notch. The natural history of infraspinatus atrophy in volleyball players.* Am J Sports Med, 1998. **26**(6):p.759–63.

152. Ferretti, A., G. Cerullo, and G. Russo, *Suprascapular neuropathy in volleyball players.* J Bone Joint Surg Am, 1987. **69**(2):p.260–3.

153. Greis, P.E., J.E. Kuhn, J. Schultheis, R. Hintermeister, and R. Hawkins, *Validation of the lift-off test and analysis of subscapularis activity during maximal internal rotation.* Am J Sports Med, 1996. **24**(5):p.589–93.

154. Chang, Y.W., R.E. Hughes, F.C. Su, E. Itoi, and K.N. An, *Prediction of muscle force involved in shoulder internal rotation.* J Shoulder Elbow Surg, 2000. **9**(3):p.188–95.

155. Gerber, C. and R.J. Krushell, *Isolated rupture of the tendon of the subscapularis muscle. Clinical features in 16 cases.* J Bone Joint Surg Br, 1991. **73**(3):p.389–94.

156. Stefko, J.M., F.W. Jobe, R.S. VanderWilde, E. Carden, and M. Pink, *Electromyographic and nerve block analysis of the subscapularis liftoff test.* J Shoulder Elbow Surg, 1997. **6**(4):p.347–55.

157. Gerber, C., O. Hersche, and A. Farron, *Isolated rupture of the subscapularis tendon.* J Bone Joint Surg Am, 1996. **78**(7):p.1015–23.

158. Tokish, J.M., M.J. Decker, H.B. Ellis, M.R. Torry, and R.J. Hawkins, *The belly-press test for the physical examination of the subscapularis muscle: electromyographic validation and comparison to the lift-off test.* J Shoulder Elbow Surg, 2003. **12**(5):p.427–30.

159. Kim, T.K., P.B. Rauh, and E.G. McFarland, *Partial tears of the subscapularis tendon found during arthroscopic procedures on the shoulder: a statistical analysis of sixty cases.* Am J Sports Med, 2003. **31**(5):p.744–50.

160. Armstrong, A., C. Lashgari, J. Menendez, S.A. Teefey, L.M. Galatz, and K. Yamaguchi, *Ultrasound evaluation of the subscapularis tendon after total shoulder arthroplasty,* in *Ninth International Congress on the Surgery of the Shoulder.* 5/4/2004: Washington, D.C.

161. Patte, D. and J. Debeyre, *Surgical treatment of ruptures of the rotator cuff of the shoulder.[French].* Chirurgie, 1983. **109**(4):p.337–41.

162. Hovelius, L., C. Akermark, B. Albrektsson, E. Berg, L. Korner, B. Lundberg, and T. Wredmark, *Bristow-Latarjet procedure for recurrent anterior dislocation of the shoulder. A 2–5 year follow-up study on the results of 112 cases.* Acta Orthop Scand, 1983. **54**(2):p.284–90.

163. Richards, R.R., A.R. Hudson, J.T. Bertoia, J.R. Urbaniak, and J.P. Waddell, *Injury to the brachial plexus during Putti-Platt and Bristow procedures. A report of eight cases.* Am J Sports Med, 1987. **15**(4):p.374–80.

4

Rotator Cuff Disease and Impingement

Rotator cuff disease is the most common condition of the shoulder for which patients seek treatment. The symptoms of rotator cuff disease increase with age almost linearly, so most people will have one episode of shoulder pain during their adult lives that will be due to rotator cuff problems. Rotator cuff disease also affects athletes and active individuals regardless of age and activity level, and this underscores that there are several possible etiologies of rotator cuff problems.

Exactly what causes rotator cuff problems has been debated for several centuries, and the debate is far from over. New knowledge has begun to question old dogma and to create new theories of why rotator cuff disease occurs and how it produces symptoms. Consequently, a review of the history of the concepts of rotator cuff disease serves to illustrate that the exact etiology of this condition is not known. Knowledge of the pathophysiology of rotator cuff disease is essential to understanding the variability of the complaints of the patient and why the examination continues to be challenging for this common condition.

There is increasing evidence that rotator cuff problems are a multifactorial disease. The most accepted theory in the past 40 years has been on of "impingement," as popularized by Neer.[1] There is increasing evidence, however, that rotator cuff disease may not be due to impingement alone. There is also some evidence that impingement between structures may occur in different ways and in different areas than previously understood. The anatomy of the rotator cuff was described in Chapter 3.

■ Background

Who first used the term *rotator cuff* is not obvious in the literature. The first description of its rupture, however, is by Smith in 1834.[2] He described seven cases of tears in the rotator cuff in specimens obtained by grave robbing.

He described many of the variations of rotator cuff pathology recognized today, ranging from small tears involving the subscapularis to massive degenerative tears with an associated biceps tendon dislocation.

Codman[3] revolutionized the knowledge about the musculotendinous cuff, or rotator cuff. In his book, he summarized his 25 years' experience with rotator cuff disease. He recommended early operative repair for complete cuff tears and is credited with the first cuff repair, in 1909. Other authors noted that the lesions of the rotator cuff seemed to be degenerative with age, but the exact etiology was uncertain.

■ Theories of Rotator Cuff Disease

There are several current theories regarding the etiology of rotator cuff pathology. These include degeneration of the tendon due to senescence, tearing of an avascular area of the tendons, impingement, tears due to anterior shoulder instability, tears due to trauma, and tears due to superior instability associated with superior labrum anterior to posterior (SLAP) lesions. Some physicians would suggest that tears of the rotator cuff may be due to any of these or to several mechanisms at once. It is likely that some of these mechanisms are associated or related to each other, such that one cause is linked closely to another. For example, Pettersson[4] suggested that normal tendons rarely tear due to traumatic mechanisms, whereas tendons that have been affected by age are weaker (and thereby abnormal) and subject to tearing more easily with sudden stress.

There is significant evidence that rotator cuff tears are due in part to senescence of the tendons with age.[1,3,5–11] There is no doubt that the incidence of rotator cuff pathology and tears increases with age. This is supported by cadaveric studies, radiological imaging studies, and patient case series. The cadaveric studies are summarized in **Table 4–1**. Imaging studies using arthrography,

complaints, they found that 35 patients had a full-thickness rotator cuff tear, and 70% had a type III acromion. It should be noted, however, that their study did not delineate definitive criteria for each acromial shape. Although they proved an association between acromial shape and rotator cuff pathology, they did not establish causality.

These criticisms were to form the basis of a controversy that continues to the present day. A study by Bright et al[51] evaluated the inter- and intraobserver reliability of Bigliani et al's classification system. The supraspinatus outlet views of 40 patients were reviewed twice, 4 months apart, by six reviewers. For each of the two readings, all observers agreed only 18% of the time, and Bright et al suggested that more definitive criteria are needed to distinguish and classify the acromion. A study by Jacobson et al[52] reported similar results.

Several subsequent researchers attempted to duplicate the findings of Morrison and Bigliani.[50] Aoki et al[53] developed a technique of measuring the slope of the acromion with a lateral radiograph in the plane of the scapula. Their investigations of bleached skeleton shoulders revealed that the acromial spur and narrowing of the supraspinatus outlet are associated with a flatter acromial slope. This supported Neer's original statement implicating the increasing slope of the acromion in the impingement syndrome.[1] Edelson and Taitz[54] found that the length of the acromion plays an important role in the development of degenerative changes and associated cuff problems. Nicholson et al[55] demonstrated on a review of 420 scapulae that spur formation of the anterior acromion was an age-related process such that individuals younger than 50 years of age had less than one quarter the prevalence of those older than 50 years of age. The status of the rotator cuffs of these shoulders was unknown.

Ozaki et al[7] studied the histology of the acromial undersurface in 200 cadavers and found that rotator cuff tears that did not extend to the bursal surface were associated with normal acromial histology, whereas those that extended to the bursal surface were associated with pathologic changes. Fukuda et al[56] also concluded that most cuff tears are related to tendon degeneration and that acromial changes are secondary to pathology of the bursal side of the cuff. Although the above studies indicate a strong association between aging and the presence of cuff tears, it is unclear whether the changes in acromial morphology were caused by or resulted from the cuff defects, or whether both were the consequences of an aging rotator cuff.

> Studies of acromial shape support the concept that acromial spurs are not the only factor in the development of rotator cuff disease and that the change of acromial shape may be a result of shoulder stress.

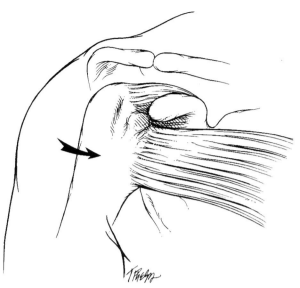

FIGURE 4–7 With the arm in flexion and internal rotation, the lesser tuberosity and bicipital groove (hatched area) come into contact with the acromion and coracoacromial arch.

Coracoid Impingement

Coracoid impingement as a source of shoulder pain was first described by Goldthwait in 1909.[57] He suggested that the subcoracoid bursa could be irritated by compression between the coracoid and the humeral head (**Fig. 4–7**). He also noticed that the size and shape of the coracoid may be an explanation of why the impingement occurred in some individuals and not in others; however, Codman did not agree with this concept, and it did not receive much attention in the literature for many years.

Gerber et al[58] can be credited with resurrecting the concept that the coracoid may be a source of contact between the rotator cuff and the coracoid as a source of pain. They called this entity "subcoracoid impingement," because they felt that the subcoracoid space was bounded by the acromion superiorly, the coracoid anteriorly, and the coracoacromial ligament anterolaterally. They noticed that patients who had anterior shoulder pain had a previous surgical procedure for instability known as a Trillat procedure. In a Trillat procedure, the coracoid is osteotomized and rotated so that it juts out in front of the joint. This operation had as its rationale the idea that the bone would prevent anterior instability of the shoulder by acting as a bony block. In some patients who had this operation, the researchers identified a loss of internal rotation, tenderness over the tip of the coracoid, and anterior shoulder pain that could radiate down the arm.

Gerber el al[58] suggested that the pain of coracoid impingement often could radiate such that it would have the appearance of a cervical radiculopathy. These patients typically would have a negative Neer impingement sign in flexion, suggesting that the impingement did not occur in flexion because the humeral head could clear the coracoid; however, placing the arm in a Kennedy-Hawkins impingement position (forward flexion to 90 degrees and internal rotation) was found to reproduce the pain in many patients.

Gerber et al[58] and Dines et al[59] suggested that injection of local anesthetic into the subcoracoid space may help in making the diagnosis of coracoid impingement. Gerber et al[58] found that injecting the subacromial bursa also may be necessary to distinguish between coracoid impingement and subacromial impingement, but they did not report upon the accuracy of the injections or upon the clinical effectiveness of these injections in making the diagnosis. They also suggested that despite computed tomography (CT) scanning, sometimes the diagnosis could not be definitely made until the time of surgery, when the arm could be placed into internal rotation and flexion, demonstrating impingement of the structures to the coracoid.

Gerber et al[58] felt that there were several possible clinical scenarios where coracoid impingement may occur; these included idiopathic, iatrogenic, and posttraumatic forms. The first, or idiopathic, form was found in individuals with no previous injuries or surgeries where the condition was felt to be due to a prominent coracoid process. In their series of 37 shoulders, 4 were felt to have the idiopathic form. In those patients the diagnosis was made upon clinical examination and confirmed with CT scanning. In one of these patients, isolated removal of the tip of the coracoid relieved the pain and produced a normal shoulder. In the other three patients the tip of the coracoid and the coracoacromial ligament were removed, and two had a standard anterior acromioplasty.

Dines et al[59] reported on eight patients with symptoms of coracoid impingement; four had an idiopathic form. In their series the patients' pain was improved with osteotomy of the coracoid, removal of the tip, or removal of the outer 1.5 cm of the coracoid. Ferrick[60] reported on one patient with idiopathic coracoid impingement who did well with only 6 months of follow-up after distal coracoid excision. He concluded that subcoracoid impingement was uncommon but should be considered in patients who have anterior shoulder pain, especially if the pain is not relieved with treatment of subacromial impingement.

In a subsequent study, Gerber et al[61] found that in normal volunteers the distance between the coracoid and the humeral head depended on the rotation of the humeral head. They found that with the arm at the side, the humeral head was closest to the coracoid when the arm was in internal rotation (8.7 ± 2.4 mm) versus neutral or external rotation. Next, Gerber et al studied the shoulders using CT with the arm in a position simulating coracoid impingement: flexed (90 to 100 degrees), horizontally forward flexed (90 to 115 degrees), and fully

internally rotated. They found that the distance between the humeral head and the coracoid decreased to 6.8 ± 2.9 mm (range 2.5 to 13 mm) with the arm in this position; this was statistically different from the distance when the arm was at the side. They also described other measures of the relationship between the glenoid, coracoid, and proximal humerus that may further delineate the relationships that would predispose an individual to coracoid impingement.

Friedman et al[62] subsequently measured the coracohumeral distance with the arm in maximal internal rotation using MRI in symptomatic and unsymptomatic shoulders. They found that in normal shoulders the coracohumeral distance average was 11 mm (range 4 to 17 mm), whereas in symptomatic patients it was 5.5 mm (range 0 to 1 mm).

Both Gerber et al[58] and Patte[63] emphasized that bony impingement between the humerus and the coracoid could not be demonstrated due to the interposition of soft tissue in the subcoracoid space. These structures in the subcoracoid space included the subscapularis tendon; the joint capsule, including the superior and middle glenohumeral ligaments; the articular cartilage of the humeral head; and the biceps tendon. Valadie et al[64] studied cadavers with the shoulder in flexion and internal rotation, such as seen with a Kennedy-Hawkins sign. They found that the subscapularis tendon was deformed by the coracoid in one of four specimens.

The role of the subscapularis in filling the subcoracoid space was not supported by a study by Nove-Josserand et al,[65] who measured the coracohumeral distance using CT scanning in 206 patients with rotator cuff tears. They found that the distance was the same in patients with an isolated subscapularis tear (9 mm) as it was in patients with tears of the supraspinatus and infraspinatus (9 ± 2 mm); however, the coracohumeral distance was statistically smaller in patients who had combined tears of the infraspinatus, supraspinatus, and subscapularis. Nove-Josserand et al concluded that the coracoid probably was not a factor in isolated subscapularis tendon tears. They also suggested that a tear of the subscapularis tendon was necessary with tears of other tendons to produce narrowing of the coracohumeral head distance.

The second cause of coracoid impingement was felt to be iatrogenic after a Trillat procedure or after posterior glenoid osteotomies. Gerber et al[58] suggested that in 56 Trillat procedures that his group had performed, symptoms of coracoid impingement were common. They felt that the humeral head was making contact with the coracoid and that it could cause pain and loosening of the screw used to secure the coracoid in position.

Another cause of iatrogenic coracoid impingement was found by Gerber et al[58] in two patients who had previous posterior glenoid osteotomies for posterior shoulder instability. In those patients, the persistent anterior shoulder pain was relieved by coracoidplasty. The researchers speculated that changes in the glenoid tilt may have predisposed the humeral head to abut the coracoid. Dines et al[59] reported one case of coracoid impingement due to a posterior glenoid osteotomy. In our personal experience, anterior shoulder pain is a frequent occurrence after posterior capsular shifts for posterior instability; however, all of those patients had resolution of the pain with time, and the exact etiology of the anterior shoulder pain could not be established.

The third cause of coracoid impingement could be posttraumatic, where deformities are created that can produce impingement symptoms. In their[58] series of patients, one patient had a proximal humeral malunion after an anterior fracture-dislocation of the shoulder, and a second had malunion after a three-part fracture of the humeral head. Both were successfully treated with a shortening procedure of the coracoid. Another patient who apparently did not undergo surgery had symptoms of coracoid impingement after a proximal humeral rotational osteotomy for persistent anterior shoulder instability. Dines et al[59] reported one case of a malunion of a lesser tuberosity fracture that caused coracoid impingement.

Gerber et al[58] also suggested that impingement upon the coracoid could occur with processes that might enlarge the greater tuberosity. They reported two cases of calcific deposits that caused impingement upon the coracoid; one was in the supraspinatus tendon. Patte[63] suggested that another cause of coracoid impingement could be an increase in the size of the contents of the subcoracoid space. This increase in volume could be due to an isolated tear of the subscapularis tendon with subsequent dislocation of the long head of the biceps tendon, scar formation after tearing of the coracohumeral ligament, or calcification of the subscapularis tendon. He also suggested that laxity due to partial tears of the supraspinatus may lead to a "functional" impingement upon the coracoid. Ko et al[66] reported a case of a ganglion cyst arising from the subscapularis tendon as a cause of coracoid impingement.

> The exact pathophysiology of coracoid impingement remains unknown, and criteria for making this diagnosis remain unclear.

Internal Impingement

The concept of internal impingement was introduced by Walch et al[67] in 1992. They described contact of the rotator cuff to the posterior and superior glenoid when the arm is placed in an abducted and externally rotated position (**Fig. 4–8**). They noted this contact in patients undergoing diagnostic arthroscopy of the shoulder by placing the arm into this position with the arthroscope in

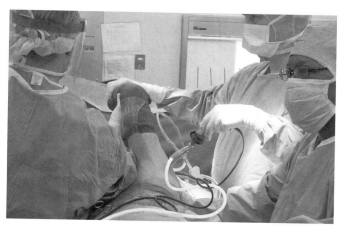

FIGURE 4–8 Internal impingement of the shoulder was initially described during arthroscopic evaluation of the shoulder with the arm in abduction and externally rotated.

a posterior portal. Their patients included 17 athletes; all but 1 played a throwing sport. None of their patients had signs of anterior shoulder instability, and all had pain posteriorly and superiorly with the arm in abduction and external rotation.

At the time of arthroscopy, 14 of the patients had pathology of the rotator cuff, 12 had lesions of the posterosuperior labrum, and 8 had osteochondral lesions higher up on the humeral head than a typical Hill-Sachs lesion. Of the rotator cuff tears, 10 involved partial tears of the supraspinatus, of which three were type I Ellman tears and the rest were type II. Walch et al[67] classified the partial-thickness cuff tears according to the Ellman classification,[68] where the normal tendon is considered 10 to 12 mm thick. According to this classification, a grade I partial tear is less than 3 mm deep. A grade 2 lesion is 3 to 6 mm deep but does not exceed one half of the thickness of the tendon. Lesions more than 6 mm in depth are grade 3 partial cuff tears (**Table 4–4**). These tears can be on the articular surface, on the bursal surface, or within the tendon. The tears within the tendon are not visible from the surface and occur in the interstitial layers of the tendon. In addition, three tears involved the infraspinatus (of which two were type I Ellman tears and one was type II).

Walch et al[67] suggested that this was a new type of impingement that was distinctly different from the Neer

TABLE 4–4 Ellman Classification of Partial Rotator Cuff Tears

Location	Grade
Partial-thickness tear	I: < 3 mm deep
Articular surface	II: 3–6 mm deep
Bursal surface	III: > 6 mm deep
Interstitial	

Ellman H. Arthroscopic subacromial decompression: analysis of one- to three-year results. Arthroscopy. 1987;3(3):173-81.

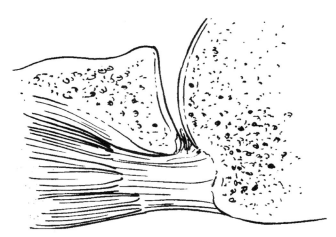

FIGURE 4–9 A drawing of the contact of the greater tuberosity of the humerus and of the rotator cuff tendon to the superior glenoid with the arm in abduction and external. This type of contact was originally called internal impingement. (Adapted with permission from Jobe F, ed. Operative Techniques in Upper Extremity Sports Injuries. St. Louis: Mosby, 1996:170, Fig. 7–6B.)

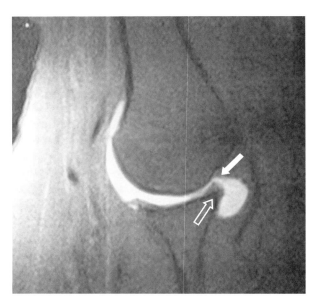

FIGURE 4–10 Internal impingment of the rotator cuff (closed arrow) on the glenoid (open arrow) with the arm in abduction can be demonstrated with magnetic resonance imaging enhanced with gadolinium (oblique coronal view).

impingement and from F. Jobe's[69] theory of instability causing cuff pathology (**Fig. 4–9**). Although they also suggested that the contact of the rotator cuff to the posterior and superior glenoid that they observed may be physiological (i.e., normal), they postulated that in the throwing or overhead athletes, partial tears of the rotator cuff were due to this repetitive contact of the rotator cuff to the posterior and superior glenoid.

Further evidence of this type of contact was supplied by subsequent anatomic, radiological, and clinical studies. C. Jobe[70] reported on cadavers that were fixed in abduction and external rotation and found that the posterosuperior labrum was deformed by the greater tuberosity.

Radiographic studies also demonstrated that this contact could be visualized with MRI arthrography.[70,71] Tirman et al[71] studied eight competitive athletes (seven baseball players and one volleyball participant) with shoulder pain who were found to have internal impingement arthroscopically using MRI (**Fig. 4–10**). The researchers concluded that MRI-arthrograms were more sensitive for internal impingement and for detecting undersurface rotator cuff tears and posterosuperior labrum lesions. They found that the infraspinatus tendon was more commonly involved with partial tears in this group than were supraspinatus tears. They suggested that these patients had anterior instability based on the examination under anesthesia, but there were no Bankart or Hill-Sachs lesions found at the time of arthroscopy.

The first report to suggest that internal impingement may be associated with anterior instability was by Liu and Boynton[72] in 1993, which described a patient with posterosuperior impingement arthroscopically who had signs of increased laxity and possible anteroinferior instability. Davidson et al[73] in 1995 reported on internal impingement in two patients who were professional pitchers with anterosuperior and posterosuperior shoulder pain associated with throwing. They found partial tears of the posterior supraspinatus, posterosuperior labrum lesions, and diminutive Inferior Glenohumeral Ligaments (IGHLs) in both patients.

Davidson et al[73] speculated that the partial cuff tears were due to contact of the rotator cuff to the posterosuperior labrum. They suggested that this phenomenon could occur in patients with no instability, and in these cases "hyperangulation" of the proximal humerus in abduction and external rotation as seen in overhead athletes allowed the greater tuberosity to impact upon the glenoid. The second way this contact could occur was when the IGHL was lax; this laxity would allow increased anterior translation and contact of the greater tuberosity to the posterior and superior glenoid. Davidson et al[73] also speculated that scapular malpositioning may contribute to this condition, but it was not specifically studied in their two patients.

This concept of internal impingement was expanded later by C. Jobe,[70] who suggested that it may be seen not only in overhead athletes but also in patients whose occupations involved abduction and external rotation of the shoulder. Although Jobe's series included two greater tuberosity fractures that did not undergo arthroscopy, in the eight patients in the series who underwent arthroscopy, there was damage in seven patients to the rotator cuff, the superior labrum, or the posterior

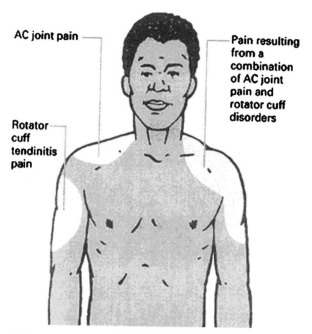

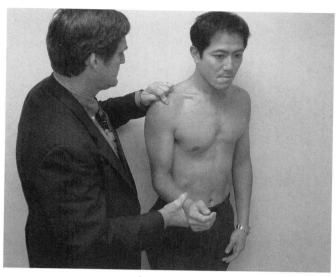

FIGURE 4–15 When palpating for the supraspinatus insertion on the tuberosity, the arm should be at the side, and the area just beyond the edge of the acromion should be palpated.

FIGURE 4–14 The distribution of rotator cuff pain is typically in the deltoid area, and pain from the acromioclavicular (AC) joint pathology is typically on top of the shoulder. The distribution of pain can overlap if both problems are present. (Adapted with permission from McFarland EG, Hobbs WR. The active shoulder: AC joint pain and injury. Your Patient & Fitness 1998;12(4):23–27.)

the patient. We prefer to stand in front of the patient to be able to see his or her facial expressions. Palpation should be firm but not hard enough to produce pain from pressing on the periosteum of the bone. If there is doubt, then the other side can be palpated for comparison. The patient's arm should be in internal rotation and resting at the side.

The supraspinatus attachment is anterior to the acromion and may be more easily palpated by externally rotating the shoulder a few degrees (**Fig. 4–15**). The insertion continues past the anterolateral edge of the acromion along the greater tuberosity. The infraspinatus can be palpated lateral to the posterior joint line where it attaches to the tuberosity. Nobahara[88] and others have suggested that the teres minor can be palpated just inferior to the infraspinatus, but there is little to distinguish the two muscles except the relative proximity of the two.

It is important to try to distinguish tenderness in the posterior shoulder joint from tenderness in the infraspinatus insertion. This can be difficult due to the overlying deltoid muscle (**Fig. 4–16**). Patients with posterior and superior joint line tenderness may have a SLAP lesion or a strain of the infraspinatus. Posterior joint line tenderness also may be seen in patients with degenerative arthritis or a frozen shoulder. Nobahara[88] suggests that posterior joint line tenderness in the middle of the joint and at the

infraspinatus insertion is suspicious for a partial cuff tear in this area. He calls this syndrome the infraspinatus tendon partial (ITP) tear lesion.

Nobuhara[88] has described palpating the latissimus dorsi tendon insertion by following the muscle belly inferior to the axilla until you feel the tendinous portion. It is helpful to elevate the arm to ~60 degrees and to ask the patient to try to rotate the arm internally. He suggests that the tendon can then be palpated at its attachment to

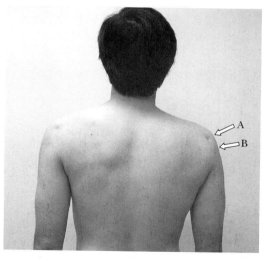

FIGURE 4–16 When palpating the posterior shoulder joint, tenderness is a nonspecific sign. More superior tenderness may indicate a superior labrum anterior to posterior (SLAP) lesion, arrow (A) whereas tenderness in the middle portion of the joint may be due to pathology of the infraspinatus or other structures arrow (B).

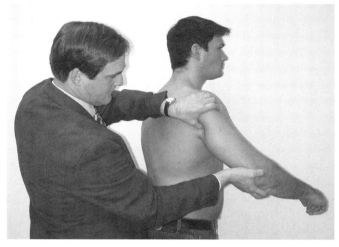

FIGURE 4–17 Nobuhara's method of palpating for latissimus dorsi tendon tenderness just beneath the axilla. The arm is elevated to 60 degrees and slightly internally rotated, and the tendon should be palpated at the insertion on the humerus.

the proximal humerus (**Fig. 4–17**). Tenderness in this area is a necessary criterion for the diagnosis of latissimus syndrome, which is discussed further in Chapter 3.

Tenderness around the shoulder girdle tends to be a non-specific finding because many structures overlap. We know of no studies that validate that tenderness in one location is highly correlated with damage to one individual structure; however, local tenderness is important in helping the clinician localize the general source of pain in the shoulder. Tenderness should be considered an adjunct to other portions of the examination of the shoulder for rotator cuff disease.

> Tenderness around the shoulder is not specific for rotator cuff pathology, but it can give the examiner an idea of the general location of the pathology.

Crepitus and the Abrasion Sign

Many physicians have suggested that rotator cuff disease can cause crepitus.[1,24,89] Yocum[89] suggested that the location of crepitus can be determined by careful palpation, but he did not study this observation. Crepitus can have multiple causes in the shoulder, including fracture, cuff tendinitis, biceps tendinitis, frozen shoulder, glenohumeral arthritis, AC arthritis, and scapular snapping syndrome. Crepitus is common after surgical procedures of the shoulder, and its exact cause is unknown. Crepitus after shoulder surgery has been speculated to be due to scar formation between structures or to irregularities of the bursa after surgery. We tell patients that painless crepitus is usually not significant provided the examination and evaluation are otherwise negative for the above disorders.

Matsen et al[90] described what they called the "abrasion" sign due to crepitus. With the arm elevated 90 degrees, the

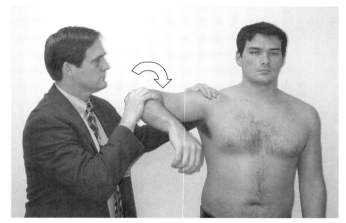

FIGURE 4–18 The abrasion sign is performed with the arm in 90 degrees of flexion and then subjected to slight internal and external rotation. A positive sign is indicated by crepitus.

shoulder is moved with slight internal and external rotation (**Fig. 4–18**). If this causes painful crepitus that reproduces the patient's symptoms, then it is considered indicative of rotator cuff. Matsen et al did not specify whether this was a partial- or full-thickness tear of the tendon.

There have been no studies to establish the validity or accuracy of this sign. Our experience has been that crepitus is a nonspecific sign, even when it is painful. Crepitus is also quite common after surgical procedures, and although the cause is speculative, it could be due to suture material, scar in the subacromial space, or a recurrent tear of the rotator cuff.

> Crepitus around the shoulder can be due to a variety of conditions, and painless crepitus typically is not clinically significant.

"The Rent" Sign: Palpation of a Tendon Defect

The ability to palpate a defect in the rotator cuff was first suggested by Codman in 1934.[3] He suggested that by palpating just anterior or lateral to the acromion, it was possible in some cases to feel a defect in the supraspinatus tendon; however, the ability to perform this assessment depends on the bulk of the deltoid muscle.

Lyons and Tomlinson[91] evaluated the transdeltoid palpation for the diagnosis of rotator cuff tear in 42 patients by correlating clinical palpation of the rent with the size of the tear found at surgery. They found clinical palpation to have a sensitivity, specificity, and diagnostic accuracy of 91, 75, and 88%, respectively.

Wolf and Agrawal[92] sought to evaluate the rent test because they felt that the small sample size in the Lyons and Tomlinson study may have contributed to results that they considered too low. Hence they evaluated the rent test in 109 patients using the technique as originally

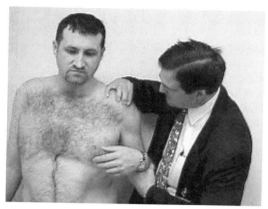

FIGURE 4–19 The rent sign is the ability to feel a rent in the rotator cuff.

described by Codman.[3] Palpation was performed anterior to the anterior margin of the acromion, and the examiner would then palpate through the deltoid. The patient was asked to relax, allowing the arm to dangle freely. While positioned behind the patient, the examiner held the patient's forearm with the elbow flexed to allow rotational control to maneuver the arm while the examiner's other hand was used for palpation (**Fig. 4–19**). The arm was gently maneuvered into full extension. Internal and external rotation was used to palpate the rotator cuff tendons.

In the presence of a tear, both an eminence and a rent were palpable. The tear was palpated as the arm was brought in and out of full extension and internally and externally rotated. The eminence represented the prominent greater tuberosity in the presence of a full-thickness rotator cuff tear. The rent is the soft tissue defect created by the rotator cuff that avulsed from the tuberosity. The size of the tear can be appreciated by palpating the anterior and posterior margins of the cuff tear and the presence of an avulsed edge. Failure to palpate an avulsed edge was considered a sign of significant retraction of the tendon edge. Wolfe and Agrawal recommended that the examination be performed bilaterally to appreciate the anatomy of the uninvolved shoulder and to compare it with the symptomatic side.

Furthermore, Wolfe and Agrawal found that transdeltoid palpation had a sensitivity of 95.7% and a specificity of 96.8% for the diagnosis of full-thickness rotator cuff tear. The positive and negative predictive values for transdeltoid palpation were 95.7% and 96.8%, respectively. Overall, the diagnostic accuracy of transdeltoid palpation was 96.3%; however, it should be noted that the examiners were not blinded and that there was no control group.

The above studies suggest that transdeltoid palpation requires some experience to be used reliably. We have not found this to be an easy test to perform in a majority of patients. There are several reasons for this inability to

feel rents or tears in the rotator cuff tendons. First, the large muscle envelope makes reliable palpation of structures deep to the muscle difficult. Second, the tuberosities themselves produce lumps and irregularities that can be mistaken for tears, particularly if there is tenderness there. Scar formation or previous fractures can make palpation of the cuff difficult. Third, most tears occur on the undersurface of the rotator cuff, and palpation of partial- or nearly full-thickness defects has not proven possible in our experience.

A review of the existing literature finds that the studies suggesting palpation is possible have several methodological problems that do not justify their conclusions. Our personal experience is that palpation of rotator cuff defects is nearly impossible and not diagnostic for rotator cuff tears.

Palpation of rotator cuff defects is typically not possible.

Dawbarn's Sign

Dawbarn's sign was described in 1906 and is based on the premise that as the arm is elevated, the bursa and painful rotator cuff will pass beneath the acromion, where it will no longer be painful.[93] This test is performed by first palpating the shoulder for tender areas around the anterior and lateral acromion. The patient's arm is then passively elevated until it rests on the examiner's shoulder. If the tenderness is due to subacromial bursitis, the tender area should be beneath the acromion. As a result, the area cannot be palpated by the examiner, and there should be no pain with palpation of the shoulder in this position. Dawbarn[93] suggested that this test does not abolish the tenderness on palpation from any of the other causes of pain in this region.

The validity of this test has never been studied. Its clinical usefulness and accuracy also have never been studied. Nobuhara's text[88] mentions the use of this test, but it was not studied clinically by him.

Neer Impingement Sign

The Neer impingement sign was first described by Neer[1] in 1972; it has been misinterpreted to be the *sine qua non* of rotator cuff disease (**Fig. 4–20**). His original article suggests that with forward elevation, with the arm in either internal or external rotation, the anterior rotator cuff passes under the leading edge of the acromion at around 80 degrees. Neer suggested that excrescences on the undersurface of the anterior acromion may impinge on the cuff. This sign was initially described for stage I impingement, where the patient had edema and hemorrhage of the tendon. Neer later clarified this and suggested that the impingement sign can be positive in all three stages of impingement, from bursitis to full-thickness tears.[10]

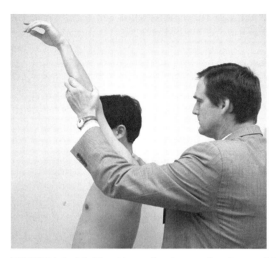

FIGURE 4–20 The Neer sign is passive forward flexion of the arm, which should produce anterior or lateral shoulder pain.

According to Neer, the impingement sign was nonspecific and could produce pain from a variety of conditions. These included stiffness, anterior instability, arthritis, calcific tendinitis, and some bone lesions.[10]

The impingement sign was also used as an adjunct to the impingement test, where lidocaine is injected into the subacromial space. If the rotator cuff is the source of the pain, then the impingement sign should be eliminated after injection of steroid.[94] Neer commented that if pain was not relieved, then the source of the pain must be coming from somewhere else.[10]

The Neer sign is performed with the examiner standing behind the patient, who is seated. The examiner uses one hand to stabilize the shoulder to prevent scapular rotation. The other is used to elevate the patient's arm in flexion until pain is reached. Although Neer never specified, most diagrams suggest that the patient's arm be elevated with the palm down and the arm in internal rotation. Pain is typically produced around 120 degrees of elevation.[1] This sign was initially described for stage I impingement, where the patient had edema and hemorrhage of the tendon.

The accuracy of the Neer impingement sign has been the subject of several studies (**Table 4–5**). These studies suggest that Neer was correct in his assessment that the impingement sign is a nonspecific test of shoulder pain. Calis et al[95] used pain relief with an injection of local

TABLE 4–5 Summary of the Reports in the Literature on the Diagnostic Accuracy of the Commonly Used Tests for Impingement Syndrome

Study	Severity of Disease	Diagnostic Test	Sensitivity (%)	Specificity (%)	PPV (%)	NPV (%)	DA (%)
Leroux, et al. (1995)[96]	Impingement syndrome	Neer	89.0				
		Hawkins	87.0				
		Yocum	78.0				
Calis et al. (2000)[95]	Impingement syndrome	Neer	88.7	30.5	75.9	52.3	72.0
		Hawkins	92.1	25.0	75.2	56.2	72.8
		Horizontal adduction	82.0	27.7	73.7	38.4	66.4
		Speed	68.5	55.5	79.2	41.6	64.8
		Yergason	37.0	86.1	86.8	35.6	51.2
		Painful arc	32.5	80.5	80.5	32.5	46.4
		Drop arm	7.8	97.2	87.5	29.9	33.6
MacDonald et al. (2000)[97]	Bursitis	Neer	75.0	47.5	36.0	82.9	
		Hawkins	91.7	44.3	39.3	93.1	
		Neer or Hawkins	95.8	41.0	39.0	96.0	
		Neer and Hawkins	70.8	50.8	36.2	81.6	
	Rotator cuff pathosis	Neer	83.3	50.8	40.0	88.6	
		Hawkins	87.5	42.6	37.5	89.7	
		Neer or Hawkins	87.5	37.7	35.6	88.5	
		Neer and Hawkins	83.3	55.7	42.6	55.7	
	Bursitis or rotator cuff tear	Neer	77.0	62.5	70.0	71.4	
		Hawkins	88.9	60.0	71.4	82.8	
Naredo et al. (2002)[101]	Supraspinatus lesion	P/E	79.3	50.0	95.8	14.2	
	Impingement	P/E	65.0	72.7	81.2	53.3	
	Tendinitis	P/E	72.2	38.4	61.9	50.0	
	Supraspinatus tear	P/E	18.7	100.0	100.0	53.5	
Smith-Teunis (2003)[153]	Tendinitis	P/E			43.0	9.0	
		P/E and MRI			65.0	7.0	
	PRCT	P/E			13.0	19.0	
		P/E and MRI			32.0	18.0	
	FRCT	P/E			89.0	43.0	
		P/E and MRI			88.0	27.0	

*Source: Adapted with permission from Park H. Diagnostic accuracy of clinical tests for the different degrees of subacromial impingement syndrome. JBJS (A) 07A:1446–1455, 2005.

0A, diagnostic accuracy; FRCT, partial rotator cuff tear; MRI, magnetic resonance imaging; NPV, negative predictive value; P/E, physical examination; PPV, positive predictive value; PRCT, partial rotator cuff tear.

patients, but they could only speculate regarding the relationship of these lesions to a painful arc.

Calis et al[95] studied the painful arc sign and found that the sensitivity was low (33%), the specificity was 81%, the positive predictive value was 80.5%, the negative predictive value was 32.5%, and the overall accuracy was 46.4%. They also examined the accuracy of the painful arc for rotator cuff pathology, which was graded using MRI criteria (**Table 4–5**). They found that its accuracy was similar for any grade of rotator cuff pathology.

In our study (**Table 4–6**) of the painful arc sign, when evaluating its accuracy for rotator cuff pathology of any degree, it was found to be more sensitive than Calis et al's study (74%), but the specificity was essentially the same (81%) as that reported by them. We also found that for rotator cuff pathology of any type, it had the highest overall accuracy of any of the signs for rotator cuff pathology; however, when further evaluated for the degree of rotator cuff pathology, the painful arc was found to have an overall accuracy for impingement with no cuff tears of 49%, for partial cuff tears of 49%, and for full-thickness tears of 68% (**Table 4–6**). These findings reflect the highly variable presentation of patients judged to have rotator cuff pathology.

> The painful arc sign should raise suspicion of rotator cuff pathology, and it has importance when combined with other tests of rotator cuff disease.

A painful arc can be present in patients with other diagnoses. In our cohort of 1200 patients, it was positive in 71% of patients with rotator cuff disease of any type, 75% of patients with osteoarthritis, 64% of patients with impingement, 25% of patients with instability, 50% of patients with AC arthritis, and 46% of patients with frozen shoulders. Although a painful arc is a helpful test for making the diagnosis of rotator cuff tears, it should be considered a nonspecific test for shoulder pathology.

> The painful arc sign can be positive in a high percentage of patients with conditions other than rotator cuff disease.

Coracoid Impingement Sign

The coracoid impingement sign was first suggested by Gerber et al[58] in 1985, when they noted that a Kennedy-Hawkins impingement sign would produce pain anteriorly in the region of the coracoid. They suggested that with the arm in flexion to 90 degrees and internal rotation, pain may be produced by coracoid impingment on the rotator cuff.

Dines et al[59] further refined this test by suggesting that more internal rotation than reported by Gerber et al was

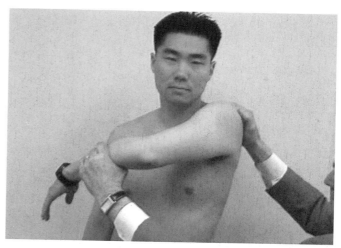

FIGURE 4–25 The coracoid impingement sign is a modification of the Kennedy-Hawkins impingement sign.

needed to produce impingement of the cuff to the coracoid (**Fig. 4–25**). They called testing the arm in this position the "coracoid impingement sign." They emphasized that a patient with coracoid impingement should have a negative Neer impingement sign.

There are no studies evaluating the accuracy of this sign. There are probably several reasons for this. First, the arm position tested is very similar to a Kennedy-Hawkins sign, so if the test is positive, it is difficult to know if the pain is due to a Neer (i.e., "outlet") type of impingement or to impingement of the tendons on the coracoid. Second, coracoid impingement does not appear to have a distinct pain pattern distinguishing it from other forms of impingement. Third, the diagnosis of coracoid impingement has been hampered by a paucity of studies that convincingly demonstrate that surgery is effective. The largest series of patients with coracoid impingement is from Dines et al,[59] who operated on eight shoulders. Recently, the diagnosis of coracoid impingement has had a resurgence with the advent of arthroscopic techniques for removing portions of the coracoid.[102,103]

Despite this new enthusiasm for the diagnosis of coracoid impingement, it is our opinion that this diagnosis should be made with caution. There is little information available about the accuracy of specific physical examination findings for this diagnosis. Although injections have been suggested to aid in the diagnosis, there have been no studies evaluating the accuracy of injections into the coracoid or subcoracoid spaces. Because there is often an extension of the joint beneath the coracoid, it is likely that injections in this area can enter the joint. Injections into this area also can enter the subacromial space and the bicipital sheath, so it is possible that this injection is not specific. Tenderness on examination of the coracoid is also a nonspecific sign in our experience, but it should be present to consider the diagnosis.

> Coracoid impingement has not been demonstrated convincingly to be a distinct clinical entity, and the examination for this condition has not been validated.

Speed's Test

Speed's test was initially described as being diagnostic for biceps tendinitis[104,105] and is discussed in detail in Chapter 6; however, several studies have assessed the utility of this physical examination finding for rotator cuff pathology (**Tables 4–5, 4–6, 4–7**).[84,95,106] The sign is performed with the arm flexed 90 degrees, horizontally extended 15 degrees, and with the forearm supinated (palm up). The patient is asked to resist a downward force applied by the examiner; this should produce pain into the biceps region (**Fig. 4–26**).

This test also can cause pain into the front of the shoulder or in other locations, which is important when evaluating the studies that examine its usefulness for rotator cuff disease. No study, including our own, asked the patient to distinguish between pain in the front of the shoulder and pain exclusively in the biceps area. As a result, the Speed's test had a sensitivity of 68.5% in the study by Calis et al[95] and 38% in our study[84] (**Table 4–6**) for rotator cuff tears of any kind. The overall diagnostic accuracy for the Speed's test for rotator cuff pathology was 65% in the Calis et al study, and in our study, 65% for tendinitis only, 67% for partial tears of the rotator cuff, and 62% for full-thickness tears (**Table 4–6**). The overlap of symptoms for this test makes it difficult to recommend it as diagnostic for either rotator cuff or biceps tendon pathologies (see Chapter 6).

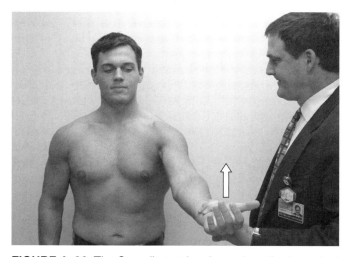

FIGURE 4–26 The Speed's test has been described as a test for biceps tendon pathology.

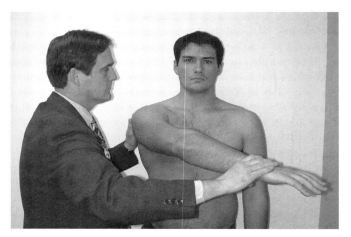

FIGURE 4–27 The Whipple test has been suggested to help make the diagnosis of partial rotator cuff tears.

> The Speed's test can be positive in a large percentage of patients with rotator cuff disease, but it is not diagnostic for rotator cuff pathology.

Whipple Test

This test has been ascribed to Terry L. Whipple, M.D., an orthopaedic surgeon who made significant contributions to the field of shoulder and arthroscopic surgery. This test was described by Savoie et al[107] in 2000, and it is meant to confirm the diagnosis of partial undersurface tearing of the supraspinatus tendon (**Fig. 4–27**). This entity is often found in conjunction with superior labrum abnormalities, a condition that Savoie and colleagues called SLAC (*s*uperior *l*abrum, *a*nterior *c*uff).

The Whipple test is performed with the patient sitting. The arm is flexed 90 degrees and then adducted until the hand is opposite the other shoulder. The physician pushes downward on the arm, and the patient resists the downward pressure. A positive test is one that elicits pain in the shoulder or down the arm. In the study by Savoie et al of 40 patients using this test, all 40 had a partial-thickness tear of the supraspinatus (100% sensitivity).

This test has had no other independent evaluation of its validity or accuracy. In our experience, it is not specific for partial rotator cuff tears, but studies of its accuracy are underway. It is unlikely that this test can distinguish between partial- and full-thickness rotator cuff tearing, but further study is needed before the exact role of the Whipple test can be determined.

Neer Impingement Test (Diagnostic Injection)

In 1972, Neer[1] first reported the usefulness of injection lidocaine into the subacromial space to determine if the pain of a Neer sign (passive flexion of the arm) was coming from the subacromial bursa. He later suggested that if pain was not improved by the injection, then other sources of the pain should be considered.[94] Since that time, numerous clinicians have suggested the diagnostic and therapeutic efficacy of injection of local anesthetic and corticosteroids into the subacromial space.[87,108–115]

Because an injection of local anesthetic was considered by Neer to be diagnostic, a critical evaluation of its place in the evaluation of the shoulder was felt to be warranted. There are two critical issues. First, does the injection into the subacromial space actually enter the subacromial space? Second, what is the diagnostic accuracy of this test?

These issues are important because the clinical effectiveness of injections of corticosteroids into the subacromial space for supraspinatus tendinitis has been reported in one study to be 82% (14 of 17 patients).[116] Darlington and Coomes[117] found that patients with rotator cuff pathology had significant decreases in pain with resisted abduction compared with similar patients with no treatment; however, Withrington et al[118] utilized a double-blinded comparison of steroid injection for supraspinatus tendinitis versus a placebo of saline and found no differences in the groups at 2 and 8 weeks.

The variable results of these studies can be explained in part by the difficulty of injecting the correct location. In a study involving 12 cadavers using an aqueous dye visible to the eye, after dissecting the 24 shoulders Partington and Broome[119] found that a subacromial injection was successful in 83%. In the shoulders where the dye was found to hit the subacromial space, 15 had other structures hit by the injection (deltoid muscle $n = 4$, rotator cuff tendon $n = 7$, AC joint $n = 3$, glenohumeral joint $n = 2$).

Yamakado[120] studied the accuracy of a subacromial injection in 56 shoulders in patients who had impingement syndrome. He injected the subacromial space with lidocaine, corticosteroids, and radiographic contrast material simultaneously, then examined the location of the dye using plain radiographs immediately after the injection. He found that 70% reached the subacromial bursa, 21% were in the deltoid muscle, 4% were in the glenohumeral joint, and 5% were subcutaneous. Pain relief was the same in patients who had evidence of injection into the bursa compared with those who had injections that were intradeltoid.

Bergman and Fredericson[121] used MRI to evaluate the location of a subacromial injection of lidocaine and a corticosteroid in six patients. They found that the injection missed the subacromial space in one patient, that in three patients a portion of the injection was in the subcutaneous tissues, and that in one patient the fluid tracked up the trapezius fascia. Both of these studies suggest that a diagnostic injection into the subacromial space may not localize the pathology as originally suggested by Neer.[1] These studies also may explain the variability in the clinical results of studies of the efficacy of corticosteroid injections for rotator cuff pathology.

> Subacromial injections will hit the subacromial space in ~80% of subjects.

It is important, however, to distinguish between pain relief immediately after a subacromial injection and pain relief that occurs days later. When injecting an anesthetic agent with corticosteroids into the subacromial space, if rotator cuff disease with accompanying subacromial bursitis is causing the patient's pain, it is commonly believed that the patient should have immediate relief of that pain due to the local anesthetic. If a patient does not get immediate pain relief, then other causes of the shoulder pain should be considered, such as a frozen shoulder or cervical disk disease.

It is not uncommon for patients to have no immediate pain relief but to say that their pain relief began several days after the injection. This delayed relief is most likely due to absorption of the steroids into the bloodstream. We have noticed this phenomenon particularly in patients who have degenerative arthritis of the shoulder or who have stiff shoulders. Though not diagnostic, in patients who do not get immediate relief with a cortisone shot into the subacromial space but who do get delayed pain relief, diagnosis other than rotator cuff disease should be suspected.

How to Do a Subacromial Injection

It is important to be able to define the anatomy of the shoulder when performing injections into the subacromial space. We recommend exposing the entire shoulder complex rather than just pulling up a sleeve or stretching a collar to reach the shoulder. Important landmarks are the posterolateral angle of the acromion, the AC joint, and the anterolateral acromion. To open the subacromial space, the patient is asked to sit on the side of the table with the arm hanging down unsupported (**Fig. 4–28**). The weight of the arm will open the subacromial space only if the patient is relaxed; we recommend palpating the deltoid prior to the injection to ascertain that the patient is relaxed.

The injection should be done sterilely, so the skin should be prepared with either alcohol or iodinated solutions. One hand should be sterile; and a gloved hand is recommended. We recently observed one physician who prepped his own finger instead of the shoulder to be able to palpate for the subacromial space accurately, but this technique is left to the discretion of the physician.

When injecting the shoulder for therapeutic reasons, it is recommended that the anesthetic agent be mixed with the corticosteroid and that they be injected together. This ensures that if the patient's pain is relieved, the corticosteroid is by definition in the proper location. If one

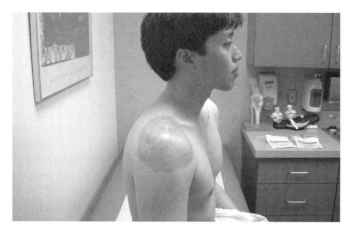

FIGURE 4–28 When performing a subaxromial injection, it is helpful to have the patient sit so that the weight of the arm will help open the subacromial space.

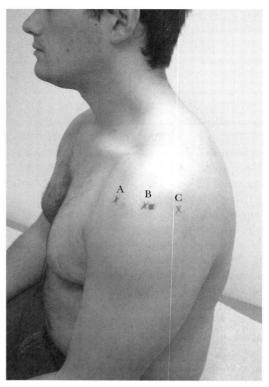

FIGURE 4–29 The subacromial space can be injected anteriorly (A), laterally (B), or posteriorly (C).

injects the two agents separately, there is no assurance that the second injection will duplicate the location of the first. Although the volume of anesthetic that is the optimum to inject into the subacromial space is unknown, we know from arthroscopy that it is a large potential space. Thus we recommend injecting a total of 10 cc of combined anesthetic and corticosteroid. The rationale is that this will allow the two agents to reach the most locations in the subacromial space. Once the subacromial space is entered, the fluid should go in very easily without resistance. If resistance is felt as the needle goes in or if the fluid does not go in easily, then there should be concern that the needle is in a solid structure, such as the rotator cuff tendons, and the needle should be redirected. We use a 22-gauge needle that is 1.5 cm in length. The patient is advised to sit up straight and let the arm hang in a relaxed position.

There are several locations to inject the subacromial space, and each has its advantages and disadvantages. The three locations are anteriorly, laterally, and posteriorly in relationship to the acromion (**Fig. 4–29**). The posterior injection site is in the soft spot just below the posterolateral edge of the acromion. It has the advantage of being easy to locate, but it has the disadvantage of being farthest away from pathology in the anterior aspect of the shoulder, such as an anterior tear of the supraspinatus tendon or biceps tendon pathology.

The anterior location has the advantage of being directly over the biceps tendon in the proximal bicipital groove and over the anterior supraspinatus; however, these structures are relatively superficial, and care must be taken not to inject into the tendon. In addition, the coracoacromial ligament and anterior acromial spurs may make it difficult to reach the subacromial space.

The lateral or anterolateral injection site has the advantage of easy access to the subacromial space and of being able to inject anteriorly or posteriorly (**Fig. 4–30**).

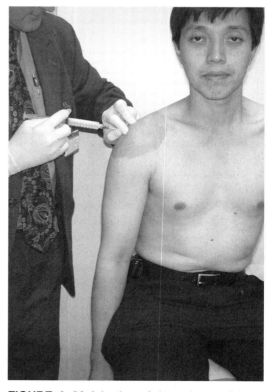

FIGURE 4–30 Injection of the subacromial space through a lateral site allows the anterior portion of the space to be reached.

This position allows fluid to easily reach the anterior portions of the subacromial space and the bicipital groove. The disadvantage is that the lateral acromion may angle down and make it difficult to reach the subacromial space. If the patient contracts his or her muscles or is not relaxed, this injection site can be difficult because the subacromial space may be compressed by the humeral head against the acromion.

We use the lateral injection site the most and explain to the patient that the needle is place laterally but that the medicine is going where their pain is located anteriorly. If the pain is posterior, we use a posterior injection site. We rarely use the anterior site, but it can be effective in experienced hands. After the injection we carefully observe the patient for vasovagal symptoms. If there is any concern, we have the patient assume a supine position for a brief time after the injection.

We typically warn the patient that there may be pain once the local anesthetic wears off. The patient is told to ice the shoulder for 20 to 30 minutes every 2 hours if necessary, and to ice the shoulder daily for a few days for 20 to 30 minutes if it is sore. Patients are told that the shoulder may be sore for a few days, and that they should consider the use of acetaminophen for pain. In patients who have adverse reactions to the shot, we will occasionally give them pain medication (usually a light narcotic) in case they have more severe reaction to the injection later. One study demonstrated a slight increased use of pain medication in the first few days postinjection in patients who had a subacromial cortisone shot compared with a control group of patients who were injected with saline, but the differences were not statistically significant.[117]

Patients are warned about potential side effects, including pain and loss of motion briefly after the injection. Diabetic patients are warned that the injection may cause an increase in their blood sugar levels and that they should monitor the levels closely. Infections are very uncommon after cortisone shots and are typically seen in patients who are immunocompromised. Vitiligo can be seen after injections of the AC joint, but in our experience this condition, after a subacromial injection of corticosteroid, is rare in the lateral shoulder.

■ Strength Testing for Rotator Cuff Disease

A more detailed analysis of strength testing and tests for strength testing of the rotator cuff are in Chapter 3. This section will discuss these tests as they relate to rotator cuff disease and to making the diagnosis of rotator cuff disease. The major complaints of patients with rotator cuff dysfunction are pain, loss of motion, and loss of strength. All three of these complaints can be due to causes that are not related to the rotator cuff

and should be excluded with a careful history and examination.

Drop Arm Sign

The drop arm sign was initially described by Codman[3] in 1934. In a case of complete rupture of the tendon of the supraspinatus, he observed that the patient was unable to start abduction, but when the arm was passively abducted to ~140 degrees, the patient, by a strong contraction of the deltoid, could prevent the arm from falling for an instant; however, the slightest downward pressure made it drop to the side.

A drop arm sign is now defined as an inability to hold the arm up at or above the shoulder against gravity. It can be performed in two different ways. The first way to perform a drop arm sign is to passively elevate the patient's arm to 90 degrees of abduction and ask the patient to hold it there (**Fig. 4–31**). If the patient cannot hold it there, then it is considered a positive test. A second way to perform this test is to ask the patient to elevate the arm fully to 140 to 160 degrees, then ask him or her to bring the arm down very slowly. As the arm approaches the horizontal position, the patient will be unable to hold it against gravity. If the patient drops the arm, then it is considered a positive test.

A drop arm sign can be positive for several reasons; these etiologies include weakness or pain due to any cause. This can include neurological diseases, nerve injury, and rotator cuff pathology. As a result, it is a sensitive but not specific cause for rotator cuff pathology. This test has been studied by Park et al.,[100] who found that in full-thickness rotator cuff tears, the sensitivity was 35% and the specificity 88%. In cases of partial tears, however, the test had a sensitivity of only 14% (**Table 4–6**).

Murrell and Walton[98] performed a prospective study of 23 clinical tests of the shoulder in a cohort of 400 patients with and without rotator cuff tears. They found that the

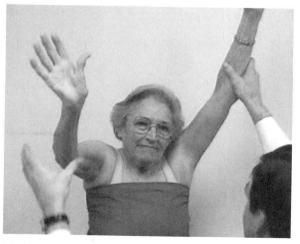

FIGURE 4–31 The drop arm sign is positive when the subject cannot hold the arm elevated against gravity.

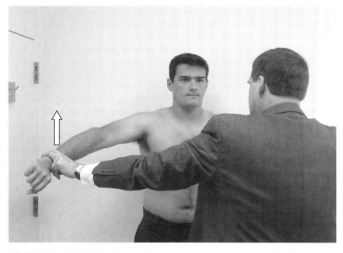

FIGURE 4–32 Testing of the supraspinatus with the arm abducted and the thumbs down is known as the Jobe sign or the "empty can" position.

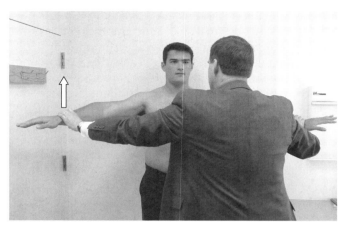

FIGURE 4–33 Testing of the supraspinatus can be performed with the arm in neutral rotation with the thumb parallel to the floor.

drop arm sign was highly specific (98%) for rotator cuff tears; however, its sensitivity was only 10% in the rotator cuff tear group, which reinforces the finding that some patients with rotator cuff tears can have excellent motion and strength.

In summary, the drop arm sign is a significant finding that typically indicates either severe pathology in the shoulder or that the patient has pain inhibiting the ability to hold the arm up in space. A painless drop arm sign can be seen with paralysis of any cause or with massive rotator cuff tears. Patients with a positive drop arm sign should be examined carefully for an etiology for this finding.

Jobe Sign

Strength testing of the supraspinatus can be done in a variety of ways, as discussed in Chapter 3. F. Jobe

popularized testing the supraspinatus with the arm in abduction of 90 degrees in the scapular plane.[122] He recommended testing the muscle with the arm in maximum internal rotation, which has been called the "empty can" position (**Fig. 4–32**). The patient is asked to resist abduction, and the examiner then pushes downward on the elbow or the wrist. This test can be performed accurately with the arm in neutral (**Fig. 4–33**) and with the thumb up ("full can" position) (**Fig. 4–34**).

We typically examine the patient first by pushing down on the elbow because it does not produce as much pain as when testing is done by pushing down on the wrist (**Fig. 4–35**). If the patient is not weak after testing by pushing on the elbow, we then push on the wrist with the

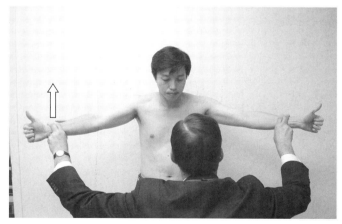

FIGURE 4–34 Electromyogram (EMG) studies show that the Jobe sign can be equally effective in testing the supraspinatus tendon and is known as the "full can" position.

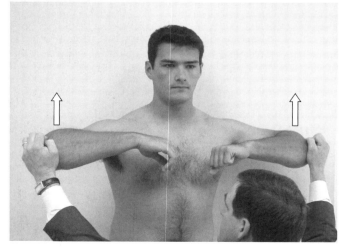

FIGURE 4–35 The strength of the supraspinatus can be performed with the elbow flexed when the patient has pain.

elbows extended, which puts more stress on the supraspinatus. A positive test is when the patient cannot resist the examiner and the arm gives away. Weakness can be graded using scales discussed in Chapter 3. Pain with resisted abduction is considered by some to be indicative of rotator cuff pathology.

Weakness in abduction is an important test for detecting rotator cuff tears. If weakness with supraspinatus testing is used as a sign of rotator cuff pathology, it is found that several pathologies can produce a positive test (**Table 4–6**). Park et al.[100] found that weakness in abduction is fairly specific (89.5%) for rotator cuff pathology (tendinitis, partial tears, or full tears). However, it is not a very sensitive test (44.1%), because many patients with rotator cuff tendinitis or even full-thickness tears can exhibit good strength in manual muscle testing.

Weakness in abduction is a better test for detecting full-thickness tears (52%) than it is for rotator cuff tendinitis (sensitivity 25%) or partial-thickness rotator cuff tears (sensitivity 32%) (**Table 4–6**). In addition, weakness in abduction has more importance for detecting rotator cuff disease when it is combined with other tests, as discussed later.

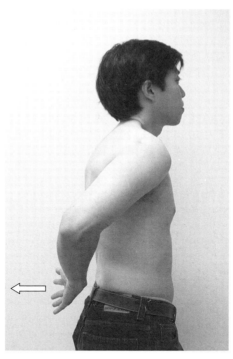

FIGURE 4–36 The lift-off test determines the strength of the subscapularis tendon.

Infraspinatus Strength Testing

Infraspinatus strength testing is performed by having the patient hold his or her arm to the side and then resist external rotation (see Chapter 3). A positive test occurs when the patient cannot resist external rotation; this can be due to pain or weakness. It is important when performing this test that the patient keep the elbows close to the side and not substitute other muscles.

Infraspinatus testing tests the infraspinatus primarily, and the patient should be examined for atrophy in the infraspinatus fossa. In patients with rotator cuff disease, however, it is unusual to have isolated infraspinatus pathology. As a result, a study by Park et al[100] found that infraspinatus weakness was sensitive for rotator cuff tears in only 50% of those patients with full-thickness tears, but it was fairly specific (84%) for full-thickness cuff tears. This means that patients can be weak in external rotation due to pain alone or to other pathologies. This test has its best utility when combined with other tests, as discussed below.

Lift-off Sign

The lift-off sign was described first by Gerber and Krushell[123] in 1991 and was considered specific for the subscapularis muscle and tendon.[124] The test was performed by asking the patient to maximally internally rotate the arm up the back, with the back of the hand against the back (**Fig. 4–36**). The patient was then asked to lift the arm off the back. An inability to lift the arm off the back was considered sensitive and specific for a subscapularis tendon tear; however, Gerber and Krushell cautioned that the test could be performed only in patients without stiffness because they would not be able to rotate the arm up the back. Subsequent EMG studies further supported the findings of Gerber and Krushell that the lift-off was a valid test of subscapularis function.[124–127] Findings from these studies are discussed further in Chapter 3.

The clinical usefulness of this test was also described by Gerber and Krushell[123] when they confirmed that the lift-off sign was positive in all of their patients with full-width, full-thickness subscapularis tendon tears (sensitivity 100%); however, there have been no studies of the specificity, overall accuracy, or likelihood ratios of this test in a large cohort of patients. The usefulness of the lift-off sign for partial-thickness, partial-width subscapularis tendon tears was studied using 314 patients from our shoulder database.[128] In that study there was no correlation between a partial subscapularis tear and a positive lift-off sign. We did not study a subscapularis lag sign, as discussed below. Further study of the overall accuracy of the lift-off test must be performed. In addition, the relationship between a positive lift-off sign and the function of the shoulder warrants further study.

Lag Signs

Lag signs were first described by Hertel et al[129] in 1996; these are the inability of the arm to maintain a certain position when there is weakness in a particular muscle group. In these tests the arm is placed in a particular position that puts the muscle at a disadvantage, and the patient is asked to hold the arm in that position. If the position cannot be maintained, then it is considered a sign that the muscle is weak or the tendon is torn.

External Rotation Lag Sign

The external rotation lag sign (ERLS) was described by Hertel and Gerber et al[129] as a test used to evaluate the integrity of the supraspinatus and the infraspinatus. This test is performed with the subject seated with his or her back to the physician. It can be performed with the patient standing. The arm is held at the side with slight abduction of 20 degrees and supported by the examiner. The examiner holds the patient's arm at the elbow, and with the other hand holds the patient's wrist. The arm is then placed into maximal external rotation and then allowed to relax 5 degrees of external rotation to avoid recoil of the arm into internal rotation (**Fig. 4–37**). The patient is then asked to maintain that position while the examiner lets go of the forearm.

A positive test is when the arm falls into internal rotation and cannot maintain an externally rotated position (**Fig. 4–38**). The degree of lag can be measured with a goniometer within the nearest 5 degrees. The opposite extremity should be examined for comparison. The authors note that the accuracy of this test may be affected by capsular contracture that limits external rotation of the arm.

Hertel et al[129] studied this test in a consecutive case series of 100 patients who underwent surgery for rotator cuff disease. They found the ERLS was positive in all patients ($n = 11$) who had a tear of the supraspinatus and

infraspinatus, and in 15 of 16 patients who had massive rotator cuff tears that included the supraspinatus, infraspinatus, and subscapularis tendons. They also found that the ERLS was less sensitive but more specific than the Jobe strength test at detecting supraspinatus and infraspinatus tears. The ERLS infrequently produced false-positive results, which the authors speculate is due to the lack of pain with this test that may affect the accuracy of the Jobe test and other provocative tests for rotator cuff disease.

Drop Sign

The drop sign was also described by Hertel et al[129] and is used for detecting tears of the infraspinatus tendon. It should be noted that this test is markedly different from the drop arm sign described by Codman,[3] which was meant to be primarily a test of the integrity of the supraspinatus tendon. The drop sign was performed with the subject seated and with the examiner behind the subject. This test can be performed with the patient standing. The physician should passively elevate the arm in the plane of the scapula to 90 degrees of elevation. The examiner should support the arm at 90 degrees of elevation with one hand and hold the wrist of the patient with the other. The arm is then maximally externally rotated without causing pain (**Fig. 4–39**). The patient is asked to hold the arm in that position as the examiner releases the hand holding the wrist. The test is positive if the arm falls back into internal rotation (**Fig. 4–40**). The degree of the lag or falling into internal rotation can be measured to the nearest 5 degrees.

In their study of 100 patients with rotator cuff disease, Hertel et al[129] found that the drop sign was negative in patients with no cuff tear or with partial supraspinatus tears. The drop sign was positive in 50% of the patients with massive rotator cuff tears, which included the supraspinatus, infraspinatus, and subscapularis tendons. In patients with only a supraspinatus and infraspinatus tear, the test was positive in only 40% of patients. The study demonstrated

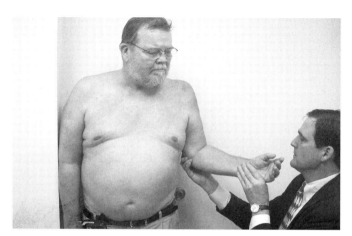

FIGURE 4–37 The external rotation lag sign is performed by externally rotating the arm with the arm at the side and asking the patient to hold that position.

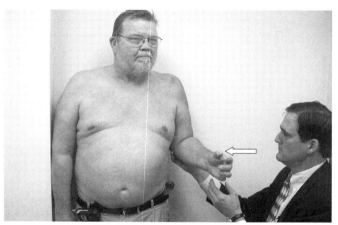

FIGURE 4–38 The external rotation lag sign is positive if the arm falls back into internal rotation.

27. Matsen, F.A., 3rd, S.C. Thomas, and C.A. Rokwood, *Anterior glenohumeral instability*, in *The Shoulder*, F.A. Matsen, 3rd, Editor. 1990, W.B. Saunders: Philadelphia. p.562–622.

28. Andrews, J.R. and J.R. Dugas, *Diagnosis and treatment of shoulder injuries in the throwing athlete: the role of thermal-assisted capsular shrinkage.* Instr Course Lect, 2001. 50:p.17–21.

29. Nelson, B.J. and R.A. Arciero, *Arthroscopic management of glenohumeral instability.* Am J Sports Med, 2000. 28(4):p.602–614.

30. Alvarez, C.M., R. Litchfield, D. Jackowski, S. Griffin, and A. Kirkley, *A prospective, double-blind, randomized clinical trial comparing subacromial injection of betamethasone and xylocaine to xylocaine alone in chronic rotator cuff tendinosis.* Am J Sports Med, 2005. 33(2): p.255–262.

31. Gotoh, M., K. Hamada, H. Yamakawa, K. Yanagisawa, M. Nakamura, H. Yamazaki, Y. Ueyama, N. Tamaoki, A. Inoue, and H. Fukuda, *Interleukin-1-induced subacromial synovitis and shoulder pain in rotator cuff diseases.* Rheumatology (Oxford), 2001. 40(9):p.995–1001.

32. Armstrong, J.R., *Excision of the acromion in the treatment of the supraspinatus syndrome. Report of ninety-five excisions.* J Bone Joint Surg, 1949. 31B:p.436–442.

33. Hammond, G., *Complete acromionectomy in the treatment of chronic tendinitis of the shoulder.* Am J Orthop, 1962. 44-A:p.494–504.

34. Hammond, G., *Complete acromionectomy in the treatment of chronic tendinitis of the shoulder. A follow-up of ninety operations on eighty-seven patients.* J Bone Joint Surg Am, 1971. 53(1):p.173–180.

35. McLaughlin, H.L., *Lesions of the musculotendinous cuff of the shoulder. The exposure and treatment of tears with retraction. 1944.* Clin Orthop, 1994(304):p.3–9.

36. Moseley, H.F., *Shoulder lesions.* 3rd ed, ed. H.F. Moseley. 1969, Edinburgh and London: E&S Livingstone.

37. Yamanaka, K., H. Fukuda, K. Hamada, and M. Mikasa, *Incomplete thickness tears of the rotator cuff.* Orthop Traumatol Surg (Tokyo), 1983. 26:p.713.

38. Petersson, C.J. and C.F. Gentz, *Ruptures of the supraspinatus tendon. The significance of distally pointing acromioclavicular osteophytes.* Clin Orthop Relat Res, 1983(174):p.143–148.

39. Zuckerman, J.D., F.J. Kummer, F. Cuomo, J. Simon, and S. Rosemblum, *The influence of coracoacromial arch anatomy on rotator cuff tears.* J Shoulder Elbow Surg, 1992. 1:p.4–14.

40. Kessel, L. and M. Watson, *The painful arc syndrome. Clinical classification as a guide to management.* J Bone Joint Surg Br, 1977. 59(2): p.166–172.

41. Watson, M., *The refractory painful arc syndrome.* J Bone Joint Surg Br, 1978. 60–B(4):p.544–546.

42. Inman, V.T., J.B. Saunders, and L.C. Abbott, *Observation of the function of the shoulder joint.* J Bone Joint Surg, 1944. 26A:p.1–31.

43. Johansson, J.E. and T.W. Barrington, *Coracoacromial ligament division.* Am J Sports Med, 1984. 12(2):p.138–141.

44. Weiner, D.S. and I. Macnab, *Superior migration of the humeral head. A radiological aid in the diagnosis of tears of the rotator cuff.* J Bone Joint Surg Br, 1970. 52(3):p.524–527.

45. Bernageau, J., *Roentgenographic assessment of the rotator cuff.* Clin Orthop, 1990(254):p.87–91.

46. Prato, N., S. Bianchi, E. Schiaffini, M. Oliveri, and G. Gambaro, *The Leclercq test in diagnosis of tear in the rotator cuff.* Chir Organi Mov, 1991. 76(1):p.73–76.

47. Grashey, R., *Atlas Typischer Rontgenfilder*, ed. R. Grashey. 1923, Munchen: Lehman.

48. Rockwood, C.A. and K.L. Jensen, *X-Ray evaluation of shoulder problems*, in *The Shoulder*, F.A. Matsen III, Editor. 1998, W.B. Saunders: Philadelphia. p.220–225.

49. Bigliani, L.U., D. Morrison, and E.W. April, *The morphology of the acromion and its relationship to rotator cuff tears.* Orthop Trans, 1986. 10:p.228.

50. Morrison, D.S. and L.U. Bigliani, *The clinical significance of variations in acromial morphology.* Orthop Trans, 1987. 11:p.234.

51. Bright, A.S., B. Torpey, D. Magid, T. Codd, and E.G. McFarland, *Reliability of radiographic evaluation for acromial morphology.* Skeletal Radiol, 1997. 26(12):p.718–721.

52. Jacobson, S.R., K.P. Speer, J.T. Moor, D.H. Janda, S.R. Saddemi, P.B. MacDonald, and W.J. Mallon, *Reliability of radiographic assessment of acromial morphology.* J Shoulder Elbow Surg, 1995. 4(6):p.449–453.

53. Aoki, M., S. Ishii, and M. Usui, *The slope of the acromion and rotator cuff impingement.* Orthop Trans, 1986. 10:p.228.

54. Edelson, J.G. and C. Taitz, *Anatomy of the coraco-acromial arch. Relation to degeneration of the acromion.* J Bone Joint Surg Br, 1992. 74(4):p.589–594.

55. Nicholson, G.P., D.A. Goodman, E.L. Flatow, and L.U. Bigliani, *The acromion: morphologic condition and age-related changes. A study of 420 scapulas.* J Shoulder Elbow Surg, 1996. 5(1):p.1–11.

56. Fukuda, H., K. Hamada, and K. Yamanaka, *Pathology and pathogenesis of bursal-side rotator cuff tears viewed from en bloc histologic sections.* Clin Orthop, 1990(254):p.75–80.

57. Goldthwait, J.E., *An anatomic and mechanical study of the shoulder joint, explaining many of the cases of painful shoulder, many of the recurrent dislocations, and many of the cases of brachial neuralgias or neuritis.* Am J Orthop Surg, 1909. 6(4):p.579–606.

58. Gerber, C., F. Terrier, and R. Ganz, *The role of the coracoid process in the chronic impingement syndrome.* J Bone Joint Surg Br, 1985. 67(5): p.703–708.

59. Dines, D.M., R.F. Warren, A.E. Inglis, and H. Pavlov, *The coracoid impingement syndrome.* J Bone Joint Surg Br, 1990. 72(2):p.314–316.

60. Ferrick, M.R., *Coracoid impingement. A case report and review of the literature.* Am J Sports Med, 2000. 28(1):p.117–119.

61. Gerber, C., F. Terrier, R. Zehnder, and R. Ganz, *The subcoracoid space. An anatomic study.* Clin Orthop Relat Res, 1987(215): p.132–138.

62. Friedman, R.J., P.M. Bonutti, and B. Genez, *Cine magnetic resonance imaging of the subcoracoid region.* Orthopedics, 1998. 21(5): p.545–548.

63. Patte, D., *Classification of rotator cuff lesions.* Clin Orthop, 1990(254):p.81–86.

64. Valadie, A.L., 3rd, C.M. Jobe, M.M. Pink, E.F. Ekman, and F.W. Jobe, *Anatomy of provocative tests for impingement syndrome of the shoulder.* J Shoulder Elbow Surg, 2000. 9(1):p.36–46.

65. Nove-Josserand, L., et al, *Coracohumeral space and rotator cuff tears.* J Bone Joint Surg, 2000. 82-B (Suppl III):p.290.

66. Ko, J.Y., C.H. Shih, W.J. Chen, and R. Yamamoto, *Coracoid impingement caused by a ganglion from the subscapularis tendon. A case report.* J Bone Joint Surg Am, 1994. 76(11):p.1709–1711.

67. Walch, G., P. Boileau, E. Noel, and S. Donell, *Impingement of the deep surface of the supraspinatus tendon on the posterior superior glenoid rim: An arthroscopic study.* J Shoulder Elbow Surg, 1992. 1(5):p.238–245.

68. Ellman, H., *Diagnosis and treatment of incomplete rotator cuff tears.* Clin Orthop, 1990(254):p.64–74.

69. Jobe, F.W., R.S. Kvitne, and C.E. Giangarra, *Shoulder pain in the overhand or throwing athlete. The relationship of anterior instability and rotator cuff impingement.* Orthop Rev, 1989. 18(9):p.963–975.

70. Jobe, C.M., *Superior glenoid impingement. Current concepts.* Clin Orthop, 1996(330):p.98–107.

71. Tirman, P.F., F.W. Bost, G.J. Garvin, C.G. Peterfy, J.C. Mall, L.S. Steinbach, J.F. Feller, and J.V. Crues, 3rd, *Posterosuperior glenoid impingement of the shoulder: findings at MR imaging and MR arthrography with arthroscopic correlation.* Radiology, 1994. 193(2):p.431–436.

72. Liu, S.H. and E. Boynton, *Posterior superior impingement of the rotator cuff on the glenoid rim as a cause of shoulder pain in the overhead athlete.* Arthroscopy, 1993. 9(6):p.697–699.

73. Davidson, P.A., N.S. Elattrache, C.M. Jobe, and F.W. Jobe, *Rotator cuff and posterior-superior glenoid labrum injury associated with increased glenohumeral motion: a new site of impingement.* J Shoulder Elbow Surg, 1995. 4(5):p.384–390.

74. Jobe, C.M., *Posterior superior glenoid impingement: expanded spectrum.* Arthroscopy, 1995. 11(5):p.530–536.

75. Jobe, C.M., *Superior glenoid impingement.* Orthop Clin North Am, 1997. 28(2):p.137–143.

76. Iannotti, J.P. and E.D. Wang, *Avulsion of the supraglenoid tubercle: A variation of the SLAP lesion.* J Shoulder Elbow Surg, 1992. 1: p.26–30.

77. Jobe, C.M. and J.P. Iannotti, *Limits imposed on glenohumeral motion by joint geometry.* J Shoulder Elbow Surg, 1995. 4(4):p.281–285.

78. Halbrecht, J.L., P. Tirman, and D. Atkin, *Internal impingement of the shoulder: comparison of findings between the throwing and nonthrowing shoulders of college baseball players.* Arthroscopy, 1999. 15(3):p.253–258.

79. McFarland, E.G., C.Y. Hsu, C. Neira, and O. O'Neil, *Internal impingement of the shoulder: a clinical and arthroscopic analysis.* J Shoulder Elbow Surg, 1999. 8(5):p.458–460.

80. Edelson, G. and C. Teitz, *Internal impingement in the shoulder.* J Shoulder Elbow Surg, 2000. 9(4):p.308–315.

81. Riand, N., C. Levigne, E. Renaud, and G. Walch, *Results of derotational humeral osteotomy in posterosuperior glenoid impingement.* Am J Sports Med, 1998. 26(3):p.453–459.

82. Burkhart, S.S., C.D. Morgan, and W.B. Kibler, *Shoulder injuries in overhead athletes. The "dead arm" revisited.* Clin Sports Med, 2000. 19(1):p.125–158.

83. Struhl, S., *Anterior internal impingement: An arthroscopic observation.* Arthroscopy, 2002. 18(1):p.2–7.

84. Kim, T.K., McFarland, E.G., *Internal Impingement of the Shoulder in Flexion.* Clin Orthop Related Res, 2004(421):p.112–119.

85. McFarland, E.G., et al. *Relationship of symptoms with a positive Neer sign to rotator cuff contact to the superior glenoid.* in *8th International Congress on Surgery of the Shoulder.* 2001. Cape Town, Africa.

86. Kinchen, M., et al. *Three dimensional computer simulation of shoulder impingement.* in *American Academy of Orthopaedic Surgeons.* 1999. Anaheim, CA.

87. Gerber, C., R.V. Galantay, and O. Hersche, *The pattern of pain produced by irritation of the acromioclavicular joint and the subacromial space.* J Shoulder Elbow Surg, 1998. 7(4):p.352–355.

88. Nobuhara, K., *The Shoulder: It's function and clinical aspects.* 2003, Singapore: World scientific publishing.

89. Yocum, L.A., *Assessing the shoulder. History, physical examination, differential diagnosis, and special tests used.* Clin Sports Med, 1983. 2(2):p.281–289.

90. Matsen III, F.A., C.T. Arntz, and L. S.B., *Rotator cuff, in The shoulder,* in *Editor 1990,* F.A.I. Matsen, Editor. 1990, W.B. Saunders: Philadelphia. p.755–839.

91. Lyons, A.R. and J.E. Tomlinson, *Clinical diagnosis of tears of the rotator cuff.* J Bone Joint Surg Br, 1992. 74(3):p.414–415.

92. Wolf, E.M. and V. Agrawal, *Transdeltoid palpation (the rent test) in the diagnosis of rotator cuff tears.* J Shoulder Elbow Surg, 2001. 10(5): p.470–473.

93. Dawbarn, R., *Subdeltoid Bursitis: A pathognomonic sign for its recognition.* Boston Med Surg J, 1906. 154:p.691.

94. Neer, C.S., 2nd and R.P. Welsh, *The shoulder in sports.* Orthop Clin North Am, 1977. 8(3):p.583–591.

95. Calis, M., K. Akgun, M. Birtane, I. Karacan, H. Calis, and F. Tuzun, *Diagnostic values of clinical diagnostic tests in subacromial impingement syndrome.* Ann Rheum Dis, 2000. 59(1):p.44–47.

96. Leroux, J.L., E. Thomas, F. Bonnel, and F. Blotman, *Diagnostic value of clinical tests for shoulder impingement syndrome.* Rev Rhum Engl Ed, 1995. 62(6):p.423–428.

97. MacDonald, P.B., P. Clark, and K. Sutherland, *An analysis of the diagnostic accuracy of the Hawkins and Neer subacromial impingement signs.* J Shoulder Elbow Surg, 2000. 9(4):p.299–301.

98. Murrell, G.A. and J.R. Walton, *Diagnosis of rotator cuff tears.* Lancet, 2001. 357(9258):p.769–770.

99. Hawkins, R.J. and P.E. Hobeika, *Impingement syndrome in the athletic shoulder.* Clin Sports Med, 1983. 2(2):p.391–405.

100. Park, H.B., A. Yokota, H.S. Gill, G. El Rassi, and E.G. McFarland, *Diagnostic Accuracy of Clinical Tests for the Different Degrees of Subacromial Impingement Syndrome.* Accepted for publication in JBJS 07A:1446–1455, 2005.

101. Naredo, E., P. Aguado, E. De Miguel, J. Uson, L. Mayordomo, J. Gijon-Banos, and E. Martin-Mola, *Painful shoulder: comparison of physical examination and ultrasonographic findings.* Ann Rheum Dis, 2002. 61(2):p.132–136.

102. Karnaugh, R.D., J.W. Sperling, and R.F. Warren, *Arthroscopic treatment of coracoid impingement.* Arthroscopy, 2001. 17(7):p.784–787.

103. Lo, I.K. and S.S. Burkhart, *Arthroscopic coracoplasty through the rotator interval.* Arthroscopy, 2003. 19(6):p.667–671.

104. Holtby, R. and H. Razmjou, *Accuracy of the Speed's and Yergason's tests in detecting biceps pathology and SLAP lesions: comparison with arthroscopic findings.* Arthroscopy, 2004. 20(3):p.231–236.

105. Bennett, W.F., *Specificity of the Speed's test: arthroscopic technique for evaluating the biceps tendon at the level of the bicipital groove.* Arthroscopy, 1998. 14(8):p.789–796.

106. Zlatkin, M.B. and F.S. Falchook, *Magnetic resonance pathology of the rotator cuff.* Top Magn Reson Imaging, 1994. 6(2):p.94–120.

107. Savoie, F.H., 3rd, L.D. Field, and S. Atchinson, *Anterior superior instability with rotator cuff tearing: SLAC lesion.* Orthop Clin North Am, 2001. 32(3):p.457–461, ix.

108. Blair, B., A.S. Rokito, F. Cuomo, K. Jarolem, and J.D. Zuckerman, *Efficacy of injections of corticosteroids for subacromial impingement syndrome.* J Bone Joint Surg Am, 1996. 78(11):p.1685–1689.

109. Valtonen, E.J., *Subacromial betamethasone therapy. I. The effect of subacromial injection of betamethasone in cases of painful shoulder resistant to physical therapy.* Ann Chir Gynaecol Fenn Suppl, 1974. 188:p.5–8.

110. White, R.H., D.M. Paull, and K.W. Fleming, *Rotator cuff tendinitis: comparison of subacromial injection of a long acting corticosteroid versus oral indomethacin therapy.* J Rheumatol, 1986. 13(3):p.608–613.

111. Kerlan, R.K. and R.E. Glousman, *Injections and techniques in athletic medicine.* Clin Sports Med, 1989. 8(3):p.541–560.

112. Speed, C.A., *Disease of the rotator cuff. Consider subacromial injection therapy.* Bmj, 1993. 307(6918):p.1559.

113. Eustace, J.A., D.P. Brophy, R.P. Gibney, B. Bresnihan, and O. FitzGerald, *Comparison of the accuracy of steroid placement with clinical outcome in patients with shoulder symptoms.* Ann Rheum Dis, 1997. 56(1):p.59–63.

114. Zuckerman, J.D., M.A. Gallagher, C. Lehman, B.S. Kraushaar, and J. Choueka, *Normal shoulder proprioception and the effect of lidocaine injection.* J Shoulder Elbow Surg, 1999. 8(1):p.11–16.

115. Naredo, E., F. Cabero, P. Beneyto, A. Cruz, B. Mondejar, J. Uson, M.J. Palop, and M. Crespo, *A randomized comparative study of short term response to blind injection versus sonographic-guided injection of local corticosteroids in patients with painful shoulder.* J Rheumatol, 2004. 31(2):p.308–314.

116. Hollingworth, G.R., R.M. Ellis, and T.S. Hattersley, *Comparison of injection techniques for shoulder pain: results of a double blind, randomised study.* Br Med J (Clin Res Ed), 1983. 287(6402):p.1339–1341.

117. Darlington, L.G. and E.N. Coomes, *The effects of local steroid injection for supraspinatus tears.* Rheumatol Rehabil, 1977. 16(3):p.172–179.

118. Withrington, R.H., F.L. Girgis, and M.H. Seifert, *A placebo-controlled trial of steroid injections in the treatment of supraspinatus tendonitis.* Scand J Rheumatol, 1985. 14(1):p.76–78.

119. Partington, P.F. and G.H. Broome, *Diagnostic injection around the shoulder: hit and miss? A cadaveric study of injection accuracy.* J Shoulder Elbow Surg, 1998. 7(2):p.147–150.

120. Yamakado, K., *The targeting accuracy of subacromial injection to the shoulder: an arthrographic evaluation.* Arthroscopy, 2002. 18(8):p.887–891.

121. Bergman, A.G. and M. Fredericson, *Shoulder MRI after impingement test injection.* Skeletal Radiol, 1998. 27(7):p.365–368.

122. Moseley, J.B., Jr., F.W. Jobe, M. Pink, J. Perry, and J. Tibone, *EMG analysis of the scapular muscles during a shoulder rehabilitation program.* Am J Sports Med, 1992. 20(2):p.128–134.

123. Gerber, C. and R.J. Krushell, *Isolated rupture of the tendon of the subscapularis muscle. Clinical features in 16 cases.* J Bone Joint Surg Br, 1991. 73(3):p.389–394.

124. Greis, P.E., J.E. Kuhn, J. Schultheis, R. Hintermeister, and R. Hawkins, *Validation of the lift-off test and analysis of subscapularis activity during maximal internal rotation.* Am J Sports Med, 1996. 24(5):p.589–593.

125. Jobe, F.W., J.E. Tibone, J. Perry, and D. Moynes, *An EMG analysis of the shoulder in throwing and pitching. A preliminary report.* Am J Sports Med, 1983. 11(1):p.3–5.

126. Tokish, J.M., M.J. Decker, H.B. Ellis, M.R. Torry, and R.J. Hawkins, *The belly-press test for the physical examination of the subscapularis muscle: electromyographic validation and comparison to the lift-off test.* J Shoulder Elbow Surg, 2003. 12(5):p.427–430.

127. Stefko, J.M., F.W. Jobe, R.S. VanderWilde, E. Carden, and M. Pink, *Electromyographic and nerve block analysis of the subscapularis liftoff test.* J Shoulder Elbow Surg, 1997. 6(4):p.347–355.

128. Kim, T.K., P.B. Rauh, and E.G. McFarland, *Partial tears of the subscapularis tendon found during arthroscopic procedures on the shoulder: a statistical analysis of sixty cases.* Am J Sports Med, 2003. 31(5):p.744–750.

129. Hertel, R., F.T. Ballmer, S.M. Lombert, and C. Gerber, *Lag signs in the diagnosis of rotator cuff rupture.* J Shoulder Elbow Surg, 1996. 5(4):p.307–313.

130. Walch, G., A. Boulahia, S. Calderone, and A.H. Robinson, *The 'dropping' and 'hornblower's' signs in evaluation of rotator-cuff tears.* J Bone Joint Surg Br, 1998. 80(4):p.624–628.

131. Hertel, R., S.M. Lambert, and F.T. Ballmer, *The deltoid extension lag sign for diagnosis and grading of axillary nerve palsy.* J Shoulder Elbow Surg, 1998. 7(2):p.97–99.

132. Goutallier, D., J.M. Postel, J. Bernageau, L. Lavau, and M.C. Voisin, *Fatty muscle degeneration in cuff ruptures. Pre- and postoperative evaluation by CT scan.* Clin Orthop, 1994(304):p.78–83.

133. Lehman, C., F. Cuomo, F.J. Kummer, and J.D. Zuckerman, *The incidence of full thickness rotator cuff tears in a large cadaveric population.* Bull Hosp Jt Dis, 1995. 54(1):p.30–31.

134. Yamada, H. and F. Evans, *Strength of biological materials.* 1972, Williams & Wilkins: Baltimore.p.67–70.

135. Bakalim, G. and M. Pasila, *Surgical treatment of rupture of the rotator cuff tendon.* Acta Orthop Scand, 1975. 46(5):p.751–757.

136. Hawkins, R.J., G.W. Misamore, and P.E. Hobeika, *Surgery for full-thickness rotator-cuff tears.* J Bone Joint Surg Am, 1985. 67(9):p.1349–1355.

137. Brown, J.N., S.N. Roberts, M.G. Hayes, and A.D. Sales, *Shoulder pathology associated with symptomatic acromioclavicular joint degeneration.* J Shoulder Elbow Surg, 2000. 9(3):p.173–176.

138. Sher, J.S., J.W. Uribe, A. Posada, B.J. Murphy, and M.B. Zlatkin, *Abnormal findings on magnetic resonance images of asymptomatic shoulders.* J Bone Joint Surg Am, 1995. 77(1):p.10–15.

139. Milgrom, C., M. Schaffler, S. Gilbert, and M. van Holsbeeck, *Rotator-cuff changes in asymptomatic adults. The effect of age, hand dominance and gender.* J Bone Joint Surg Br, 1995. 77(2):p.296–298.

140. Tempelhof, S., S. Rupp, and R. Seil, *Age-related prevalence of rotator cuff tears in asymptomatic shoulders.* J Shoulder Elbow Surg, 1999. 8(4):p.296–299.

141. Worland, R.L., D. Lee, C.G. Orozco, F. SozaRex, and J. Keenan, *Correlation of age, acromial morphology, and rotator cuff tear pathology diagnosed by ultrasound in asymptomatic patients.* J South Orthop Assoc, 2003. 12(1):p.23–26.

142. Goldberg, B.A., R.J. Nowinski, and F.A. Matsen, 3rd, *Outcome of nonoperative management of full-thickness rotator cuff tears.* Clin Orthop, 2001(382):p.99–107.

143. Hawkins, R.H. and R. Dunlop, *Nonoperative treatment of rotator cuff tears.* Clin Orthop, 1995(321):p.178–188.

144. Samilson, R.L. and W.F. Binder, *Symptomatic full thickness tears of rotator cuff. An analysis of 292 shoulders in 276 patients.* Orthop Clin North Am, 1975. 6(2):p.449–466.

145. Kessler, K.J., A.E. Bullens-Borrow, and J. Zisholtz, *LactoSorb plates for rotator cuff repair.* Arthroscopy, 2002. 18(3):p.279–283.

146. Cofield, R.H., J. Parvizi, P.J. Hoffmeyer, W.L. Lanzer, D.M. Ilstrup, and C.M. Rowland, *Surgical repair of chronic rotator cuff tears. A prospective long-term study.* J Bone Joint Surg Am, 2001. 83-A(1):p.71–77.

147. Gartsman, G.M., M. Khan, and S.M. Hammerman, *Arthroscopic repair of full-thickness tears of the rotator cuff.* J Bone Joint Surg Am, 1998. 80(6):p.832–840.

148. Budoff, J.E., R.P. Nirschl, and E.J. Guidi, *Debridement of partial-thickness tears of the rotator cuff without acromioplasty. Long-term follow-up and review of the literature.* J Bone Joint Surg Am, 1998. 80(5):p.733–748.

149. Liu, S.H., *Arthroscopically-assisted rotator-cuff repair.* J Bone Joint Surg Br, 1994. 76(4):p.592–595.

150. Levy, H.J., J.W. Uribe, and L.G. Delaney, *Arthroscopic assisted rotator cuff repair: preliminary results.* Arthroscopy, 1990. 6(1):p.55–60.

151. Norwood, L.A., R. Barrack, and K.E. Jacobson, *Clinical presentation of complete tears of the rotator cuff.* J Bone Joint Surg Am, 1989. 71(4):p.499–505.

152. Ellman, H., G. Hanker, and M. Bayer, *Repair of the rotator cuff. End-result study of factors influencing reconstruction.* J Bone Joint Surg Am, 1986. 68(8):p.1136–1144.

153. Smith-Teunis, C.B., J.W. Xerogeanes, and R.J. Hawkins. *Accuracy of Rotator Cuff Diagnosis on the Basis of Physical Examination with and without MRI.* in *29th Annual AOSSM Meeting.* 2003. San Diego, CA. July 20–23, 2003.

5

Instability and Laxity

One of the most common shoulder conditions is instability of the glenohumeral joint. Shoulder instability continues to be a significant problem for athletic and active individuals, but it can be seen in any age group due to trauma. The concepts of instability continue to evolve, and the physical examination changes with these concepts. In clinical practice, however, shoulder instability presents one of the most difficult diagnostic areas as a result of a variety of factors. First, our knowledge of the anatomy and the biomechanics of shoulder function as it relates to stability continues to increase and change. Second, the examinations for instability are good for diagnosing some types of instability but not others. For example, the anterior apprehension test for anterior shoulder instability is fairly accurate for the patient with traumatic anterior instability, but its usefulness is less clear in the throwing athlete who does not have true subluxations or dislocations. The overhead athlete who has pain in the shoulder and who may have some form of shoulder instability continues to be a diagnostic dilemma.

This chapter summarizes the existing examination findings for instability and interprets their meaning, clarifies the difference between laxity and instability, and discusses the examination of the shoulder in light of evolving concepts of instability.

■ History of the Concepts of Instability

Instability at one time was a seemingly straightforward concept for the clinician. If the humeral head came out of the socket and stayed there, then the patient was thought to have a shoulder dislocation. If the humeral head went part of the way out but then went back into the joint, it was considered a subluxation. Over the past few years the normal anatomy has become better appreciated, and the complexity of shoulder instability has become apparent (**Figs. 5–1, 5–2, 5–3**).

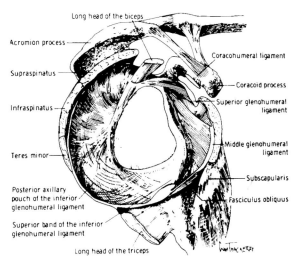

FIGURE 5–1 Ligament anatomy of the shoulder when viewed from the side (sagittal view). (Adapted with permission from Turkel SJ, Panio MW, Marshall JL, et al. Stabilizing mechanisms preventing anterior dislocation of the glenohumeral joint. 1981;63:1209.)

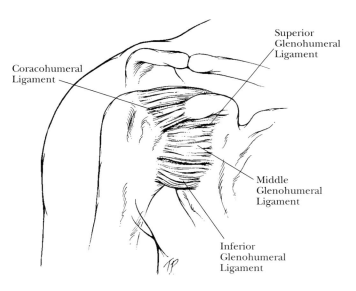

FIGURE 5–2 Ligament anatomy of the shoulder from the front (coronal view).

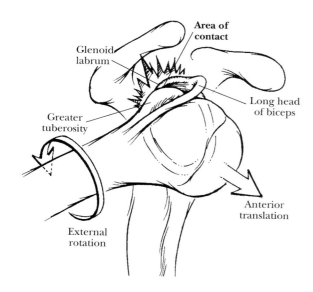

FIGURE 5–3 There are numerous variations of the superior labrum and middle glenohumeral ligaments. (Adapted with permission from Rao AG, KT, Chronopoulos E, McFarland EG. Anatomical variants in the anteroposterior aspect of the glenoid labrum: a statistical analysis of seventy-three cases. J Bone Joint Surg Am 2003;85(4):653–659.)

Initially, it was unclear which structures in the shoulder were damaged when the shoulder became unstable from traumatic causes. Perthes and Bankart[1,2] both defined the pathology as a disruption of the labrum attachments to the glenoid, and subsequent studies demonstrated that there often is some form of capsular failure associated with labrum detachments (**Fig. 5–4**).

Rowe and Zarins[3] in 1981 widened the concept of instability when they described the "dead arm" syndrome. They evaluated 60 shoulders where the patients complained of sudden, sharp, and paralyzing pain with the arm

in an abducted and externally rotated position. This pain and heaviness of the arm could be caused by any activity in which the arm was used over shoulder level, including overhead work, tennis, swimming, and baseball. After the episode of pain the arm could be weak or "dead" for hours or days. Some of Rowe and Zarins' patients had experienced a blow with the arm in abduction and external rotation, such as that seen in football and basketball players. In their cohort of patients, 26 patients with 27 shoulders injured could recall a sensation that the shoulder had distinctly come out of the socket. The other 32 patients with 33 shoulders injured did not feel a subluxation and complained only of the symptoms mentioned above. At the time of surgery, 32 shoulders (64%) had Bankart lesions, and the remainder had only capsular laxity.

Consequently, Rowe and Zarins[3] can be given credit for the concept of occult instability, where the patient did not feel a subluxation or dislocation of the humeral head out of the socket, but whose symptoms were due to some form of instability of the shoulder. These patients were unaware that they were actually having subluxations or near subluxations of the joint.

Rowe and Zarins were the first to suggest that the treatment of this condition was to perform only a capsular shift in cases where there was no Bankart lesion. Interestingly, 20 (54%) of their patients were felt to have a large rotator cuff interval, which they repaired with sutures. Of the patients who had their dominant arm operated upon, 64% were able to return to overhead work or sports with no limitation. Of the eight patients whose shoulders were judged to be damaged from forceful baseball pitching, four (50%) returned to their previous level of throwing, and four did not.

This concept was further expanded and popularized in the 1980s by Dr. Frank Jobe and colleagues,[4] who postulated that the etiology of pain in overhead athletes was

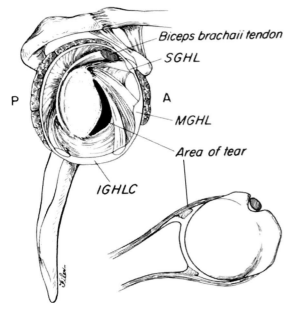

FIGURE 5–4 A Bankart lesion is detachment of the anteroinferior labrum from the glenoid rim. (Adapted with permission from Warner JP, Caborn DNM. Overview of shoulder instability. Crit Rev Phys Rehabil Med 1992;4:145–198.)

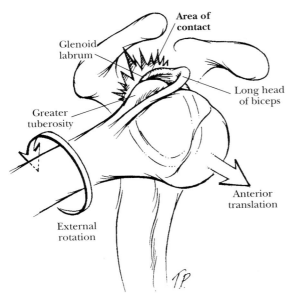

FIGURE 5–5 Hyperangulation of the humerus was postulated by Dr. Frank Jobe to lead to labrum and rotator cuff pathologies.

rotator cuff tendinitis due to instability. Whereas the throwing or overhead athlete felt only pain or a dead arm, the symptoms were produced by repetitive injury to the anterior restraining structures of the shoulder, specifically the anteroinferior glenohumeral ligament. Jobe et al theorized that the shoulder of throwing athletes and those athletes involved in overhead sports sustained significant stress to the ligaments when the arm was in an abducted and externally rotated position. This repetitive microtrauma to the ligaments resulted in their elongation. As the ligaments stretched, the rotator cuff impinged on the anterolateral acromion and produced pain (**Fig. 5–5**).

Upon examination of the patient, Jobe et al noticed that the shoulders felt loose and that placing the arm in a position of abduction and external rotation reproduced the pain. If nonoperative treatments failed, they recommended that an anterior capsular shift be performed to tighten the anteroinferior ligament complex. Jobe et al[5] reported that this capsular shift procedure resulted in 68% of athletes capable of returning to throwing at their previous level for at least 1 year.

As a result of this work, shoulder pain in athletes was felt by many subsequent clinicians to be due to this form of occult instability, where the athlete did not feel overt subluxations or dislocation. In this syndrome, the only symptoms reported by patients included pain and the inability to perform their sport to a maximum level. The surgical treatment involves tightening the shoulder capsule that contains the ligaments, by performing a capsular shift either on the glenoid side[5] or on the humeral side[6,7] of the ligament attachments.

Other surgical techniques evolved to tighten the ligaments, including arthroscopic suturing and thermal

capsular shrinkage techniques.[8–10] The arthroscopic methods use sutures that are placed in the capsule arthroscopically to remove any redundancy in the capsule; this procedure is referred to as an arthroscopic capsular placation.[11–13] In the thermal capsular shrinkage procedures, devices are used that generate heat to shrink the ligaments. This thermal injury to the tissue initiates a healing response that may tighten the ligaments. The thermal techniques were originally described as an initial treatment for capsular laxity, but due to high recurrence rates, they are increasingly recommended as an adjunct to other methods to tighten the capsule.[14–16]

The concepts of what causes pain in the shoulder of the overhead athlete continue to evolve. Walch et al[17] in 1992 reported on internal impingement of the rotator cuff to the posterior and superior glenoid. When performing arthroscopy on the shoulders of 17 patients, Walch and colleagues could demonstrate this contact intra-articularly with the arm in abduction and external rotation. These concepts are discussed in more detail in Chapter 4. Because none of their patients seemed to be unstable upon examination, Walch et al suggested that this contact of the rotator cuff to the posterior and superior glenoid was physiological. For patients who failed nonoperative treatment, they recommended a humeral osteotomy, an operation they have since abandoned for this entity.[18]

With the advent of shoulder arthroscopy in the early 1980s, important discoveries were made about intra-articular pathology that was associated with shoulder pain and instability. In 1985, Andrews et al[19] reported on superior labrum lesions in overhead athletes; they found that the stress of throwing was somehow the etiology. Subsequently, Snyder et al[20] described four variations of superior labrum anterior to posterior (SLAP) lesions, and it became appreciated that these superior labrum detachments were found often in the overhead athlete.

F. Jobe et al[4] noted that overhead athletes at the time of arthroscopy had SLAP lesions, partial rotator cuff tears, posterior humeral head chondromalacia, and rarely Bankart lesions. They later noticed that internal impingement as described by Walch et al[17] could be seen arthroscopically in the shoulders of throwing athletes with pain. Jobe et al suggested that this contact of the rotator cuff to the posterior and superior labrum caused partial thickness cuff tears, labrum tears, or both (**Fig. 5–6**). These concepts are discussed in more detail in Chapter 6.

> Pathology seen in the shoulder of the overhead athlete may include partial rotator cuff tears, SLAP lesions, and chondromalacia on the humeral head.

Another theory of why throwing athletes have pain in the shoulder is that they have a form of superior instability. Morgan et al[21] and Burkhart et al[22] suggested that the superior labrum attachments are gradually stretched by

TABLE 5–2 Role of Glenohumeral Ligaments in Shoulder Stability

Authors	SGHL	CHL	MGHL	IGHL
Warner et al[50]	Primary restraint to inferior translation at 0° ABD & NL	No significant role for inferior translation when SGHL present	Restraint to inferior translation at 0° ABD & ER	Anterior band primary restraint to inferior translation at 45° ABD & NL; Posterior band primary restraint to inferior translation at 90° ABD & NL
Turkel et al[148]	Minor role in anterior instability	N/R*	Restraint to anterior instability at 45° ABD	Primary restraint to anterior instability at 90° ABD
Ovesen et al[48,149,150]	Restraint to posterior instability	Restraint to inferior instability; secondary role in posterior instability	Restraint to posterior instability	Posterior band restraint to posterior instability at 45–90° ABD
Basmajian et al[151]	Primary restraint to inferior translation in ADD	Primary restraint to inferior translation in ADD	N/R	N/R
O'Brien et al[45]	N/R	N/R	N/R	Restraint to anterior and posterior instability, primary stabilizer in ABD and ER
Harryman et al[49]	Significant restraint to posterior and inferior translation	Significant restraint to posterior and inferior translation	N/R	N/R
Helmig et al[152]	Restraint in inferior translation	Primary restraint to inferior translation	N/R	N/R
Ferrari et al[102]	Restraint to ER <60° ABD	Restraint to inferior translation & ER	Restraint to ER at 60° and 90° ABD	N/R
Burkhart et al[153]	Restraint to inferior translation in 0–50° ABD	Restraint to inferior translation in 0–50° ADD	Restraint to anterior instability at 45–60° ABD	Primary restraint for anterior shoulder dislocation

ABD, abduction; ADD, adduction; NL, neutral; ER, external rotation; IR, internal rotation; SGHL, superior glenohumeral ligament; CHL, coracohumeral ligament; MCHL, middle glenohumeral ligament; IGHL, inferior glenohumeral ligament; *N/R, not reported.

The exact contribution of the labrum to the concavity compression depends on the arm position and the amount of compressive load.[41] According to Matsen et al,[28] the labrum effectively deepens the socket, and it creates a bumper to resist translation (**Fig. 5–8**). The labrum doubles the anteroposterior depth of the glenoid.[42] Matsen et al[28] calculated that this mechanism provides up to 60% of the force resisting translation of the humerus on the glenoid. Lippitt et al[43] demonstrated that excision of the glenoid labrum reduces the stability of the glenohumeral joint through the concavity compression mechanism by ~20%. Thus, in a shoulder with a labral lesion, the concavity compression mechanism may be compromised, so that there are increased translations of the humeral head on the socket with shoulder motion.

In the normal shoulder, Matsen et al[28] suggested that the majority of compression forces are provided by the rotator cuff muscles (subscapularis, supraspinatus, infraspinatus, teres minor), and this compression of the humeral head into the glenoid provides stability to the joint. Though controversial, some have suggested that the biceps tendon may provide some stability to the glenohumeral joint with the arm in certain positions. As a result, it has been suggested that patients with instability of the shoulder through the concavity compression mechanism can increase the security of the gleno-humeral joints by strengthening the rotator cuff muscles. Clinically, the concavity compression mechanism can be compromised in patients with shoulder muscle weakness, torn rotator cuff tendons, labral tears, or glenoid defects.[28]

The next major restraints to shoulder motion are the capsular ligaments (**Table 5–2**). Biomechanical studies have indicated that the major restraint to anterior translation of the humeral head upon the glenoid with the arm at the side is the anterior capsule.[26] With the arm in an abducted and externally rotated position, the anterior band of the inferior glenohumeral ligament is the major restraint to instability of the joint. The second major restraint to translation in this position is the anterior glenoid labrum. Once the anterior structures fail, the next structures to undergo deformation include the posterior capsule. This injury to the opposite side of the primary direction of instability is referred to as the "circle concept" of shoulder stability (**Fig. 5–12**).[44]

The major restraint to posterior excursion is the posterior capsule when the arm is at the side or when the arm is in front of the body. In one biomechanical study, for a posterior dislocation to occur with the arm in this position, the anterosuperior capsule also had to be incised from the 12 to the 3 o'clock position.[45–48] Furthermore, Harryman et al[49] demonstrated with the

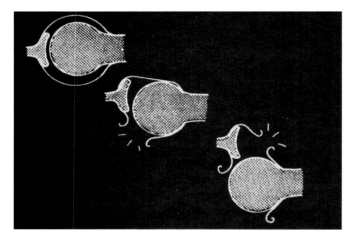

FIGURE 5–12 The circle concept of shoulder instability suggests that for severe excursion of the humeral head to occur, the ligaments opposite the side of the direction of translation will also eventually fail. (Adapted with permission from Pagnini MJ, Warren RF. Stabilizer of the glenohumeral joint. J Shoulder Elbow Surg 1994;3:173–190.)

arm in an adducted position that the rotator cuff interval (anterosuperior capsule) was the primary restraint of the inferior and posterior translation of the humeral head. With the arm in a position of adduction, flexion, and internal rotation, the glenohumeral joint did not dislocate posteriorly. In the adducted arm in the external rotation position, the middle glenohumeral ligament has the primary role in preventing inferior subluxation of the humeral head.[50]

The major restraints to inferior translation have been found to be dependent on shoulder position. Warner et al[50] demonstrated that the primary capsuloligamentous constraint to inferior humeral subluxation in the abducted position is the posterior band of the inferior glenohumeral ligament. At 45 degrees of abduction, the anterior band of the inferior glenohumeral ligaments becomes the primary restraint to inferior translation in either a neutral or an internally rotated position; when the arm is in an externally rotated position, the posterior band is the primary restraint of the inferior glenohumeral ligament. At 90 degrees of abduction, the posterior band of the glenohumeral ligament is the primary restraint to inferior translation in external rotation, and the anterior band is the primary restraint to inferior translation in internal rotation.[50]

The major structures that prevent superior subluxation and instability of the humeral head depend on which direction is being considered. Some authors suggest that there is a difference between straight superior subluxation and anterosuperior subluxation.[21,51–53] The major restraint to superior migration of the humeral head is the supraspinatus tendon. When the supraspinatus tendon is torn, the next restraints to superior migration become the acromion and the acromioclavicular (AC) joint. Some patients with massive rotator cuff tears can have migration of the humeral head superiorly to the point of causing erosion of the AC joint.[54–56]

The major restraints to anterior and superior subluxation include the coracoacromial ligament, the rotator cuff interval tissue, and the anterior edge of the acromion.[57–59] Although the coracoacromial ligament has been implicated as a culprit in the etiology of rotator cuff disease, there is increasing evidence that it serves an important function as a restraint to the humeral head as the arm is elevated. This function is increased when the rotator cuff tendons are torn and no longer keep the humeral head centered in the glenoid. This anterior and superior subluxation of the humeral head has become recognized as a common cause of disability in patients with massive rotator cuff tears, after failed rotator cuff repairs, and after hemiarthroplasty for proximal humerus fractures.

The "Zero" or "Loose Packed" Position

The resting position of the shoulder has been described as the position in which the shoulder capsule is the most lax. It is supposed that this position would be where the greatest translations of the shoulder can occur due to small concavity-compressive forces.[60] This has also been called the "loose packed" position. This position has been recommended for assessing joint laxity and for evaluating restrictions that may cause pain.[60,61]

This position should not be confused with the position of the arm at rest when the arm is at the side. Based on observation and experience, the zero or loose packed position has been reported to be in the plane of the scapula and around 55 to 70 degrees of abduction of the arm (i.e., the humerus in relation to the thorax)[60,61] (**Fig. 5–13**). There have been several studies that have evaluated shoulder joint laxity based on arm position. Debski et al,[62] using robotic manipulators in a cadaveric shoulder model, found that anteroposterior translation of the shoulder was greatest with the arm in neutral rotation and elevated between 30 and 60 degrees in relation to the thorax.

Hsu et al[60] studied translations in a cadaver model using an instrumented testing machine. They found that the position for the greatest excursion of the humerus on the glenoid was at 40 degrees of glenohumeral abduction, which corresponds to a position of around 55 to 70 degrees of arm abduction if one were to adjust the model for scapulothoracic motion. They found that there was no one position for all specimens where there is the most laxity, but rather the loosest position overall for all specimens seemed

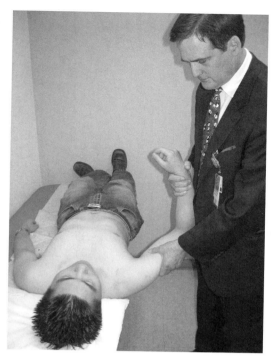

FIGURE 5–13 The position of the area where the ligaments are loosest, also known as the "loose-packed position," is with the arm abducted 50 to 60 degrees with neutral rotation as shown here.

to be around 45% of maximum arm abduction. Like other researchers they found that the joint became more constrained (i.e., had less laxity) above or below that level.

The importance of these findings is that the position where the arm is tested for laxity testing will determine how much translation is available upon examination. There is increasing evidence that the constraints to movement are dependent upon arm position and the amount of compressive force applied to the joint. These factors explain why two physicians may obtain different results when examining the same shoulder. If the movements are not tested with the arm in nearly the same position, it is likely that different results will be obtained.

> The position of the arm when testing for laxity is important when comparing results by multiple examiners or when performing serial examinations.

Laxity Testing

The shoulder is one of the most mobile joints in the body, but it is important to be able to evaluate shoulder laxity because it can help when making the diagnosis of

instability. When testing ligaments in the body to determine if they are torn, it is important to measure not only the laxity of the joint (how much excursion there is between the bones) but also the firmness of the end point of the test. If a ligament is intact, there typically is a "firm" end point with examinations that test that ligament; if it is torn, then the end point is "soft" because the ligament does not abruptly stop motion.

Unfortunately, in the shoulder it is difficult to evaluate the end point in any one direction because several parts tend to want to move at once during the examination. When trying to examine the shoulder for laxity, the scapula can move on the thorax, and the humerus can rotate at the glenohumeral joint. As a result, one cannot reliably use the presence or absence of an end point as a criterion for ligament disruption in the shoulder.

The inherent laxity of the shoulder has been measured in laboratory and clinical studies. It is important to understand how the studies are performed, because this influences the amount of laxity that can be expected in the shoulder. In the laboratory studies, the bones of the shoulder typically are placed in jigs, which hold them in place, or electromagnetic sensors are attached that will closely monitor the movement of the bones. In studies where the bones are attached to jigs, the excursion of the bones must necessarily be constrained in some direction or other.

One thing to consider when evaluating these biomechanical studies of shoulder ligament function is the effect of venting the joint on the bone movements. The shoulder capsule creates a suction effect when it is closed, and when it is vented this suction effect is lost, and the bone excursion can increase significantly.[40] Venting the joint may produce results that do not accurately reflect the normal function and motion of the shoulder joint.

Another important variable when evaluating these studies is the amount of force used to create excursion or translation of the joint. This is important because a large force will cause greater excursion, and a lesser force will produce less excursion. The amount of force used can influence the amount the bones move in both laboratory studies and in clinical studies involving measurement of laxity using surface markers or indwelling pins placed in the bones. This variability in force used to measure translation can be a factor in clinical practice because one examiner may push harder on the joint than another. This may result in one examiner measuring a large translation of the bones and another examiner measuring less translation in the same subject. The position of the bones at the time of testing in these studies is also important because it may not duplicate the clinical situation.

The results of these laxity studies are summarized in **Table 5–3**. These numbers are important to consider

TABLE 5-3 Review of the Literature on Shoulder Translation

Study	N	Population	Pathology	Age (Years)	Gender	Consciousness	Tests Performed	Body Position
Sauers et al (2001)[25]	51	Physically active, no OH athletes	Nonimpaired	22.0 + 2.8	Mixed	Awake	Instrumented load and shift	Sitting
Sauers et al (2001)[68]	25	Physically active, no OH athletes	Nonimpaired	21.9 + 2.6	Mixed	Awake	Instrumented Load & Shift	Sitting
Borsa et al (2001)[63]	20	Physically active, no OH athletes	Nonimpaired	20.9 + 3.6	Mixed	Awake	Instrumented load and shift and sulcus	Sitting
Borsa et al (2000)[154]	24	Physically active, no OH athletes	Nonimpaired	22.1 + 2.5	Males	Awake	Instrumented load and shift	Sitting
	27			22.4 + 3.1	Females			
Borsa et al (1999)[65]	20	Physically active, no OH athletes	Nonimpaired	25.1 + 5.5	Mixed	Awake	Instrumented load and shift	Sitting
Harryman et al (1992)[64]	8	Nonathletes	Nonimpaired	25–45	N/A	Awake	Manual AP drawer and sulcus	Sitting
Lippitt et al (1994)[155]	8	Patients	Nonimpaired	25–45	Male	Awake	Manual AP drawer and sulcus	Sitting
	8	Patients	TUBS	18–39	7 male, 1 female	Anesthesia	Manual AP drawer and sulcus	Beach chair
	8	Patients	AMBRI	15–37	4 male, 4 female	Anesthesia	Manual AP drawer and sulcus	Beach chair
Tillander & Norlin (2001)[156]	102	Patients	All (stable and unstable)	NR	NR	Anesthesia	Manual AP drawer and sulcus	Lateral decubitus
	102	Patients	All (stable and unstable)	NR	NR	Anesthesia	Instrumented AP drawer and sulcus	Lateral decubitus
	58	Patients	Pathologic but stable	NR	NR	Anesthesia	Instrumented AP drawer and sulcus	Lateral decubitus
	44	Patients	Unstable (31 TUBS, 13 MDI)	NR	NR	Anesthesia	Instrumented AP drawer and sulcus	Lateral decubitus
	13	Patients	MDI	NR	NR	Anesthesia	Instrumented AP drawer and sulcus	Lateral decubitus

AP Arm Position	Inferior Arm Position	Measurement Technique	Side	Force Applied	Anterior	Posterior	AP Laxity	Inferior
20° abduction in scapular plane/0° rotation	N/A	Surface linear displacement transducers (mm)	Both	67 N 89 N 111 N 134 N Avg 0–134 N Range	8.0 + 2.2 9.4 + 2.5 10.7 + 2.7 11.9 + 2.9 10.0 + 2.9 4.3 − 19.4	8.6 + 2.7 9.9 + 3.0 10.9 + 3.2 11.8 + 3.3 10.3 + 3.3 3.3 − 19.7	N/A N/A N/A N/A 20.3 + 5.3 8.4 − 37.0	N/A N/A N/A N/A N/A N/A
20° abduction in scapular plane/0° rotation	N/A	Surface linear displacement transducers (mm)	Both	67 N 89 N 111 N 134 N Range	7.5 + 2.1 8.9 + 2.3 10.2 + 2.6 11.3 + 2.8 4.3 − 17.3	9.3 + 2.2 10.7 + 2.3 11.8 + 2.4 12.7 + 2.5 4.7 − 17.5	N/A N/A N/A N/A N/A	N/A N/A N/A N/A N/A
20° abduction in scapular plane/0° rotatio	Dependent, neutral rotation	Surface electromagnetic tracking system (mm)	Both	181–203 N Range	14.5 + 2.3 10.1 − 18.7	14.0 + 2.8 7.7 − 19.3	N/A N/A	13.9 + 4.6 8.9 − 23.1
20° abduction in scapular plane/0° rotation	N/A	Surface linear displacement transducers (mm)	Both	Avg 0–134 N	8.3 + 2.2	9.6 + 2.9	N/A	N/A
			Both	Avg 0–134 N	11.4 + 2.8	10.9 + 3.5	N/A	N/A
20° abduction in scapular plane/0° rotation	N/A	Surface linear displacement transducers (mm)	Both	67 N 89 N 111 N 134 N Range	6.1 + 1.7 7.4 + 1.8 8.7 + 1.9 9.7 + 2.0 3.4 − 12.8	5.0 + 2.7 6.1 + 3.0 6.8 + 3.7 6.5 + 4.1 0.9 − 13.3	N/A N/A N/A N/A N/A	N/A N/A N/A N/A N/A
Dependent, neutral rotation	Dependent, neutral rotation	Bone-pinned electromagnetic tracking system (mm)	NR	Manual	8 + 4 (2 − 13)	8 + 6 (3 − 20)	N/A	11 + 4 (5 − 15)
Dependent, neutral rotation	Dependent, neutral rotation	Bone-pinned electromagnetic tracking system (mm)	NR	Manual	8.1 + 3.8	7.4 + 5.5	15.5 + 9.0	11.2 + 3.6
Dependent, neutral rotation	Dependent, neutral rotation	Bone-pinned electromagnetic tracking system (mm)	Symptomatic	Manual	7.9 + 3.1	11.6 + 3.7	19.5 + 6.0	11.2 + 3.1
Dependent, neutral rotation	Dependent, neutral rotation	Bone-pinned electromagnetic tracking system (mm)	Symptomatic	Manual	8.5 + 4.0	12.1 + 2.4	20.6 + 5.1	9.1 + 3.4
20° abduction, 10° flexing, 0° rotation	20° abduction, 10° flexing, 0° rotation	0–3 + (Altcheck et al, 1989)	Symptomatic	Manual	N = 102: 0 = 47, 1+ = 2 0, >2+ = 35	N = 101: 0 = 59, 1+ = 16, >2+ = 26	N/A	N = 71: 0 = 53, 1+ = 11, >2+ = 7
20° abduction, 10° flexing, 0° rotation	20° abduction, 10° flexing, 0° rotation	Bone-pinned shoulder translation tester (mm)	Symptomatic	Manual	0 = 4 + 2, 1+ = 7 + 3, >2+ = 13 + 4	0 = 4 + 2, 1+ = 8 + 3, >2+ = 12 + 4	N/A	0 = 4 + 2, 1+ = 7 + 2, >2+ = 10 + 3
20° abduction, 10° flexing, 0° rotation	20° abduction, 10° flexing, 0° rotation	Bone-pinned shoulder translation tester (mm)	Symptomatic	Manual	5 + 3	5 + 4	N/A	4 + 2
20° abduction, 10° flexing, 0° rotation	20° abduction, 10° flexing, 0° rotation	Bone-pinned shoulder translation tester (mm)	Symptomatic	Manual	12 + 5	9 + 5	N/A	7 + 3
20° abduction, 10° flexing, 0° rotation	20° abduction, 10° flexing, 0° rotation	Bone-pinned shoulder translation tester (mm)	Symptomatic	Manual	14 + 5	12 + 6	N/A	9 + 4

(*Continued*)

TABLE 5–3 *(Continued)*

Study	N	Population	Pathology	Age (Years)	Gender	Consciousness	Tests Performed	Body Position
Tibone et al (2003)[67]	27	Soccer players	Nonimpaired	18.8 (17–24)	Female	Awake	Manual AP drawer	Supine
	16	Swimmers	Nonimpaired	18.8 (17–24)	Female	Awake	Manual AP drawer	Supine
Sauers et al (2001)[69]	30	Cadaver specimens	Nonimpaired	70 + 14	Mixed	N/A	Instrumented load and shift and sulcus	Scapula rigidly fixed
Manzour et al (2001)[157]	20	Cadaver specimens	Nonimpaired	71 + 14	Mixed	N/A	Instrumented load and shift and sulcus	Scapula rigidly fixed
							Manual load and shift and sulcus	
							Manual load and shift and sulcus	
Reis et al (2003)[66]	7	Cadaver specimens	N/A	N/A	N/A	N/A	Manual a/P drawer	Rigidly fixed
Borsa et al (2004)[158]	33	Professional baseball pitchers	Nonimpaired	25 + 3	Male	Awake	Instrumented AP drawer	Sitting
Scibek et al (2002)[159]	29	13 collegiate swimmers, 16 nonswimmers	Nonimpaired	19.3 and 20.5	Females	Awake	Instrumented AP drawer	Sitting
Krarup et al (1999)[160]	20	Patients	Traumatic Anterior Instability	28 (18–57)	13 males, 7 females	Awake	Instrumented anterior drawer	Sitting
	20	Patients	Nonimpaired	34 (22–53)	10 males, 10 females	Awake	Instrumented anterior drawer	Sitting
Ellenbecker et al (2000)[161]	20	Professional baseball pitchers	Nonimpaired	21.25 + 2.31	Males	Awake	Instrumented anterior drawer	Sitting
							Instrumented anterior drawer	Sitting
							Manual anterior drawer	Supine
Pizzari et al (1999)[162]	12	Volunteers physiotherapy students	Nonimpaired	22 (19–34)	Male	Awake	Instrumented AP drawer	Prone
	16	Volunteers physiotherapy students	Nonimpaired		Female	Awake	Instrumented AP drawer	Prone

AP arm Position	Inferior arm Position	Measurement Technique	Side	Force Applied	Anterior	Posterior	AP Laxity	Inferior
90° abduction/ neutral rotation	N/A	Surface electromagnetic tracking system (mm)	Dominant Nondominant	Manual Manual	N/A N/A	N/A N/A	9.6 (5.8 − 15.1) 10.7 (5.2 − 16.7)	N/A N/A
90° abduction/ neutral rotation	N/A	Surface electromagnetic tracking system (mm)	Dominant Nondominant	Manual Manual	N/A N/A	N/A N/A	12.4 (8.9 − 15.9) 13.8 (8.8 − 17.4)	N/A N/A
20° abduction in scapular plane/0° rotation	Dependent, neutral rotation	Surface electromagnetic tracking system (mm)	Mixed	200 N	10.4 + 4.0	9.9 + 5.0	N/A	15.0 + 5.6
		Surface electromagnetic tracking system (mm)	Mixed	Manual	13.1 + 5.6	8.5 + 4.7	N/A	17.6 + 4.7
		Bone-pinned electromagnetic tracking system (mm)	Mixed	Manual	11.1 + 4.4	7.5 + 4.1	N/A	12.8 + 4.3
0° flexing/40° abduction	N/A	Surface electromagnetic tracking system (mm)	NR	Manual	9.8 + 4.0	9.7 + 5.1	N/A	N/A
	N/A	Bone-pinned electromagnetic tracking system (mm)	NR	Manual	10.1 + 3.8	11.5 + 5.1	N/A	N/A
80–120° abduction/ 20–30° flexing	N/A	Modified Hawkins (I or II)	Both	Manual	N/A	I = 49%, II = 51%	N/A	N/A
N/A	Dependent, neutral rotation	I ≤ 1 cm, II = 1–1.5 cm, III ≥ 1.5 cm	Both	Manual	N/A	N/A	N/A	I = 46%, II = 51%, III = 3%
90° abduction/ 60° external rotation	N/A	Ultrasound sonographic imaging (mm)	Dominant Nondominant	10 daN 10 daN	2.39 2.45	4.87 4.91	7.25 7.35	N/A N/A
90° abduction/ 0° rotation	N/A	Ultrasound sonographic imaging (mm)	Both	100 N	1.9 + 2.4	5.2 + 4.1	N/A	N/A
Internally rotated and fixed to body	N/A	Ultrasound sonographic imaging (mm)	Unstable Stable	90 N 90 N	4.9 + 0.6 2.1 + 0.2	N/A N/A	N/A N/A	N/A N/A
Internally rotated and fixed to body	N/A		Both	90 N	1.8 + 0.1	N/A	N/A	N/A
90° abduction/ 60° external rotation	N/A	Millimeters using stress radiography	Dominant Non-Dominant	15 daN 15 daN	1.40 + 2.14 2.07 + 2.10	N/A N/A	N/A N/A	N/A N/A
90° abduction	N/A	0 – 3+ (Altcheck et al., 1989)	Dominant Nondominant	Manual Manual	2.75 + 0.9 2.35 + 0.9	N/A N/A	N/A N/A	N/A N/A
N/A	NR	0 = 0 mm, 1+ = <5 mm, 2+ = 5–10 mm, 3+ = >1 mm	Dominant Nondominant	Manual Manual	N/A N/A	N/A N/A	N/A N/A	1.56 1.47
90° abduction/ 0° rotation	N/A	KT-1000 knee ligament arthrometer (mm)	Dominant Nondominant	67 N 67 N	N/A N/A	N/A N/A	17.1 + 3.7 18.3 + 3.7	N/A N/A
90° abduction/ 0° rotation	N/A	KT-1000 knee ligament arthrometer (mm)	Dominant Nondominant	67 N 67 N	N/A N/A	N/A N/A	22.6 + 4.6 23.8 + 4.2	N/A N/A

(Continued)

TABLE 5–3 *(Continued)*

Study	N	Population	Pathology	Age (Years)	Gender	Consciousness	Tests Performed	Body Position
Jorgensen & Bak (1995)[71]	10	Patients	Nonimpaired	25 (15–40)	5 females, 5 males	Awake	Instrumented AP drawer	Sitting
	10	Patients	Traumatic anterior instability	30 (18–49)	3 females, 7 males	Awake	Instrumented AP drawer	Sitting
	10	Overhead athletes	Pain and sensation of instability	23 (16–45)	5 females, 5 males	Awake	Instrumented AP drawer	Sitting
	10	Patients	Atraumatic MDI	24 (18–45)	9 females, 1 male	Awake	Instrumented AP drawer	Sitting
McFarland et al (1996)[77]	178	High school and college athletes	Nonimpaired	16 (13–20)	123 male	Awake	Manual posterior drawer	Supine
							Sulcus	Sitting
					55 female	Awake	Manual posterior drawer	Supine
							Sulcus	Sitting
Lintner et al. (1996)[93]	76	Division I college athletes	NR	19	32 males, 44 females	Awake	Manual AP drawer and sulcus	Supine
Warner et al. (1990)[163]	14	Orthopedic residents and PTs	Nonimpaired	27 (20–41)	Mixed	Awake	Manual AP drawer and sulcus	Supine
	10	Sports medicine clinic patients	Impingement	31 (17–47)	Mixed	Awake	Manual AP drawer and sulcus	Supine
	28	Sports medicine clinic patients	Instability	24 (16–43)	Mixed	Awake	Manual AP drawer and sulcus	Supine
Bigliani et al. (1997)[164]	72	Professional baseball pitchers	Nonimpaired	22.9 (18–28)	Male	Awake	Sulcus	NR
	76	Professional baseball position players	Nonimpaired	22.6 (16–28)	Male	Awake	Sulcus	NR
Crockett et al (2002)[165]	25	Professional baseball pitchers	Nonimpaired	18–35	Male	Awake	Manual AP drawer and sulcus	Supine
	25	Nonoverhead athlete controls	Nonimpaired	18–35	Male	Awake	Manual AP drawer and sulcus	Supine
Hawkins et al. (1996)[75]	18	Patients	Stable shoulders	30 (15–40)	11 males, 7 females	Anesthesia	Manual load and shift	Supine
	10	Patients	Recurrent anterior instability	25	6 males, 4 females			
	10	Patients	MDI	21	3 males, 7 Females			

N/A, not applicable; NR, not reported.

AP arm Position	Inferior arm Position	Measurement Technique	Side	Force Applied	Anterior	Posterior	AP Laxity	Inferior
0° abduction/ 0° rotation	N/A	Donjoy knee laxity tester (mm)	Left Right	89 N 89 N	N/A N/A	N/A N/A	2.1 + 1.7 2.1 + 1.7	N/A N/A
0° abduction/ 0° rotation	N/A	Donjoy knee laxity tester (mm)	Left Right	89 N 89 N	N/A N/A	N/A N/A	6.4 + 3.6 2.8 + 2.9	N/A N/A
0° abduction/ 0° rotation	N/A	Donjoy knee laxity tester (mm)	Left Right	89 N 89 N	N/A N/A	N/A N/A	5.8 + 2.6 3.2 + 2.0	N/A N/A
0° abduction/ 0° rotation	N/A	Donjoy knee laxity tester (mm)	Left Right	89 N 89 N	N/A N/A	N/A N/A	11.9 + 6.3 11.0 + 6.4	N/A N/A
80–120° abduction/ 20–30° flexing	N/A	Modified Hawkins (I or II)	Both	Manual	N/A	I = 35%, II = 65%	N/A	N/A
N/A	Dependent, neutral rotation	I ≤ 1 cm, II = 1–1.5 cm, III ≥ 1.5 cm	Both	Manual	N/A	N/A	N/A	I = 36%, II = 55%, III = 9%
80–90° abduction/ 10–20° flexing	Dependent, neutral rotation	0–3 + (Altcheck et al, 1989)	Both	Manual	0 = 30%, 1+ = 49%, 2+ = 21%	0 = 9%, 1+ = 37%, 2+ = 54%	N/A	0 = 25%, 1+ = 69%, 2+ = 6%
80–120° abduction/ 0–20° flexing	Dependent, neutral rotation	0–3 + (Altcheck et al, 1989)	Both	Manual	<0.5	0.5	N/A	<1+
80–120° abduction/ 0–20° flexing	Dependent, neutral rotation	0–3 + (Altcheck et al, 1989)	Symptomatic	Manual	<0.5	<0.5	N/A	<0.5
80–120° abduction/ 0–20° flexing	"Dependent, neutral rotation"	0–3 + (Altcheck et al, 1989)	Symptomatic	Manual	1.5–2+	1.5	N/A	1.5
90° abduction/ 0° rotation	N/A	Millimeters using stress radiography	Dominant	15 daN	2.08 + 2.97	N/A	N/A	N/A
			Nondominant	15 daN	2.23 + 2.41	N/A	N/A	N/A
N/A	NR	0 = 0 mm, 1+ ≤ 5 mm, 2+ = 5–10 mm, 3+ ≥ 1 mm	Dominant Nondominant	Manual Manual	N/A N/A	N/A N/A	N/A N/A	1.37 1.36
NR	NR	I = 25% head diameter, II = 50%, III ≥ 50%	Dominant Nondominant	Manual Manual	1.36 1.24	1.92 1.8	N/A N/A	1.08 0.96
NR	NR	I = 25% head diameter, II = 50%, III ≥ 50%	Dominant Nondominant	Manual Manual	1.28 1.2	1.84 1.76	N/A N/A	1.12 1.08
NR	NR	I = 25% head diameter, II = 50%, III ≥ 50%	Dominant Nondominant	Manual Manual	1.28 1.2	1.84 1.76	N/A N/A	1.12 1.08
20° abduction/ 20° flexing/ 0° rotation	20° abduction/ 20° flexing/ 0° rotation	Radiographs w/concentric rings = % head diameter	NR	Manual	17%	26%	N/A	29%
			Unstable	Manual	29%	21%	N/A	49%
			Unstable	Manual	28%	52%	N/A	46%

when determining what is normal and what is abnormal movement of the humeral head on the glenoid. The variation in results can be explained by the variability in the experimental methods of each study.

Several studies have examined shoulder laxity in cadavers. Sauers et al[68] found that, using a 200-N force in a cadaver model, the humeral head translation on the glenoid was anteriorly 11.8 mm ± 5.7 mm, posteriorly 8.6 mm ± 4.8 mm, and inferiorly 20.2 ± 7.7 mm. Reis et al[66] measured in cadavers shoulder joint translations using electromagnetic three-dimensional goniometers and compared the results with translations measured using skin sensors. They did not report the amount of force used during the translations. They found an average anterior translation of 9.8 mm, with a range of 3.7 to 14.7 mm, and an average posterior translation of 9.6 mm, with a range of 3.7 to 17.2 mm.

Clinical studies of the laxity of the shoulder joint in living human subjects (as opposed to cadaveric studies) have been performed by several researchers. Harryman et al[64] studied shoulder laxity by placing pins into the humerus and scapula of volunteers. They then moved the bones of the subjects manually with the subjects in seated and in supine positions, but they did not quantitate the amount of force used to create the translations. It is noteworthy that there was a wide range of laxities in all three directions of translation.

Two studies have evaluated the relationship of translations obtained upon physical examination to true translations of the bones as determined by rigid pin fixation into the bones. Reis et al[66] studied cadavers with sensors attached to pins placed into the glenoid and the scapula, and they compared the translations with the results using sensors placed on the skin of the same specimens (**Table 5–4**). They found the cutaneous sensors had a strong agreement with the bone sensors for anterior and posterior translations (interclass correlation coefficients of 0.81 and 0.86, respectively). They did not quantitate the amount of force used to create translations, and the

translations were performed with the specimens upright and supine.

Sauers et al[69] performed a similar study using an instrumented laxity device that applied a 200 N load to the proximal humerus of cadavers. The translations were measured with skin sensors and with electrogoniometric devices attached by pins inserted into the bones. Sauers et al found minimal differences between the skin sensor measures and those obtained by the electromagnetic sensors. Correlation coefficients were found to be good for laxity in all directions (anterior = .71, $p < .001$; posterior = .69, $p < .001$; inferior = .68, $p < .001$). Minimal differences were observed between the cutaneous and bone-pinned measurement techniques for laxity. The authors concluded that the cutaneously applied sensors are accurate for determining shoulder laxities and stiffness of the joint.

Other studies have been done in living subjects to measure shoulder translations in millimeters. Tibone et al[67] used skin sensors to study the shoulder joint translations of 43 female athletes who were either soccer players or swimmers. The subjects were tested supine, and the arm was held in a device that supported it in 90 degrees of elevation and neutral rotation. The translations were performed manually by the examiners; there was no control of the force used to move the arm on the scapula. The mean age of the athletes was 18.8 years, and both dominant and nondominant arms were tested.

The results were reported as total anteroposterior translations and not as anterior or posterior translations (**Table 5–5**). Sauers et al found that total anteroposterior translations in the swimmers' dominant shoulders (average 12.4 mm, range 8.9–15.9 mm) and nondominant shoulders (average 13.8 mm, range 8.8–17.4 mm) were statistically larger than in the dominant (average 9.6, range 5.8–15.1 mm) and nondominant (10.7 mm, range 5.2–16.7 mm) shoulders of the soccer players. The side-to-side difference for the swimmers was 0.1 to 5.3 mm and for the soccer players, 0.1 to 4.3 mm.

Sauers et al[68] used an instrumented device with a force transducer to produce translations in the shoulders of seated volunteers. They concluded that the amount of

TABLE 5–4 Translation Measurements for Seven Cadavaric Specimens

Specimen	Anterior Translation (mm)		Posterior Translation (mm)	
	Cutaneous	Rigid	Cutaneous	Rigid
1	14.67 (1.78)	14.57 (1.67)	15.28 (2.78)	13.80 (0.66)
2	13.31 (2.21)	11.34 (2.27)	17.24 (0.89)	19.95 (0.96)
3	6.76 (2.46)	4.67 (2.23)	7.81 (1.68)	10.20 (3.04)
4	12.63 (0.23)	9.63 (0.74)	4.78 (2.35)	2.92 (1.34)
5	3.72 (1.01)	6.62 (1.60)	3.76 (1.18)	10.24 (0.63)
6	7.09 (0.69)	9.05 (1.46)	7.72 (0.90)	11.01 (0.90)
7	10.62 (1.69)	14.58 (1.00)	10.96 (1.23)	12.10 (1.10)

Source: Adapted with permission from Reis MT, Tibone JE, McMahon PJ, et al. Cadaveric study of glenohumeral translation using electromagnetic sensors. Clin Orthop 2002;400:88–92.

TABLE 5–5 Total Glenohumeral Anteroposterior Translation

Subjects	Shoulder	Mean (mm)	Range (mm)
Swimmers (n = 16)	Dominant	12.4	8.9–15.9
	Nondominant	13.8	8.8–17.4
Soccer players (n = 27)	Dominant	9.6	5.8–15.1
	Nondominant	10.7	5.2–16.7

Source: Adapted with permission from Tibone,J, Lee TQ, Csintalan RP, et al. Quantitative assessment of glenohumeral translation. Clin Orthop 2002;400:93–97.

TABLE 5-6 Glenohumeral Instability According to Radiologic Findings

	Arm Position	Radiographic View	Examination Method	Criteria for Instability	
				Anterior	Posterior
Norris[74]	Abduction 90°, flexion, IR	Axillary	Manual displacement	Any displacement	Displacement >50%
Maki[70]	Abduction, NF, NR	Axillary	Manual displacement	Displacement >25%	Displacement >50%
Papilion and Shall[72]	Abduction 90°, NF, NR	Axillary	Manual displacement	Displacement >14%	Displacement >37%

IR, internal rotation; NF, neutral flexion; NR, neutral rotation.

translation depended on how much force was applied to the shoulder. They also found that posterior laxity was found greater than anterior laxity, and that a wide spectrum of laxity was found in the shoulders of asymptomatic volunteers.

Other studies attempted to measure the head translation using radiographic techniques (**Table 5-6**).[70-74] These studies vary according to the position of the arm tested, the type of radiographs taken, how the landmarks on the bones were measured, and how much force was used in the translations. The methodology used for measuring the radiographs influenced the results, so there is not a consistent measurement between studies.

■ Quantitative Measures of Laxity from the Clinical Examination

In these biomechanical studies, laxity was measured accurately in millimeters, but the best way to measure laxity in the office or operating room remains controversial. There have been three different systems for measuring shoulder laxity in clinical practice.

Translation of the Humeral Head in Millimeters

The first system for measuring how much the humeral head moves on the socket is in millimeters; this system was recommended by Hawkins et al [75] (**Fig. 5-14**). They recommended that the classification of humeral head translation be expressed in millimeters of translation over the glenoid face. In this schema, grade 0 equals no translation, grade I equals mild translation (<1 cm), grade II equals moderate translation (1-2 cm, or to the rim), and grade III equals severe translation (>2 cm, or over the rim).

Using millimeters to estimate shoulder laxity for anterior and posterior translations, to our knowledge, has never been validated as accurate. Similarly, no study has evaluated the inter- or intraobserver reproducibility of using millimeters as a measure for anterior or posterior laxity. As a result, we do not recommend this type of estimation of shoulder laxity in clinical practice.

The millimeter system has been used frequently for quantitating inferior translation of the humeral head with the sulcus sign. Commonly reported grading systems for inferior laxity using this sign include grade I (0.5-1 cm of translation), grade II (1-2.0 cm), and grade III (> 2.0 cm).[76] However, there are some studies where the sulcus sign is graded as I (0.5-1.0 cm), II (1.0-1.5 cm), and III (> 1.5 cm).[77,78] Hawkins et al[75] recommended a classification of inferior translation with sulcus testing: grade 0 (no translation), grade I (mild translation, 0-1 cm), grade II (moderate translation, 1-2 cm), and grade III (severe translation, > 2 cm).[76,79,80]

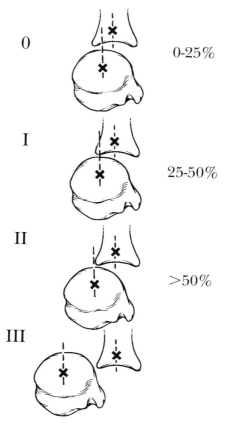

0   0-25%

I   25-50%

II   >50%

III

FIGURE 5-14 The Hawkins classification of humeral head translation suggests that the magnitude of translation can be reported by the examiner in millimeters.

None of these systems for measuring the sulcus sign has been validated using accurate methods of measuring translation, such as electrogoniometers with pins placed in bones. It should be noted that in Harryman et al's study,[64] the inferior excursion of the humeral head inferiorly was 11 mm ± 4 mm, with a range of 5 to 15 mm. They examined only normal male subjects between the ages of 25 and 45 years, so it is unclear what translations are possible in females or in subjects with instability. The only study to demonstrate inferior translations that approach 20 mm was conducted by Sauers et al[69] upon cadavers. As a result, it is likely that most grade III sulcus signs that are measured in clinical practice are actually under 2 cm of translation.

There have been only two published studies that have evaluated the intraobserver reproducibility of the grading system of sulcus signs.[78,81] In a study by Levy et al,[81] four examiners evaluated 43 athletes for a sulcus sign, then repeated the test 3 months later. The examiners included physicians with different degrees of experience, including a resident, two orthopedic sports medicine fellows, and a sports medicine attending physician. The patients were examined supine. The researchers found that the intraexaminer reproducibility for a sulcus sign was 93% for the senior surgeon (kappa > 0.5), for the fellows 91% (kappa > 0.5), 74% (kappa = 0.5), and 86% for the resident (kappa > 0.5). They found that the interobserver agreement between the attending physician and the fellows was 43% and 39%, and 64% for the resident. When they combined grades 0 and 1, there was improvement of the reproducibility to 85%, but the kappa value remained low at > 0.5. Although the reproducibility appeared to be high within one examiner, the sulcus sign was not agreed upon by different examiners.

> The sulcus sign is a measure of laxity and not instability, and it should not be graded but reported as positive or negative.

We performed a study[78] of interobserver agreement for the sulcus sign using sports medicine fellows and an attending physician who examined 88 shoulders of patients who were under anesthesia. All the fellows had been in the fellowship for 6 months before participating in the study in order to gain experience and familiarity with the grading system. The examinations were performed blinded, so that one observer did not know the results of the other examiner. There was agreement on the degree of sulcus sign 70% (range 61–87%) of the time between the fellows and the attending surgeon (kappa 0.38, range 0.12–0.76). The most agreement between the fellows and the senior surgeon was when the sulcus was grade I (80% agreement) rather than grade II

(65% agreement) or grade III (zero agreement). This study used the results of the attending physician as the gold standard because it was not possible to validate the exact amount of excursion in terms of millimeters. This study suggests that different examiners tend to disagree on inferior laxity as the amount of the laxity increases.

Only one study[80] has evaluated the usefulness of the sulcus sign in patients with shoulder instability. Tzannes and Murrell[80] reported on the sensitivity, specificity, and likelihood ratios (see appendix) of the sulcus sign for an unspecified group of patients with multidirectional shoulder instability (MDI). It should be noted that they did not define MDI in this study. They reported that a sulcus sign of under 1 cm had a sensitivity of 72% and a specificity of 85% for instability, but when the sulcus sign was over 2 cm, sensitivity went down to 28%, and specificity was 97%. These data demonstrated that using a strict criterion of 2 cm as a sign of inferior instability results in 72% of patients with MDI not being diagnosed with that condition. The authors did not validate the measures with radiographs or other techniques.

Translation of the Humeral Head in Percent Head Diameters

The second way to measure the amount of translation of the humeral head is to report the movement in terms of percent of the total head diameter.[82,83] In this classification scheme, the humeral head is said to move to the rim (grade I), over the rim less than 50% of the diameter, or over the rim 50% of the head diameter. It has been suggested by some researchers that 25% is a subluxation and 50% a dislocation.[84]

There are several difficulties with this method of gauging translation of the humeral head. First, there has been no study that validates this method of measurement and that proves that the grades actually correspond to certain percentages of head diameter. Second, humeral head diameters vary widely, and the examiner cannot really estimate the head diameter exactly. Third, Harryman et al[64] tried to validate the use of humeral head diameters as a measure of laxity. In their study of normal volunteers, they translated the shoulder and calculated the percent of humeral head translation by using normative data for humeral head diameters obtained from the literature. They found in their normal male subjects that the excursion anteriorly would have been only 35% of the humeral head and posteriorly only 35 to 39% of the humeral head. Inferior translation would have been 44% of the diameter of the humeral head on average. Harryman et al concluded that this form of measurement of translation was problematic and that the accuracy of this grading system using percent of humeral head diameters was questionable.

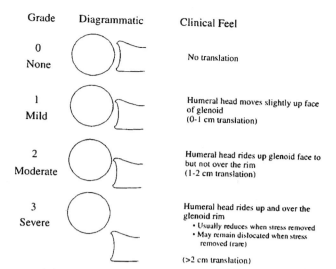

FIGURE 5–15 The Hawkins classification of instability is based upon what is felt by the examiner. (Adapted with permission from Matsen FI, Lippitt S, Sidles J, Harryman DI. Practical Evaluation and Management of the Shoulder. Philadelphia: WB Saunders; 1994.)

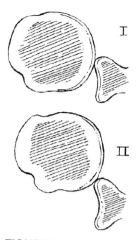

FIGURE 5–16 Studies have shown that combining translations 0 and 1 of the Hawkins classification increases the accuracy of the system. In a modified Hawkins scale, the examiner reports the translation as 1 (not over the rim), 2 (over the rim), or 3 (locks out). (Adapted with permission from McFarland EG, Campbell G, McDowell J. Posterior shoulder laxity in asymptomatic athletes. Am J Sports Med 1996;24(4):468–471.)

Translation of the Humeral Head Based on What is Felt

The third method of measuring translation of the humeral head is to describe what is felt by the examiner and not to rely on exact measures in millimeters or percentages. This classification was first described by Hawkins and Krisman[85,86] and included four grades: 0 = normal translation, I = translation of the head to the rim, II = translation of the head over the rim, and III = locks out, where the humeral head stays out of the joint when the hands are removed (**Fig. 5–15**). This method of measuring translation was adopted by the American Shoulder and Elbow Society in 1994.[87]

A similar classification was suggested by Altcheck et al,[88] but it included a comparison of the shoulder translation to the opposite shoulder. In their system, a grade I laxity indicated that there was increased translation compared with the other shoulder, but there was no subluxation or dislocation upon examination. Grades II and III laxity were the same as those reported by Hawkins and Krisman.[85,86] This classification was encumbered by the need to accurately examine both shoulders, which is not always possible. This system also assumes that symmetry is normal, but subsequent studies have demonstrated that asymmetry of translation is frequently normal.[77]

We modified the Hawkins classification to discard the grade 0 designation because "normal" translation upon physical examination was not something that could be felt or quantitated by the observer. Upon examination the examiner either will feel the head go over the rim

(grade II laxity) or will not (grade I) (**Fig. 5–16**). This modified Hawkins scale includes grade III as "locks out."

The validity of these classification systems has not been determined by biomechanical studies. None of the previously published studies using this measurement have demonstrated exactly how much translation is needed to subluxate the shoulder over the rim. Also, in some patients a click is felt when attempting to subluxate the shoulder, and it is sometimes difficult to know if that click is a subluxation or some other phenomenon, such as the labrum clicking. The intraobserver reproducibility of the Hawkins system, however, has been examined by McFarland et al[24,78] and Levy et al.[81] In the study by McFarland et al, one examiner evaluated 40 shoulders in 20 volunteers 4 weeks apart. The shoulder was evaluated using an anterior and posterior drawer as described by Gerber and Ganz.[89] In this study we used the modified Hawkins scale, where there was no grade 0 but only grades I, II, and III. Twelve shoulders were eliminated when the subjects could not relax, so only 28 shoulders were included in the study. For anterior translation the reproducibility for one examiner was 100%, and for posterior translation it was 86%. It is possible that these numbers were so high because the examiner was an experienced shoulder surgeon with a consistent technique of making the measurement.

The second study to evaluate the intraobserver reproducibility of the Hawkins scale for anterior and posterior translations was performed by Levy et al[81] on athletes at Duke University. The five examiners in this study included an attending orthopedic surgeon, two sports medicine fellows, and a resident who examined 43 athletes

2 months apart. They found that intraobserver reproducibility was only 46% (kappa < 0.5) for all examiners (range 44–50%). If grade 0 laxity was included with grade I laxity (modified Hawkins scale), then the intraobserver agreement increased to 73% (range 67–73%).

The interobserver reliability of this measure has been studied by the same groups. In the study by McFarland et al,[24,78] a modified Hawkins scale was used, and the patients were all examined under anesthesia using an anterior and posterior drawer test as described by Gerber and Ganz.[89] The four fellows agreed with the attending physician for anterior translations 69 to 89% of the time (kappa 0.41–0.73). For posterior translations, the fellows agreed with the attending physician 57 to 87% of the time (kappa 0.12–0.76). These kappa values are in the fair to poor range for interobserver agreement.

In their study, Levy et al[81] found that overall interobserver agreement was 47% if the original rating scale of Hawkins and Bokor[83] was utilized. For anterior translations, if grades 0 and 1 were equalized (a modified Hawkins scale), the overall interobserver agreement increased to 73%. Once the modified Hawkins scale was used, the fellows agreed with the attending physician 68 and 75% of the time for posterior translation, and the agreement between the attending physician and both fellows was 67% of all shoulders tested.

These studies suggest that this grading scale can be used to measure translations such that they can be communicated between observers, but these studies also suggest that comparing studies may still be difficult due to interobserver variability. It is our belief that this system has the most utility for clinical practice, but an instrumented device holds the most promise for the future.

> A modified Hawkins scale is the most valid and reproducible method for reporting laxity of the shoulder in an anterior and posterior direction.

■ Examination Techniques for Measuring Anteroposterior Laxity

Anterior and Posterior Drawer

The anterior and posterior drawer signs for measuring laxity were described by Gerber and Ganz[89] in 1984. This examination is performed with the patient supine and the examiner to the side. The subject must be relaxed, and it is recommended that the subject be placed so that the shoulder is not supported by the table. Gerber and Ganz recommended abducting the shoulder between 80 and 120 degrees.

The posterior drawer is performed by holding the patient's wrist with one hand and placing the other hand

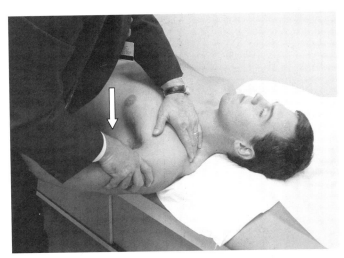

FIGURE 5–17 The posterior drawer test described by Gerber is performed with one hand stabilizing the scapula.

over the patient's shoulder so that the thumb is in the front and the fingers in the back (**Fig. 5–17**). Gerber and Ganz recommended holding the forearm with the elbow flexed, but we prefer to hold the arm at the wrist because the arm is easier to control (**Fig. 5–18**). The thumb should be placed directly over the humeral head and a posteriorly directed force applied on the humeral head. It is essential that the arm be forward flexed at the same time a posterior force is applied to allow the head to sublux posteriorly out the back of the shoulder. The fingers in the back can be used to palpate the head as it goes out the back. Pressure is then relieved from the thumb anteriorly so that there is no longer any force from the examiner keeping the shoulder subluxated out the back of the shoulder. It is then determined by the examiner if the head stays subluxated out the back of the shoulder joint with no force. If the

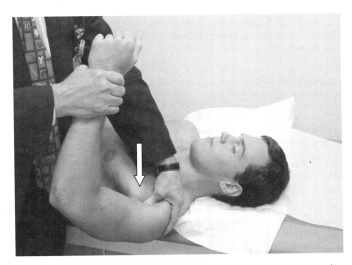

FIGURE 5–18 Posterior laxity testing of the shoulder can be performed without stabilizing the scapula.

humeral head stays subluxated out the back (i.e., "locked out"), then it is considered a grade III laxity. The head typically subluxes back into the joint on its own as the arm is extended, and the examiner can use the fingers posteriorly to feel the reduction (i.e., a grade II laxity).

We typically ask patients if the subluxation reproduces any of their symptoms. Crepitus with this maneuver is nonspecific and does not indicate either a labral tear or instability. It should be noted that in our studies of the posterior drawer that we perform the maneuver with the arm elevated ~45 to 60 degrees where the posterior capsule is the most lax.[26] This position is also called the zero "unpacked" position because it is the point at which the joint has the most mobility[90]. This discrepancy in arm position between our studies and studies using Gerber and Ganz's technique may explain the higher laxity grades reported in our studies compared with others.

> More translation of the humerus on the scapula can be obtained with the arm abducted less than 90 degrees when performing laxity testing.

The anterior drawer is more difficult because the examiner has to control scapular rotation on the thorax. The arm is abducted 80 to 120 degrees, flexed 0 to 20 degrees, and held in 0 to 30 degrees of external rotation. Gerber and Ganz[89] recommended that one hand stabilize the scapula, while the second hand holds the arm at the proximal humerus area (**Fig. 5–19**). The hand stabilizing the scapula holds the thumb on the coracoid and the fingers tightly on the scapular spine like a clamp. An anterior force is then directed on the humerus to create anterior translation.

We have modified the anterior drawer test to control rotation of the scapula (**Fig. 5–20**). The hands changed from the position used in the posterior drawer so that now

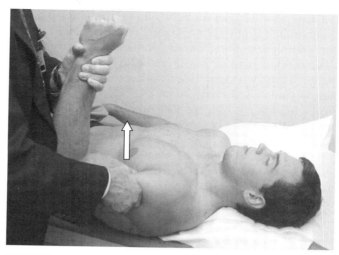

FIGURE 5–20 The anterior drawer test may obtain more excursion using the modified anterior drawer technique shown.

one hand is on the wrist and one hand is on the proximal arm of the extremity. The arm is abducted ~40 degrees and slightly internally rotated, and a slight axial load is applied to prevent the scapula from rotating. This axial load also improves the ability to feel the humeral head subluxate over the glenoid rim. The examiner then applies an anterior force and rolls the humeral head onto the chest in one motion. It is important to try to translate the whole arm and not just the humeral head, because simply pushing the head anteriorly will tighten the anterior structures and prevent subluxation. Once the head is subluxed, pressure is relieved to see if the head remains out of the socket (grade III). If the humeral head subluxes back once pressure is released, then it is a grade II translation.

> Applying a slight axial load to the humerus into the socket with an anterior drawer test makes it easier to feel the humeral head translate over the glenoid rim with laxity testing.

We are in agreement with Gerber and Ganz[89] and Emery and Mullaji,[91] who feel that shoulder laxity and translations can be appreciated better with the patient supine versus sitting. The subject is more apt to relax his or her muscles when supine than when sitting. Also, the position of the shoulder where there is the most laxity in the capsule is with the arm abducted around 45 degrees; this position is difficult to obtain with the patient sitting.

When performing the posterior drawer, if the patient has pain due to the hand placement on the proximal humerus, we recommend a modification whereby the proximal humerus is not grasped rigidly by the examiner. Instead, the arm can be held more distally, or the palm of the examining hand can be used to create a posterior force.

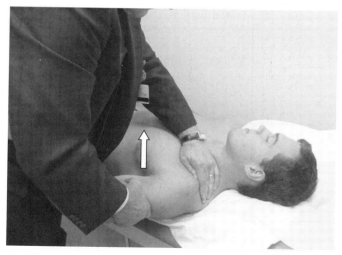

FIGURE 5–19 The anterior drawer test as described by Gerber is performed with one hand stabilizing the scapula.

The validity of this grading system of translation has not been studied, but its reproducibility and reliability have been studied and are discussed above. Several studies using this test have demonstrated that the normal shoulder typically has a grade II laxity where the humeral head can be subluxated over the rim.[24,78,92] In our study[77] of high school and collegiate athletes who never had shoulder problems, 65% of the women and 50% of the men could be subluxated over the posterior rim with this test (i.e., were a type II laxity). This emphasized that it actually is more common in that age group to have a positive posterior drawer than it is to not have one. That is, a positive posterior drawer as we perform it suggests that the ability to subluxate the shoulder over the rim is normal.

> It is normal to be able to subluxate the shoulder over the rim posteriorly in young athletic populations.

Several studies using the anterior and posterior drawer signs have demonstrated that asymmetry of shoulder laxities between the dominant and nondominant extremity is common. In our study of 178 athletes using a posterior drawer sign, we found that 10 percent had asymmetric laxities, and only in half of the subjects was the increased laxity in the dominant extremity.[77] Lintner et al[93] studied 76 collegiate athletes and found that 24 had asymmetry (31%). In 19 (79%) of the athletes, the asymmetry was due to increased laxity in the dominant extremity.

> Asymmetry of laxity of the shoulders of one patient is common and cannot be used alone as a criterion for diagnosing instability.

The results of this test can change when the patient is under anesthesia compared with when he or she is awake. The elimination of muscle forces and a totally relaxed patient without pain tend to make laxity measures increase when the patient is under anesthesia. There have been two studies that have evaluated this issue, and both demonstrate that laxity is increased by approximately one half of a grade on average in patients with traumatic, anterior instability.[94,95] However, the examiners were not blinded to the diagnosis, and they admit that, although an increase of one half of a grade of laxity may be statistically significant, it may not be clinically significant.

We conducted a study (unpublished data) of our patients who were examined under anesthesia prior to their surgical procedure. Each patient underwent an anterior and posterior drawer as described above. There was only one examiner (EGM) who performed the examination, but that examiner was not blinded to the diagnosis. Using a modified Hawkins scale, the laxities for each diagnostic group were tabulated. The results are reported in **Table 5–7**. The ability to subluxate the shoulder over the rim had a high prevalence among all groups, and laxity was seen to decrease with increasing age (**Table 5–8**).

The other important observation was that grade III laxity (where the shoulder locks out) was very uncommon, even with patients under anesthesia. Of 908 patients undergoing preoperative laxity examination by one physician (EGM) for various diagnoses, only 23 (2.5%) had grade III anterior laxity according to the modified Hawkins scale. Furthermore, only 15 patients (1.65%) had grade III posterior laxity, and 28 patients (3%) had grade III inferior laxity.

> Shoulder laxities will increase under anesthesia due to muscle relaxation, but it is uncommon for shoulders to lock out even under anesthesia.

TABLE 5–7 Preoperative Laxity under General Anesthesia in Different Patients Grouped by Diagnosis

Diagnosis	Anterior			Posterior			Inferior		
	I	II	III	I	II	III	I	II	III
Full RCT (N = 429)	97 (22.6%)	331 (77.2%)	1 (0.2%)	195 (45.5%)	232 (54.5%)	2 (0.5%)	353 (82.0%)	74 (17.5%)	2 (0.5%)
Partial RCT (N = 186)	46 (24.7%)	140 (75.3%)	0 (0%)	88 (47.3%)	98 (52.7%)	0 (0%)	145 (78%)	37 (20.0%)	4 (2.0%)
Impingement[†] (N = 186)	56 (30.1%)	130 (69.9%)	0 (0%)	90 (49.0%)	95 (51.5%)	1 (0.5%)	148 (79.5%)	36 (19.5)	2 (1.0%)
Anterior instability[‡] (N = 310)	12 (3.8%)	265 (85.7%)	33 (10.5%)	47 (15%)	262 (84.5%)	1 (0.5%)	167 (54.0%)	137 (44.0%)	9 (25.0%)
Posterior[§] instability (N = 12)	0 (0%)	12 (100%)	0 (0%)	0 (0%)	7 (58.0%)	5 (42.0%)	3 (25.0%)	9 (75.0%)	0 (0%)

Source: Data from The Johns Hopkins University Shoulder Database.

RCT, rotator cuff tear

[†]Impingement includes patients with subacromial impingement.

[‡]Anterior instability includes patients with traumatic anterior instability and occult instability.

[§]Posterior instability includes patients with traumatic and voluntary posterior instability.

TABLE 5–8 Glenohumeral Laxity by Age

Age by Decade	N	Anterior Translation n (%)			Posterior Translation n (%)			Sulcus Sign n (%)		
		Grade I	Grade II	Grade III	Grade I	Grade II	Grade III	Grade I	Grade II	Grade III
1–20	75	5 (7)	68 (91)	2 (3)	15 (20)	58 (77)	2 (3)	26 (35)	48 (64)	1 (1)
21–30	93	12 (13)	79 (85)	2 (2)	18 (19)	72 (77)	3 (3)	59 (63)	27 (29)	7 (8)
31–40	100	22 (22)	76 (76)	2 (2)	34 (34)	66 (66)	0	68 (68)	31 (31)	1 (1)
41–50	126	38 (30)	87 (69)	1 (1)	57 (45)	68 (54)	1 (1)	98 (78)	25 (20)	3 (2)
51–60	120	23 (19)	97 (81)	0	57 (48)	63 (53)	0	89 (74)	29 (24)	2 (2)
61–70	87	28 (32)	59 (68)	0	41 (47)	46 (53)	0	71 (82)	14 (16)	2 (2)
71	38	9 (24)	29 (76)	0	12 (32)	26 (68)	0	24 (63)	14 (37)	0
Total	639	134 (21)	495 (77)	7 (1)	234 (37)	399 (62)	6 (1)	435 (68)	188 (29)	16 (3)

*Source: Data from The Johns Hopkins University Shoulder Database.

Load and Shift Test

The second technique for measuring anteroposterior translation is the load and shift test, which was first described by Silliman and Hawkins[96] in 1993. In the original description, they recommended that this test be performed with the patient sitting or supine. When the patient is sitting, the examiner typically stands to the side of the subject (**Fig. 5–21**). The examiner stabilizes the scapula and shoulder by placing one hand over the top of the shoulder, and the scapula is stabilized as recommended by Gerber and Ganz[89] when performing the anterior or posterior drawer tests. The examiner places the second hand ion the proximal arm, and the arm is held in a position of 20 degrees of abduction, 20 degrees of flexion, and in neutral (or perhaps slight internal rotation).[75]

Silliman and Hawkins suggest that the shoulder be "loaded" to center the humeral head in the glenoid.[96,97] This is intended to make sure that the humeral head is concentrically reduced and to assist in the ability to feel the humeral head subluxation over the rim if it occurs. A force is then directed anteriorly by the hand on the humerus in an attempt to sublux the humeral head over

the rim. Next, the force is directed posteriorly in an attempt to subluxate the humeral head over the posterior rim.

Once this was completed, Silliman and Hawkins recommended that this examination be repeated with the patient supine.[96,97] When performing this examination with the patient supine, the arm is abducted 20 degrees and forward flexed in neutral rotation. One hand is used to grasp the proximal humerus, and the other stabilizes the arm. The authors note that this test can be painful when the proximal arm is grasped by the examiner.

The load and shift test has not been validated using biomechanical or other techniques. It is unknown exactly how much laxity is needed to feel the shoulder subluxate and under what conditions the shoulder will lock out. No biomechanical study has determined if this is the best position for testing shoulder laxity.

The only study evaluating the accuracy of this test was by Tzannes and Murrell,[80] who evaluated the sensitivity, specificity, and likelihood ratios for the load and shift test with the patient supine (**Table 5–9**). They performed the test with the arm abducted 20 degrees and also a second time with the arm abducted 90 degrees. Tzannes and Murrell supported the arm at the elbow with one hand and provided anterior and posterior forces to the proximal humerus with the other hand (**Fig. 5–22**). They also emphasized the importance of loading the humeral head first to feel the head subluxate over the glenoid rim.

Tzannes and Murrell found that the load and shift for anterior instability had as sensitivity of only 50%, but it had a specificity of 100%. The likelihood ratio (see appendix) if it was positive was over 100, which would indicate that in their cohort of unstable shoulders, the ratio would verify a diagnosis of anterior instability. If the test was negative, the likelihood ratio was less than 1, indicating that it was unlikely that the patient had anterior instability.

In their study a positive posterior load and shift test was sensitive for only 14% of patients with posterior instability, but it was 100% specific in their cohort.

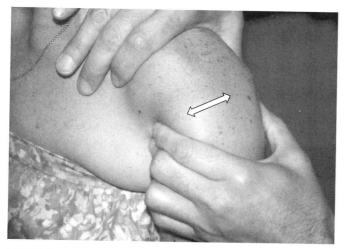

FIGURE 5–21 The load and shift test can be performed with the subject sitting (as shown) or with the subject supine.

TABLE 5-9 Validity of Clinical Tests for Shoulder Stability

Test Sensitivity	(%)	Specificity (%)	Likelihood Ratio (+)*	Likelihood Ratio (−)†
Load and shift				
Anterior	50	100	>100	0.5
Posterior	14	100	>100	0.9
Inferior	8	100	80	0.9
Sulcus sign‡				
>1 cm	72	85	5	0.3
>2 cm	28	97	9	0.7
Provocative tests				
Apprehension	NA	NA	NA	NA
Augmentation	68	100	>100	0.3
Relocation	50	100	>100	0.5
Release	92	89	8	0.1

Source: Adapted with permission from Tzannes A, Murrell GA. Clinical examination of the unstable shoulder. Sports Med 2002;32(7):447–457.
*Likelihood ratio expresses the odds that a positive test result would occur in a patient with, as opposed to a patient without, shoulder instability. A test is considered useful if a likelihood ratio is > 10.
†Likelihood ratio for a negative test result.
‡With respect to predicting multidirectional instability.
NA, not applicable.

Similarly, the likelihood ratio was over 100 if the test was positive, which means it is a helpful diagnostic test. If the posterior load and shift was negative, the likelihood ratio was less than 1, which indicates that the patient was unlikely to have posterior instability.

> Assuming the patient is relaxed for the examination, a patient with a negative anterior load and shift test is unlikely to have anterior instability, and a patient with a negative posterior load and shift is unlikely to have posterior instability.

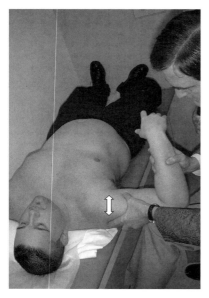

FIGURE 5-22 The load and shift test was modified by Tzannes and Murrell with the patient supine so that the subject's arm could rest on the examiner's thigh.

Our clinical experience with the load and shift test with the patient in the sitting position is different than that reported by Tzannes and Murrell. It is often difficult to stabilize the scapula with the patient sitting, and muscle relaxation is poor in our experience. With the patient supine, the load and shift has more clinical usefulness in our experience, but the ligaments of the shoulder tighten with increasing abduction. Thus increased excursions will be seen with the arm at lower degrees of elevation, such as that seen in an anterior and posterior drawer performed at 60 degrees of elevation. If the test is used to reproduce the patient's symptoms of subluxation, we feel that the subluxation can best be accomplished with the arm abducted around 50 to 60 degrees. However, we have not statistically studied this, and it may be that laxity at lower degrees of abduction does not predict the presence of instability.

Push–Pull Test

The push–pull test was described by Matsen et al[98] and was reported as a test to measure posterior laxity in the shoulder. The examiner stands at the side and places the patient's arm in 90 degrees of abduction and 30 degrees of forward flexion (**Fig. 5-23**). The examiner's other hand grasps the midhumerus and provides a posteriorly directed force. Matsen et al comment that the humerus should translate 50% of its humeral head width with this test.

Harryman et al[64] studied this test using an electromagnetic tracking device (Polhemus navigation sciences, Colchester) in volunteers and found that this test produced posterior translation 3 to 22 mm, with a mean of 9 mm. In 39% of the normal subjects, the humeral head could be felt to subluxate over the glenoid rim when the measurements were performed, but they did

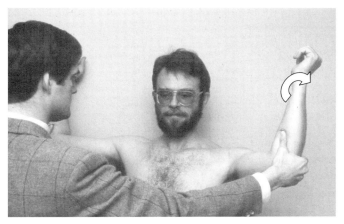

FIGURE 5–30 The anterior apprehension sign may be performed as part of the range of motion examination when testing for the degree of external rotation with the arm abducted 90 degrees.

arms abducted 90 degrees (**Fig. 5–30**). The patient is standing, and we hold both arms by the forearm. Both arms are abducted and externally rotated simultaneously, and the patient is asked to report when he or she feels pain or becomes apprehensive. This modification of the apprehension sign is helpful in the patient who has already had an apprehension test performed and who may understand what the test result is supposed to be.

When performing this test, our observation has been that apprehension does not occur at 90 degrees of elevation and 90 degrees of external rotation. In many patients there must be more abduction, more external rotation, and more arm extension (i.e., behind the plane of the body) for the test to be accurate. We also do not push anteriorly on the shoulder when performing this test because this causes pain, and it may prevent an accurate test again at a later date.

In a prospective study, (unpublished data) we considered the arm position where apprehension occurs in patients with instability prospectively. Our hypothesis was that when the test was performed without an anteriorly directed force, the position of apprehension would be greater than 90 degrees of elevation and external rotation in most patients. The degree of external rotation and abduction was measured for 18 patients who had positive apprehension test for traumatic anterior instability. Of these, 17 patients (95%) had the degree of abduction greater than 90 degrees, and 13 (72%) had external rotation greater than 90% before apprehension was felt. This suggests that some biomechanical studies that evaluate the arm in 90 degrees of abduction and 90 degrees of external rotation may not be testing the exact position where instability occurs.

Another way to perform the apprehension sign is with the patient supine.[100,3,96] The patient is brought to the

side of the table, but the scapula is supported. The arm is then externally rotated so that the table produced an anteriorly directed force on the shoulder. Lo et al[100] found that the mean external rotation before there was apprehension for patients with anterior instability was 83 degrees, for MDI 131 degrees, for posterior instability 100 degrees, and for patients with just rotator cuff tears 89 degrees.

These findings support our hypothesis that apprehension does not occur at the same position in most patients and that external rotation greater than 90 degrees may be needed to produce apprehension. Lo et al[100] found good interexaminer accuracy for the degrees of external rotation needed to produce apprehension when performing the apprehension sign supine, but they did not report the exact statistical values of the degree of agreement between examiners.

> When testing for anterior instability using the anterior drawer sign, the arm should be abducted and externally rotated as far as necessary to produce symptoms of apprehension.

There have been two studies evaluating the accuracy of the anterior apprehension sign for anterior instability. Speer et al[101] studied 100 patients with a variety of diagnoses and placed the arm in abduction of 90 degrees and external rotation of 90 degrees (**Table 5–10**). They recorded whether the patient had apprehension or pain in that position, then placed an anterior force on the shoulder and recorded whether the patient became apprehensive or had pain. They found that in patients with anterior instability, the test was positive in 63% for apprehension and that 46% had pain in this position. The incidence of pain in this position in patients with rotator cuff disease was 82%, with posterior instability 63%, AC joint disorders 80%, and osteoarthritis 60%. Speer et al did not statistically analyze the apprehension test as part of that study. They concluded that pain with

TABLE 5–10 Overall Evaluation Results of the Shoulder Relocation Test*

Diagnosis	Number Patients	N(%) with Pain	N(%) with Apprehension
Anterior instability	46	21 (45.6%)	29 (63%)
Rotator cuff tear	34	28 (82.3%)	0
Posterior instability	8	5 (62.5%)	0
Acromioclavicular disorder	5	4 (80%)	0
Osteoarthritis	5	3 (60%)	0
Instability of biceps tendon	2	2 (100%)	0
Total	100	63 (63%)	29 (29%)

Source: Adapted with permission from Speer KP, et al. An evaluation of the shoulder relocation test. Am J Sports Med 1994;22(2):177–183.
*All tests were done with 90 degrees abduction, 90 degrees external rotation.

TABLE 5–11 Results of Apprehension, Relocation, and Surprise Tests for Anterior Instability

| | Individual Test | | | | | | | | | | | |
| | Apprehension | | | | Relocation | | | | Surprise | | | |
Examiner	Sen	Spec	PPV	NPV	Sen	Spec	PPV	NPV	Sen	Spec	PPV	NPV
1	55.6	95.7	90.9	73.3	50.0	43.5	40.9	52.6	72.2	95.7	92.9	81.5
2	55.6	100.0	100.0	74.2	50.0	47.8	42.9	55.0	55.6	100.0	100.0	74.0
3	50.0	100.0	100.0	71.9	55.6	56.5	50.0	61.9	66.7	100.0	100.0	79.3
4	50.0	100.0	100.0	71.9	27.8	69.6	41.7	55.5	61.1	100.0	100.0	76.7
Mean	52.8	98.9	97.7	72.8	45.8	54.4	43.9	56.3	63.9	98.9	98.2	77.9

Source: Adapted with permission from Lo IK, et al. An evaluation of the apprehension, relocation, and surprise tests for anterior shoulder instability. Am J Sports Med 2004;32(2):301–307.

NPV, negative predictive value; PPV, positive predictive value; Sen, sensitivity; Spec, specificity.

the apprehension test was not predictive of traumatic anterior instability.

In their study of the anterior apprehension sign, Lo et al[100] had four examiners evaluate 46 patients who had several different diagnoses, including anterior instability of the shoulder. The apprehension test had a sensitivity for anterior instability for all examiners of 52% and a specificity of 98.9% for anterior instability. The positive predictive value (PPV) was 97.7%, and the negative predictive value (NPV) was 73%. The authors concluded that when pain alone was used for the diagnosis of traumatic anterior instability, the specificity of the apprehension maneuver was low; however, when apprehension was used as the criterion for a positive test, then the specificity and positive predictive value were high (**Table 5–11**).

There has been only one study evaluating the interexaminer reliability of the anterior apprehension test. Tzannes et al[108] evaluated the anterior apprehension test for interobserver reliability when the test resulted in apprehension and when the test resulted in only pain. They found the greatest agreement between examiners occurred when apprehension was used to determine if the patient was unstable rather than in pain.

The issue of pain versus apprehension constituting a positive test with an apprehension maneuver is an important one. Most practitioners feel that apprehension is a more accurate predictor of instability than pain alone with the arm abducted and externally rotated. If one uses pain alone as the criterion for instability, then the diagnosis may be made too liberally. For example, Uhorchak et al[109] performed an anterior apprehension test on 66 patients who had undergone an open Bankart procedure for traumatic, anterior shoulder instability. Only three (4.5%) patients clearly failed the operation with a recurrent subluxation or dislocation at a minimum 2-year follow-up.

However, 13 patients (20%) in their study had pain with no apprehension; an anterior apprehension maneuver was performed at the follow-up examination. The authors interpreted this pain with an apprehension sign as a failure of the operation, and they concluded that the failure rate in their group of patients with open Bankart

procedures was 24%. Based on these findings, they suggested that an open Bankart procedure had failure rates that approximated those reported for arthroscopic procedures. However, the studies by Lo et al[100] and Speer et al[101] would suggest that the use of pain as the criterion for traumatic anterior instability is not accurate in this setting and would result in overestimating the number of patients with instability.

Another variation of the apprehension sign was described by Rockwood and Wirth.[110] They recommended that the examiner stand behind a subject, who is seated on a stool. The examiner then held both arms and evaluated the amount of external rotation possible before there was pain or apprehension. Maximum external rotation was first performed with the patient's arms at the side, with the arms abducted at 45 degrees, with the arm at 90 degrees of abduction, and finally at 120 degrees of abduction. When testing at 90 and 120 degrees, only one arm was tested at a time. Rockwood and Wirth claimed that if the patient had symptoms of pain or apprehension with the arm abducted at 45 degrees, the lesion found at the time of surgery was the anterior capsule and labrum. When the symptoms occurred with the arm at 90 degrees of abduction, then the operative lesions were tears in the capsule and labrum anteriorly and inferiorly; when the symptoms occurred at 120 degrees of abduction, the lesions included the inferior capsule and extended posteriorly to the triceps attachment. Although there have been no studies to our knowledge that have confirmed these findings, other authors have suggested that laxity testing be performed at different degrees of elevation.[111]

> The anterior apprehension sign is an important test for true anterior instability when it produces apprehension, but not when it produces pain alone.

Relocation Sign

The relocation test was first described by Dr. Frank Jobe and colleagues in 1989.[4] Later, Speer et al[101] quoted Dr. Russ Warren (in a personal communication in 1992) as suggesting that the test was described by Dr. Peter Fowler in 1982. Regardless, it was Dr. Jobe who popularized the use of this test in the evaluation of the painful shoulder in overhead athletes.

Jobe's theory was that as the ligaments of the shoulder of the throwing or overhead sport athlete became stretched, the humerus could externally rotate more when the arm was elevated. This allowed the rotator cuff to impinge upon the acromion and caused classic impingement pain. This pain was typically felt to be in the anterior shoulder or into the deltoid. The ligament thought to be stretched was the anterior band of the inferior glenohumeral complex. Because the primary defect was not felt to be the rotator cuff, Jobe et al called this "secondary impingement," which meant that the rotator cuff–type pain felt by the patient was not the true, underlying cause of the pain.

The relocation test was meant by Jobe et al to reproduce this secondary impingement caused by the humeral head abutting against the acromion. The test was performed with the patient supine and with the shoulder hanging over the edge of the examining table (**Fig. 5–31**). The arm was then abducted and externally rotated into a position similar to a cocking position of a baseball player. The arm was pushed into maximum abduction and external rotation until pain was felt, and this was typically anteriorly or sometimes posteriorly. The examiner then would place the other hand on the humeral head and push posteriorly to "relocate" the humeral head. For this test to be positive, the pain had to be relieved with posterior pressure on the humeral head, which indicated that the impingement was relieved as the humeral head was pushed away from contact with other structures in the shoulder. In the

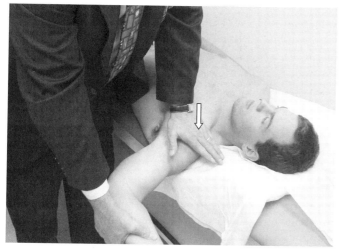

FIGURE 5–31 The relocation test described by Dr. Frank Jobe involves performing a supine anterior apprehension test, then stabilizing the humeral head with the hand once the patient reports apprehension.

treatment schema of Dr. Jobe, if the test was positive and the patient had failed nonoperative treatment, then the patient's ligaments were loose and a capsular shift was indicated to tighten up the shoulder.

While Jobe's concepts have significantly changed how we think about the shoulder of the throwing athlete, this test was not validated with anatomic or epidemiological studies. In their original description of this test, Jobe et al[4] noted that the apprehension position could produce pain in athletes with rotator cuff disease or in athletes with occult instability. With a posterior force placed against the humeral head, if the pain was improved, then it was due to occult instability, but if it was not, then it was presumably due to rotator cuff disease alone. However, like many tests there were variations of responses that remain unexplained. For example, some patients complained of increased pain with stabilization of the humeral head, and others had pain in a different location with stabilization of the humeral head.

Some patients complained of posterior and superior shoulder pain with this test, and subsequent studies by Walch et al[17] regarding internal impingement led Jobe and colleagues to alter their interpretation of the relocation test. They suggested that with the arm in the throwing position, if the patient had pain posteriorly that was relieved by posterior pressure, this was a sign that the patient had internal impingement due to the anterior inferior glenohumeral ligaments being too stretched.

As the relocation sign gained popularity, practitioners noted that the test was also helpful for patients who had overt instability patterns, such as anterior dislocations. In this case, the shoulder is placed in abduction and external rotation until the patient feels apprehensive. The humeral head is then stabilized with a posteriorly directed force, and the patient's feeling of instability goes away. Thus, when examining a patient with this test, it should be distinguished whether the patient had relief of apprehension (which represents overt instability) or just relief of pain (covert instability or internal impingement).

The utility of the relocation sign for overt or traumatic anterior instability has been the subject of several studies. As part of the same study mentioned above, Speer et al[101] evaluated the relocation test in patients with varying diagnoses with the arm abducted 90 degrees and externally rotated 90 degrees. The examiners then pushed forward on the patient's arm, as they would have during an anterior apprehension test. Patients reported whether this position of the arm gave them pain or apprehension that their shoulder would subluxate or dislocate. The examiners stabilized the head to see if the pain or apprehension went away.

The results of the relocation test for the detection of instability indicate that when the test is used to determine a sense of apprehension, it was very specific (100%) and had a positive predictive value of 100%. This means that in a patient with anterior instability, a positive relocation test indicates that the patient most likely has anterior instability of the shoulder. However, the test was only 68% specific, meaning that it will detect true anterior instability in only two thirds of patients with the disorder.

Speer et al then evaluated the relocation sign's usefulness for detecting true overt instability when the test was considered positive if the patient had pain. They found that pain was produced in this position in patients with a wide variety of diagnoses, including 82% of patients with rotator cuff disease, 63% with posterior instability, and 80% with AC disorders. In patients with true anterior instability, 67% reported pain with the arm in this position, and 87% of these had relief of the pain with a posterior force to relocate the shoulder. Speer et al concluded that the use of this test to detect true overt anterior instability using pain as the criterion is not as useful as when the test is used for determining apprehension. The sensitivity for instability when pain was the criterion was 54%, and the specificity was only 44%. The authors concluded that the relocation test for instability based on pain alone was not effective. It should be noted that they did not study its usefulness for patients who had occult instability or internal impingement.

Lo et al[100] performed a similar study by using the relocation test on 46 patients with a variety of diagnoses, including 18 patients with traumatic anterior instability. They had four examiners evaluate the patients and found that there was a high degree of agreement between the examiners for the evaluation. They also found that if the relocation maneuver was used for apprehension alone, it detected anterior instability in only 60% of the instability patients (**Table 5–12**). When using relief of apprehension as the criterion for a positive test, however, the specificity and positive predictive value of the relocation maneuver were 100% for instability, meaning that if it was a positive test, the diagnosis was reliably confirmed.

The relocation test was not as helpful for making the diagnosis of overt instability when pain was used as a criterion for a positive result. The authors noted that

patients did not uniformly report a location of pain, with pain in the instability group occurring in the shoulder anteriorly (28%), posteriorly (39%), or superiorly (33%). This study reinforces the notion that pain patterns in the shoulder are usually not specific for any one entity. Also, the incidence in pain in the other diagnostic groups was so high that the authors concluded that the test could not be used to distinguish between diagnostic groups. In the instability group, relocating the head improved the pain in only three of five patients. Lo et al concluded that for patients with traumatic overt anterior instability, the relocation test had better utility when using apprehension as the diagnostic criterion and that the use of pain as a positive test was not warranted.

Tzannes et al[108] considered the reliability of the relocation test by having four examiners evaluate a cohort of 25 patients with shoulder instability. They found that when using apprehension as a positive test, the agreement between the examiners was high (Intra Class Correlation Coefficient [ICC] = 0.71), but that it was not very high if pain was used as the diagnostic criterion (ICC = 0.31). They did not study patients with occult forms of instability or those with internal impingement symptoms.

The relocation test also has been proposed by Burkhart et al[22,112] as being an important diagnostic test for SLAP lesions. This is discussed in more detail in Chapter 6. Their study suggests that the relocation test was most sensitive (85%) and specific (68%) for posterior type II SLAP lesions (see Chapter 6, **Table 6–11**).

The apprehension sign is very accurate for anterior instability when it causes apprehension.

The apprehension sign is not accurate for anterior instability when it causes pain alone.

The apprehension and relocation signs can cause pain in patients with a variety of conditions or diagnoses and are not reliable when pain is used as a positive result.

The usefulness of these tests for occult instability in the overhead athlete is uncertain.

The relocation test may have a role in making the diagnosis of SLAP lesions.

TABLE 5–12 Evaluation of the Relocation Test Using Different Criteria for a Positive Test

Criteria	Sensitivity (%)	Specificity (%)	PPV	NPV
Pain	40.00	42.65	15.46	72.81
Pain or apprehension	45.83	54.35	43.86	56.26
Apprehension	31.94	100.00	100.00	65.28

Source: Adapted with permission from Lo IK, et al. An evaluation of the apprehension, relocation, and surprise tests for anterior shoulder instability. Am J Sports Med 2004;32(2)::301–307.

NPV, negative predictive value; PPV, positive predictive value.

Augmentation Test

The augmentation test was first described by Silliman and Hawkins[96] in 1993. This test was performed with the patient supine and the arm in an apprehension position. The patient's arm is brought into a position where it becomes apprehensive, and then an anteriorly directed force is applied. This should make the apprehension worse.

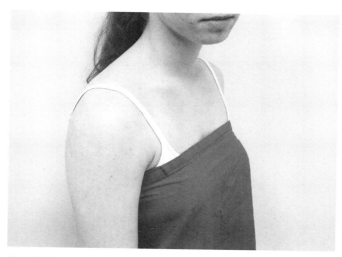

FIGURE 5–39 The resting position of a subject who can demonstrate a shoulder subluxation.

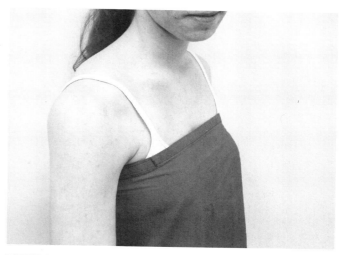

FIGURE 5–40 A subject demonstrating a posterior subluxation with the arm at the side.

overpowers the other muscles, and the shoulder subluxates or dislocates. However, this may not always be the case, and we have seen several patients with seizure disorders who sustained anterior dislocations as a result of a seizure.

Examination

Patients with acute posterior dislocations typically hold the arm in slight abduction and internal rotation (**Fig. 5–41**). External rotation is severely limited, but this is in part due to the pain and in part due to the position of the humerus. The patient should be examined carefully for neurovascular lesions.

A prominence of the humeral head posteriorly on the shoulder may not be present in acute cases due to swelling or if the individual is very muscular. In chronic cases, the prominence may be visible, but not in large individuals (**Fig. 5–42**). Under anesthesia the range of motion in external rotation is typically not as restricted because there is no pain. Patients with a reduced posterior dislocation should not have a deformity posteriorly, although some patients may be able to demonstrate the ability to subluxate and reduce the shoulder voluntarily.

Posterior Apprehension Sign

The posterior apprehension test was first described by Kessell[119] in 1982. He made the observation that patients with posterior instability would often hold their arms in

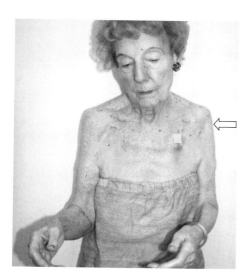

FIGURE 5–41 Appearance of a woman with a chronically locked posterior dislocation of the shoulder with her arm fixed in internal rotation.

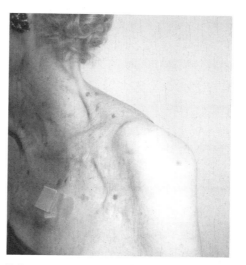

FIGURE 5–42 The prominence of the humeral head posteriorly can be seen when the patient is examined from the side.

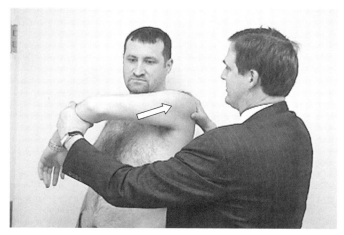

FIGURE 5–43 The posterior apprehension sign is performed by pushing posteriorly on the arm when it is in a position of flexion, adduction, and internal rotation.

flexion to 90 degrees, adducted in line with the body and in slight internal rotation (**Fig. 5–43**). He suggested that the posterior apprehension sign could be performed by placing the arm in this position and pushing posteriorly along the axis of the humerus. A positive test should produce apprehension that the shoulder will subluxate posteriorly.

However, in clinical practice we noted that the posterior apprehension test was infrequently positive in patients with posterior instability. A study was conducted using high-speed photography and skin surface markers of patients with voluntary posterior instability (see Voluntary or Demonstrable Instability).[120,121] This study revealed that the humeral head subluxation occurs with the arm abducted at an average of 94 degrees (range 0–115 degrees), 84 degrees of flexion (range 47–125 degrees), and 55 degrees of horizontal adduction[120] (**Fig. 5–44**). This is near to the position where the posterior capsule is the loosest, which some call the "zero" position.[122] After the shoulder had subluxated, the patient would adduct the arm across the body and internally rotate the extremity. This was a position where the humeral head could rest out of the glenoid with little pain.

The study demonstrated that the position interpreted by previous authors as a position of subluxation is actually the position where the subluxated shoulder rests long after it has subluxated posteriorly. There was considerable variability in the maneuvers used by the patients to subluxate their shoulders posteriorly. As a result, there was no one location that all patients subluxated their shoulders posteriorly. The consequence of this is that attempts to reproduce apprehension by placing the arm in the approximate location of subluxation were not successful. The real position of apprehension was different for each patient, and it was not the position

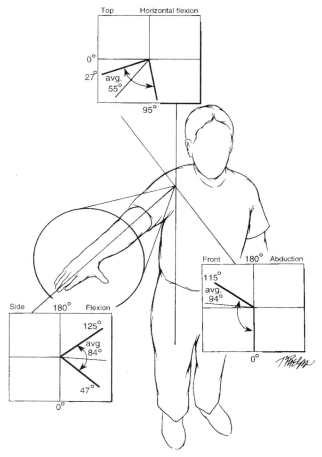

FIGURE 5–44 In patients who can demonstrate posterior subluxations, the position where the arm subluxates is not the same as that recommended for the posterior apprehension sign.

reported by Kessell[119] and numerous subsequent authors. This suggests that there is no validity to the posterior apprehension test as described.

There have been no published studies of the posterior apprehension test. Gerber and Ganz[89] mentioned that the posterior apprehension test was not consistent in detecting posterior subluxation in their patients.

We evaluated the posterior apprehension test in 12 patients who underwent a posterior stabilization for symptomatic posterior shoulder instability. (unpublished data) All patients underwent a preoperative physical examination that included a posterior apprehension sign for the presence of pain, a feeling of posterior subluxation, or apprehension that the shoulder would subluxate or dislocate posteriorly. The overall sensitivity of the test was low whether used for apprehension (42%), pain (50%), or subluxation (25%). However, the posterior apprehension test did demonstrate high specificity when it was positive (for apprehension 99%, for pain 86%, and for subluxation 98%).

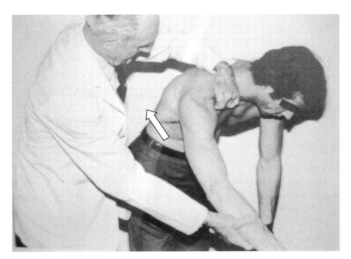

FIGURE 5–45 Test for posterior shoulder instability, with the patient standing as shown. (Adapted with permission from Rowe C. Leffert RD. Dislocation of the shoulder. In: The Shoulder. New York: Churchill Livingstone; 1988:165–291.)

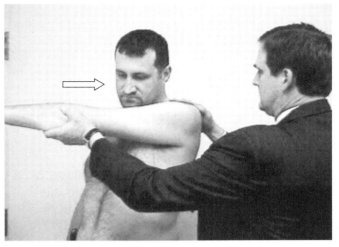

FIGURE 5–46 O'Driscoll and colleagues described a method for distinguishing impingement pain from pain produced with posterior instability when this maneuver was performed. (Adapted with permission from O'Driscoll SW, Evans DC. Contralateral shoulder instability following anterior repair: an epidemiological investigation. J Bone Joint Surg Br 1991;73(6):941–946.)

> The posterior apprehension test is rarely positive, but when it is, the patient will usually have posterior instability.

Rowe Test for Posterior Instability

Rowe[115] described a test that was similar to the posterior apprehension sign (**Fig. 5–45**). The patient was examined standing or supine. The arm was placed in forward elevation of 90 degrees and internal rotation. An axial load was applied posteriorly along the axis of the humerus. A positive test was apprehension for posterior instability or for pain posteriorly. The validity of this test has not been established, and there are no studies of its clinical application. We do not use this test in our practice and cannot comment upon its usefulness.

Posterior Apprehension Test for Pain

This test was described by O'Driscoll and Evans[123] in 1991 and included the use of a diagnostic injection to differentiate posterior instability pain from impingement pain. The arm was forward flexed and internally rotated, similar to a Kennedy-Hawkins impingement sign (see Chapter 4) (**Fig. 5–46**). The patient should then report pain in the shoulder. Because the pain could be due to the rotator cuff or to posterior instability, an injection of local anesthetic into the subacromial space was done. If the pain was relieved, then it was presumed that the pain was due to rotator cuff tendinitis or other rotator cuff pathologies. If the pain was not relieved, then the pain was proposed to be due to posterior instability.

There have been no studies of the validity or the clinical usefulness of this test. However, it is unlikely that

this test can be very specific for posterior instability. In our experience posterior shoulder pain in this arm position can be due to frozen or stiff shoulders, SLAP lesions, degenerative arthritis, and multiple other causes. Another difficulty with this test is that it requires an injection into the subacromial space in patients who otherwise would not need it for rotator cuff–type symptoms. Further study of this test is needed before its use can be recommended.

Jerk Test

The jerk test was described by Matsen et al.[98] In this test the arm was brought into flexion, adduction, and internal rotation. The examiner uses one hand to provide an axial force along the humerus to promote posterior subluxation (**Fig. 5–47**). The examiner should feel a sudden

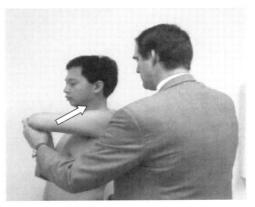

FIGURE 5–47 In the jerk test, the arm is flexed and adducted to produce a subluxation. The arm is then extended to cause the humeral head to reduce back into the glenoid.

"jerk" as the humeral head subluxates over the glenoid rim posteriorly. The examiner then extends the patient's arm away from the body toward the original position. As the arm goes beyond the neutral position, a second "jerk" may be felt as the humeral head reduces. This test has not been validated nor studied in the existing literature. Kim et al[124] reported on 31 patients with posterior shoulder instability and a multidirectional component, and they suggested that all of them had a positive jerk test (100% specificity).[125] They did not have a control group, and they did not state who did the examinations.

From our personal experience, however, it is very unusual for this test to be positive in patients with posterior instability. Though it may be specific, we do not feel that it is sensitive for that entity. The exact location that the joint subluxes posteriorly in most patients with posterior instability is highly variable, so finding the exact location to produce a subluxation is difficult. In our practice this test has occasionally been positive in a patient who has a demonstrable or voluntary component to his or her instability, but often the patient subluxes the humerus actively, and it is not accomplished passively by the examiner.

Posterior Subluxation Test (Miniaci Test)

This test was described by Clarnette and Miniaci[126] in 1998. It is a variation of the "clunk" or "jerk" sign. This can be performed with the patient sitting or supine. The arm of the patient is brought into flexion of 90 degrees, adducted across the body, and internally rotated (**Fig. 5–48**). The examiner places one hand behind the

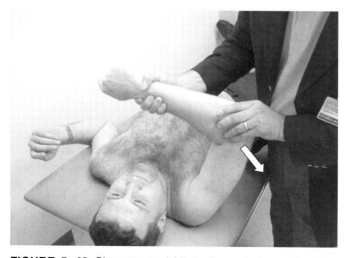

FIGURE 5–48 Clarnette and Miniaci's posterior subluxation test is similar to the jerk test because it uses arm positioning to allow the examiner to feel the posteriorly subluxated humeral head reduce back into the socket. (Adapted with permission from Clarnette RG, Miniaci A. Clinical exam of the shoulder. Med Sci Sports Exerc 1998;30(4 Suppl): S1–S6.)

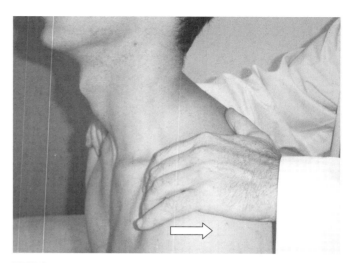

FIGURE 5–49 The Fukada test for posterior shoulder instability is performed with the patient standing and posterior laxity measured with one hand. (Adapted with permission from Neer C. Dislocations. In: Neer C, ed. Shoulder Reconstruction. Philadelphia: WB Saunders; 1990:273–362.)

patient's shoulder to feel for the relationship of the humeral head to the glenoid rim as the arm is adducted. The arm is then extended and brought back to its original position. As this is done, the examiner should feel a clunk as the humeral head reduces. This test has not been validated nor has it been studied for its clinical application.

Fukada Test

The first mention of the Fukada test was by Neer[6] in 1990, then by Cooper and Brems[82] in 1992. The test is performed with the patient sitting and the examiner behind the subject (**Fig. 5–49**). The examiner places a thumb of each hand on the scapular spines, with the fingers anteriorly on the humeral head. The examiner then pushes the proximal humerus posteriorly to create posterior translation. This test is usually done on both shoulders at once to compare the two sides. The validity of this test has not been previously documented, and its clinical usefulness has not been studied. We do not have extended experience with this test, but we have found it difficult to perform because the scapula is not easily stabilized by one hand.

Push–Pull Test

The push–pull test was described by Matsen et al[98] and is a variant of a load and shift test, with the patient supine (**Fig. 5–23**). The examiner stands to the side, and the patient's arm is placed in 90 degrees of abduction and 30 degrees of flexion. The examiner holds the patient's wrist with one hand and uses the other hand to direct a

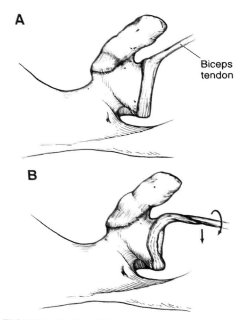

A

Biceps
tendon

B

FIGURE 6–15 (A,B) The peel-back mechanism of SLAP lesions is due to torsional forces upon the labrum. (Adapted with permission from Morgan CD, Burkhart SS, Palmeri M, Gillespie M. Type II SLAP lesions: three subtypes and their relationships to superior instability and rotators cuff tears. Arthroscopy 1998;14(6):553–565.)

the cocking phase of throwing, the biceps tendon is rotated superiorly on the glenoid, and there is tension on the biceps anchor. This twisting motion of the biceps tendon stresses the labrum attachments, and eventually the labrum begins to "peel" off the posterosuperior glenoid (**Fig. 6–15**).

It is also possible that injury to the biceps attachment is due to a combination of anteroinferior glenohumeral instability and tension in the biceps by other mechanisms. Morgan et al[16] suggested that a torsional mechanism may be the primary cause of the superior labrum failure, or that it may be a secondary contributing cause once the lesion has been initiated by the "tension overload" mechanism as described by Andrews et al.[14] Andrews et al supported the idea that superior labrum lesions are due to a combination of twisting and pulling, which they compared to "pulling weeds." Once the superior labrum is torn, this results in the increased shoulder laxity observed in athletes upon examination and at the time of surgery.

This increased laxity due to superior labrum lesions has been called a form of "superior" instability by some authors and an "anterior pseudolaxity" by others.[30] The more likely explanation is that these labrum abnormalities do effect glenohumeral translations in many subtle ways, including in an anteroinferior and possibly an anterosuperior direction; however, the exact mechanism continues to be elusive, and this inexact understanding

of the mechanism producing SLAP lesions affects our understanding of the physical examination and our treatment strategies.

The first evidence that the superior labrum may affect the biomechanics of the shoulder comes from a clinical study that found that some presumably normal labrum variants are associated with more superior labrum fraying and labrum detachments.[7] The exact mechanism by which those variations lead to pathologies could not be determined because it was an observational study.

Schulz et al[32] studied the effect of the presence of a sublabral hole in the superior labrum upon the density of the glenoid bone in cadavers. They found no difference in the bone densities and concluded that simple sublabral holes alone did not affect stability of the shoulder. This conclusion is supported by a study by Pagnani et al,[33] who evaluated the effect of an isolated release of the anterosuperior labrum upon translations of the shoulder. They found that there was no effect on translations until a larger release of the labrum attachments was performed. This release had to include the attachments of the middle glenohumeral ligament anteriorly, the biceps attachment to the superior glenoid tubercle, and the superior labrum attachments anteriorly and posteriorly.

Biomechanical studies, however, do support the possibility that superior labrum pathology contributes to anterior, inferior, and possibly superior laxities. Pagnani el al[33] demonstrated that once a complete lesion of the biceps anchor was produced (i.e., a type II SLAP lesion), there were significantly increased translations of the shoulder in an inferior-superior direction and in an anteroposterior direction. McMahon et al[34] found similar results when a superior labrum detachment was created in a cadaver model, and the effects on shoulder joint translations were studied with a robotic device. They found significant increases in anterior and inferior translations with either a partial or full detachment of the superior labrum complex, which indicates that the superior labrum complex may contribute to shoulder instability in some way.

Burkhart and Morgan[35] have suggested clinically that when a SLAP lesion is repaired arthroscopically, the laxity of the shoulder is decreased. The drive-through sign, which is performed by trying to push the arthroscope through the joint under arthroscopy, has been demonstrated to be an indication of laxity of the shoulder and not of overt instability.[36] Burkhart and Morgan[35] found that the drive-through sign was eliminated in patients who underwent a SLAP repair, supporting the idea that the superior labrum complex influences anterior and inferior shoulder laxities.

It may be that the biceps tendon attachment is important for shoulder function only in certain circumstances, such as when performing overhead sports or strenuous activities. Isolated rupture of the biceps tendon is clinically tolerated in many individuals. Surgical procedures on the biceps tendon would also question that the biceps tendon serves a significant role in the function of the shoulder. There have been many who suggest that the biceps is a vestigial structure that can be released from its attachments to the superior glenoid (called a tenotomy) or tenodesed to the proximal humerus (where the tendon is sutured to the bone to maintain tension in the biceps muscle) with impunity.[17,37]

Both biceps tenotomy and biceps tenodesis have been found to produce few to no deficits in shoulder function postoperatively. Gill et al.[38] in 2001 reported the clinical follow-up of 30 patients who underwent arthroscopic release of the biceps for bicipital tenosynovitis, dislocation, or partial rupture of the biceps tendon. Most (90%) of their patients returned to the same level of sports with minimal or no pain. Osbahr et al.[39] in 2002 compared the clinical results of 80 patients who underwent biceps tenotomy and 80 patients who underwent biceps tenodesis. They did not find a significant difference between the two groups in terms of anterior shoulder pain, muscle spasm, or cosmetic deformity. These studies would suggest that one could live and function quite well without the long head of the biceps tendon attached to the superior glenoid.

Several studies would suggest, however, that biceps tenotomy or tenodesis may be associated with some dysfunction of the biceps muscle, particularly in its superior portion. A study by West et al.[40] found that 25% of their patients with tenotomy of the long head of the biceps tendon continued to have cramping and pain in the superior biceps muscle region. This compared with patients in their study who had tenodesis who did not experience either of these complications (0%). Neither group complained of shoulder weakness or dysfunction, whereas the tenotomy group was less likely to return to their previous level of activity. Despite that observation, shoulder scores between the two groups did not differ, which suggests that the shoulder can function perfectly well without the long head of the biceps.

None of these studies have demonstrated that removing the biceps tendon from the shoulder joint affects its function or its stability. No study has shown that a biceps tenotomy or tenodesis produces shoulder instability. It may be that the biceps tendon functions as a stabilizer in only select patient groups; however, it is safe to assume that, like most other structures in the body, the long head of the biceps tendon is there for a reason, and that resection should not be performed without some concern.

The Biceps Tendon and Shoulder Pain

Another quandary involves the relationship of the biceps tendon pathology to pain in the shoulder. The biceps tendon as a source of pain has been supported by the observation that the pain that precedes a biceps tendon rupture is typically gone once the tendon tears.[41] This concept is supported by the fact that biceps tenolysis can be an effective procedure for the relief of pain in the anterior shoulder that is believed to be due to biceps tendon pathology.[42]

Some physicians have suggested, however, that anterior shoulder pain due to isolated biceps tendinitis is not common. In 1972 Neer[43] commented that because the biceps tendon was so commonly involved in impingement (rotator cuff) disease, "we now consider it unwise to operate upon the biceps tendon alone without having considered the possibility of a concomitant element of subacromial impingement" (p. 49). Especially in patients older than 40 years of age, Neer suggested that any biceps surgery should be accompanied by an anterior acromioplasty and coracoacromial ligament release. He felt that impingement of the rotator cuff and the biceps tendon upon the acromion was the cause of the biceps pain and pathology and that they typically occurred together.[43,44]

It has been suggested by some physicians that pain in the region of the biceps tendon is actually referred pain from rotator cuff pathology or other sources.[23,43] Becker and Cofield[45] found that of patients who had an isolated biceps tenodesis, 15% required further surgery, usually an acromioplasty, to eliminate their pain.

Some of the uncertainty about the diagnosis of isolated biceps pathology relates to the lack of a distinctive pain pattern associated with biceps tendon pathology. There is little doubt that lesions of the biceps tendon are capable of producing pain. A study by Soifer et al[46] of the distribution of nerve pain fibers in the shoulder was highest in the bursa, followed by the biceps tendon and the rotator cuff. It has been supposed by most physicians that the pain produced by biceps pathology radiates down the front of the shoulder in the region of the biceps tendon (**Fig. 6–16**), but this has never been convincingly established by any injection studies or other methods.[41]

Part of the challenge is that pain of rotator cuff pathology typically radiates into the anterior and lateral shoulder just like biceps pathology. Also, signs upon examination of impingement that involve internal rotation (i.e., Kennedy-Hawkins sign) of the arm can produce pain in the deltoid and anterior aspect of the shoulder, so this pattern of pain could be due either to the biceps or to the rotator cuff in patients who have both problems. What exactly causes the pain in either the Kennedy-Hawkins sign or with the coracoid impingement sign has not been determined, and the degree that biceps pathology contributes to the pain typical of impingement has not been established.

There are several cadaveric studies suggesting that arm positions that have been felt to compress the rotator cuff may also cause impingement of the biceps tendon. Valadie et al[47] in a study of cadaver shoulders found that with a Kennedy-Hawkins impingement sign (flexion and internal rotation), the biceps tendon made contact with the coracoacromial ligament in two of four specimens.

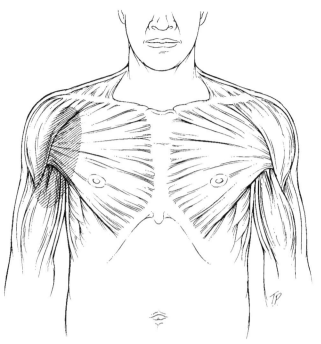

FIGURE 6–16 Biceps tendon pathology may cause pain to radiate down the front of the arm, but this is not specific to the biceps tendon.

Another study by Burns and Whipple[48] using cadaver dissections also suggested that the biceps made contact with the coracoacromial ligament with the arm in flexion and internal rotation.

Using three-dimensional electrogoniometers in a cadaver model, we simulated a Hawkins impingement sign,

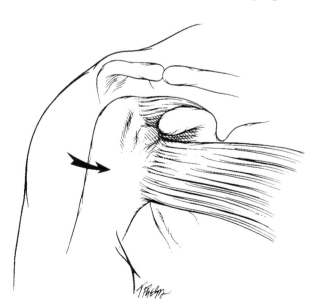

FIGURE 6–17 Coracoid impingement occurs when the arm is flexed and internally rotated so that the lesser tuberosity and bicipital groove make contact with the coracoid, coracoacromial ligament, and superior glenoid.

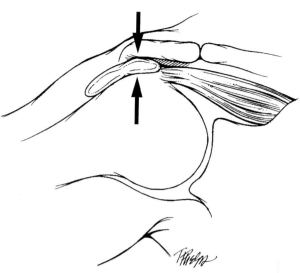

FIGURE 6–18 Subacromial impingement occurs when the arm is elevated and the greater tuberosity makes contact with the acromion.

which places the arm in flexion and internal rotation. This study found that the bicipital groove and lesser tuberosity made contact with the coracoacromial ligament as the arm was placed into internal rotation (Fig. 6–17). Likewise, a Neer impingement sign was performed (flexion of the arm), and the lateral edge of the acromion had very close proximity to the lateral edge of the bicipital groove (Fig. 6–18). This study supported the cadaveric studies above, which would suggest that in certain positions the biceps tendon could be an integral part of the impingement process.

■ Biceps Tendon Instability

Instability of the biceps tendon has received increasing attention due to the ability to evaluate arthroscopically the biceps and its pulley system. The most comprehensive evaluation of the spectrum of biceps instabilities was by Walch et al.[49] They described three distinct clinical presentations that included biceps subluxations out of the bicipital groove, dislocations of the tendon out of the groove, and intra-articular dislocations of the biceps tendon.

Frank subluxation of the biceps tendon out of the bicipital groove has been reported by many authors, including Meyer.[3] It is now known that full subluxation of the biceps tendon out of the bicipital groove is most commonly associated with partial or complete subscapularis tendon ruptures.[50] In their study, which included 25 patients who averaged 54 years of age, Walch et al[49] found that subluxations were almost always associated with supraspinatus tears and tears of the upper subscapularis.

Walch et al also found that dislocations of the tendon over the lesser tuberosity but not into the joint were associated with tears of the supraspinatus and infraspinatus tendons, and the average age of the patients with this pathology was 63 years of age. Complete intra-articular dislocations of the biceps tendon into the shoulder joint were found in patients with an average age of 56 years, and the pathology included extensive and massive rotator cuff tears. The symptoms of biceps subluxations or dislocations have been postulated to include shoulder pain and perhaps a clicking about the shoulder.[51]

Several physical examination methods of producing biceps tendon instability in the intertubercular groove have been described. All involve circumduction of the arm with rotation, which produces a painful click or pop along the anterior shoulder. The accuracy of these examinations unfortunately has never been evaluated. Walch et al[49] in their 71 cases of biceps subluxation or dislocation noted that they never saw classical signs of biceps instability such as clicking or jerking. Because all of their patients had some coexisting rotator cuff pathology, they found that their patients had symptoms more consistent with rotator cuff disease than with instability of the biceps tendon. Finally, clicks around the shoulder are nonspecific, and it is difficult to ascribe a click to a specific pathology such as biceps instability.[28]

■ The Challenge of Diagnosing SLAP Lesions

The last area of controversy involves the diagnosis of SLAP lesions upon physical examination. The accuracy of the physical examination findings for SLAP lesions is an important issue not only for making the diagnosis of these lesions but also for following the results of treatment, whether it is medical or surgical.

There are several reasons the examination of SLAP lesions is difficult. First, there has been a controversy about how the labrum functions and how it produces symptoms. Many physicians have proposed that the labrum functions much like the meniscus in the knee, and that it would produce symptoms similar to the meniscus, specifically pain, locking, a click, or any combination of these symptoms. As a result, many physical examination tests or signs are meant to provoke either pain or a click with motion.

Studies have shown, however, that a click in the shoulder is nonspecific and can be due to a variety of pathologies.[28,52] In our study of SLAP lesions, there was no difference in the incidence of clicks between patients who had SLAP lesions versus those who did not have SLAP lesions, which means that a click does not distinguish a patient with a SLAP lesion from one who does not have a SLAP lesion.

Another misconception is that the labrum can becomes trapped within the shoulder joint like a bucket handle tear of the meniscus in the knee. In our experience, a "trapped" labrum tear is rare, and when it is seen in a patient, it is typically due to a type III or IV labrum tear. Type III and IV labrum lesions are a minority of SLAP lesions in most series (**Table 6–1**).

The second reason SLAP lesions are difficult to diagnose is that there are many mechanisms that can produce SLAP lesions, so the patient's history may not be helpful in making the diagnosis. These mechanisms include a fall upon the extremity with an outstretched arm, work-related injuries, shoulder dislocation, and overuse due to overhead sports or work.

Maffet et al[15] reported on the mechanisms of injury to the shoulders in 67 patients diagnosed with SLAP lesions. Sixty-six percent of their patients had traction injuries to their arms (**Table 6–2**). This was most commonly traction in an inferior direction, such as when two people were lifting an object and one let go suddenly. Maffet et al reported that 13% of their patients had sustained a traumatic shoulder dislocation associated with their SLAP lesion. Snyder et al[12] reported that a fall on an outstretched hand was the most common mechanism of SLAP lesions; however, Maffet et al reported that only 8% of their patients' SLAP lesions were associated with a fall on an outstretched arm (**Table 6–2**).

One difficulty with many of these studies is that they include patients with other shoulder problems in addition to a SLAP lesion. When there are multiple pathologies present in a patient, it is difficult to ascribe symptoms to just one pathology. There is only one study of "isolated" SLAP lesions with no other shoulder pathologies. Snyder et al[12] reported on 23 patients diagnosed arthroscopically

TABLE 6–1 Incidence of SLAP Lesions in the Literature

Study	Number of Patients	Incidence of Types of SLAP (%)					
		All Patients	I	II	III	IV	Other	Non-I*
Snyder et al[12]	700	4	11	41	33	15	–	3.4
Maffet et al[15]	712	17	59	22	2	2	16	11.8
Snyder et al[89]	2375	6	21	55	9	10	5	4.7
Tomonobu et al[90]	305	23	17	4.6	0.3	0.7	–	5.6
Handelberg et al[91]	530	6	10	53	6	3	29	5.5
Kim[52]	544	26	74	21	0.7	4.3	–	6.7

SLAP, superior labrum anterior to posterior.
*Percent of SLAP lesion which is not type I lesion in entire group

TABLE 6–2 The Mechanism of Injury in 67 Patients Diagnosed with SLAP Lesion

Mechanisms	%
Fall onto shoulder	15
Lifting heavy object	13
Traumatic dislocation	13
Insidious onset	9
Sudden anterior traction	8
Abduction and external rotation	8
Fall onto outstretched arm	8
Gradual with repetitive lifting	6
Motor vehicle accident	6
Sudden upward traction	3
Unknown mechanism during sports	1
Lateral traction	1

Source: Adapted with permission from Maffet MW, Gartsman GM, Moseley B. Superior labrum–biceps tendon complex lesions of the shoulder. Am J Sports Med 1995;23(1):93–98.

SLAP, superior labrum anterior and posterior.

to have an isolated SLAP lesion with no other shoulder pathology. In that cohort of patients they found that a compression force applied to the shoulder as a result of a fall onto an outstretched hand was the most common mechanism of isolated SLAP lesions.

In their group with isolated SLAP lesions, the second most common mechanism of injury was a traction on the arm.[12] This mechanism was seen as a result of sudden pull on the arm or as a result of repetitive motion due to overhead sports activity. The authors concluded that SLAP lesions could be caused by a compression force on the superior joint surface or by traction forces.

The last mechanism of injury postulated to produce SLAP lesions is that they are due to impingement or "internal contact" of the greater tuberosity upon the superior glenoid and labrum when the arm is in an abducted and externally rotated position.[12,36,53–55] The association between SLAP lesions and repetitive overhead activities has been described in many studies,[14,56,57] but the exact mechanism whereby this motion creates SLAP lesions is not entirely known.

Walch et al[55] first reported this "internal impingement" phenomenon in a cohort of patients who had undergone arthroscopy of the shoulder. None of the patients had a history of trauma, and 12 of the 17 patients involved in overhead sports had a SLAP lesion. They suggested that the contact or impingement of the greater tuberosity upon the posterior and superior glenoid caused the labrum to tear in this area; however, in a study of patients undergoing arthroscopy with a variety of shoulder conditions, we found that contact occurred in 74% of patients.[58] This is in agreement with Walch and colleagues, who speculated that this "internal contact" was physiological, and that it produced symptoms due to other factors such as repetitive motion or laxity.

Biomechanical studies seem to support that SLAP lesions can occur as a result of a variety of mechanisms.

Bey et al[27] studied the etiology of superior labrum detachments using a cadaver model. They found that inferior subluxation of the shoulder resulted in type II SLAP lesions in seven of eight specimens, and they concluded that traction on the biceps as seen with anterior and inferior instability could result in biceps tendon detachments.

In contrast, a cadaver model was used by Clavert et al[59] to demonstrate that a fall on an outstretched arm can result in SLAP lesions. In this model the humerus was elevated and an axial load applied so that the greater tuberosity contacted the superior glenoid rim. The axial load was applied so that it simulated a forward fall or a fall with the hand behind the body (or backward fall). The forward fall position of the humerus resulted in five SLAP lesions in five shoulders, whereas the posterior fall position resulted in only two SLAP lesions in five specimens.

The third reason that SLAP lesions are difficult to diagnose is that they typically occur with other shoulder pathologies. In most series in the literature, isolated SLAP lesions with no other pathology typically varied from 1[60] to 12%[52] of all SLAP lesions. Of 139 patients diagnosed with a SLAP lesion at our institution between 1992 and 2000, 123 patients (88%) were found to have associated intra-articular pathology (**Table 6–3**).

As a result, a large part of the difficulty in studying SLAP lesions is that they rarely occur without other shoulder pathology, and this coexisting shoulder problem could be the cause of the symptoms ascribed to the SLAP lesion. Because isolated SLAP lesions are uncommon as an isolated finding at the time of arthroscopy, it is difficult to say convincingly that the symptoms can be

TABLE 6–3 Associated Pathology and SLAP Lesions (Percentages)

Associated Lesions	Type I	Type II	Types III and IV
Supraspinatus tears	67	59	43
Partial-thickness supraspinatus tear	49	40	43
Full-thickness supraspinatus tear	19	21	0
Infraspinatus tears	6	4	0
Partial-thickness infraspinatus tear	5	0	0
Full thickness infraspinatus tear	1	3	0
Subscapularis tears	21	20	25
Partial-thickness subscapularis tear	20	20	0
Full-thickness subscapularis tear	2	0	0
Bankart lesion	17	31	71
Hill-Sacks lesion	26	35	57
Humeral head osteoarthritis	23	31	14
Glenoid osteoarthritis	18	14	14

Source: Data from The Johns Hopkins University Shoulder Database.

SLAP, superior labrum anterior and posterior.

TABLE 6–4 Examination Findings in Patients with SLAP Lesions and No SLAP Lesions from Commonly Used Tests*

Physical Examination Findings	Descriptive Comparison*			Statistical Comparison, p Value[†]		
	No SLAP (N = 457)	Type I (N = 119)	Type II (N = 39)	No SLAP Versus Type I	No SLAP Versus Type II	Type I Versus Type II
Compression rotation test	52/207 (25%)	15/67 (22%)	5/26 (19%)	>.2	>.2	>.2
Anterior slide test	50/294 (17)	12/87 (43)	2/33 (6)	>.2	.103	>.2
Active compression test	130/297 (44)	49/91 (51)	18/33 (55)	.091	>.2	>.2
Speed's test	107/382 (28)	46/109 (42)	10/36 (28)	**.005**	>.2	.124
Apprehension test	93/404 (23)	16/114 (14)	8/36 (22)	**.038**	>.2	>.2
Relocation test	50/210 (24)	11/64 (17)	8/26 (31)	>.2	>.2	.153
Neer impingement sign	263/438 (60)	77/119 (51)	20/39 (51)	>.2	>.2	.136
Hawkins impingement test	274/435 (63)	87/119 (73)	26/39 (67)	**.040**	>.2	>.2
Painful arc sign	117/242 (48)	41/72 (57)	16/30 (53)	>.2	>.2	>.2
Drop arm sign	88/367 (24)	26/101 (26)	8/34 (24)	>.2	>.2	>.2
AC adduction test	104/381 (27)	30/105 (29)	11/34 (32)	>.2	>.2	>.2

Source: Unpublished data from The Johns Hopkins University Shoulder Database.

*The data are given as the proportion of subjects with a positive result in patients who underwent each test, with the percentage in parentheses.

[†]Statistical significance among the three groups was determined for the differences in proportions of the positive tests in each test, and significant numbers ($p < .05$) are given boldface[92].

AC, overall accuracy; SLAP, superior labrum anterior to posterior.

ascribed to the SLAP lesion. When coexisting pathology has been surgically treated along with a SLAP lesion, it is difficult to know which operation solved the problem; likewise, if the procedure fails, it is important to know whether it was the SLAP repair that failed or not.

The distribution of the type of SLAP lesions may also be age related. When patients with a variety of diagnoses are included, type II SLAP lesions appear to have different etiologies depending on the age of the patient[52]. Type II SLAP lesions in patients under the age of 40 were more commonly associated with a diagnosis of instability and the presence of a Bankart lesion, whereas those in patients over the age of 40 were associated with a diagnosis of rotator cuff disease and osteoarthritis of the shoulder[52]. Type I SLAP lesions are more clearly a degenerative phenomena, but it is possible that some type II SLAP lesions are related in some fashion to senescence of shoulder tissues.

Another reason SLAP lesions are difficult to diagnose is that the pain pattern produced by them is not specific. Patients may complain of pain "deep in the shoulder," and although this pattern of pain may be seen with SLAP lesions, it is not specific. Berg and Ciullo[61] suggested that SLAP lesion pain should radiate down the biceps tendon in the front of the shoulder. Several tests upon physical examination suggest that pain with this characteristic "deep in there" quality is diagnostic for a SLAP lesion, but one study has demonstrated that the pain pattern produced with several tests for SLAP lesions is highly variable among patients with SLAP lesions[28].

Analysis of our data would suggest that most SLAP lesions cannot be accurately defined with any of the tests currently available. It is common for patients with SLAP lesions to have positive examination signs typical of other disease processes, such as rotator cuff tendinitis or shoulder instability. Several studies have commented on the overlap of the physical examination of patients with SLAP lesions and other shoulder problems[28,52]. It is not uncommon for a patient with a SLAP lesion to have positive physical findings for other entities, such as a positive Neer or Hawkins impingement sign.

We evaluated the accuracy of commonly used physical examination tests for shoulder pathology upon patients with and without SLAP lesions (**Table 6–4**)[52]. The prevalence of positive findings was similar between patients with no SLAP lesions and those with SLAP lesions. It was not uncommon for a patient with a SLAP lesion to have multiple tests for other shoulder entities positive upon physical examination.

Parentis et al[62] performed a similar study on 132 consecutive patients undergoing shoulder arthroscopy. All of the patients underwent a physical examination preoperatively that included several common shoulder tests. In their cohort there were 23 patients who had type II SLAP lesions. The researchers found that, though sensitive for SLAP lesions, most of these tests were not specific for SLAP lesions (**Table 6–5**).

It should be noted, however, that a legitimate criticism of both our study and the study by Parentis et al is that neither evaluated isolated SLAP lesions. It may be that in cases

TABLE 6–5 Specificity and Sensitivity of different Tests in Patients with SLAP II Lesions

Test	Specificity	Sensitivity
Yergason's test	92.7*	13.0
Pain provocative test	89.9	17.4
Anterior slide test	83.5	13.0
Crank test	82.6	8.7
Speed's test	67.9	47.8*
Relocation test	51.4	43.5*
Neer test	51.4	47.8*
Active compression test	48.6	65.2*
Hawkins test	30.3	65.2*

Source: Adapted with permission from Parentis MA, Mohr KJ, ElAttrache NS. Disorders of the superior labrum: review and treatment guidelines. Clin Orthop 2002(400):77–87.

*$p < .05$

SLAP, superior labrum anterior and posterior.

TABLE 6–6 Preoperative Physical Examination in 23 Patients with Isolated SLAP Lesions

Finding	Number of Patients	% of Study Group
Impingement (Neer test)	12	52
Popping/snapping	10	43
Anterior apprehension	9	39
Impingement (Hawkins test)	8	35
Resisted supraspinatus	8	35
Biceps tension	8	35
Resisted external rotation	2	9
Adduction compression	2	9
Tenderness	2	9
Compression rotation	1	4
Relocation	1	4

Source: Adapted with permission from Stenson WB, Snyder SE, Karzel RP, Banas MP, Rahal SE. Long-term clinical follow-up of isolated SLAP lesions of the shoulder. Arch Am Acad Orthop Surg 1997;1(1):61–64.

SLAP, superior labrum anterior and posterior.

where there are only SLAP lesions (and no other existing shoulder pathology), these clinical examinations are more accurate. It should be remembered that most SLAP lesions occur with other shoulder pathologies, so our study and the Parentis et al study represent "real life" when examining the shoulders of most patients. Stenson et al[60] did attempt to evaluate isolated SLAP lesions in a cohort of 2375 shoulder arthroscopies. They found only 23 patients (1%) with no other pathologies at the time of arthroscopy. When they analyzed this group, they found that the most common presentation was similar to rotator cuff symptoms (**Table 6–6**).

Lastly, the literature regarding SLAP lesions should be interpreted by clinicians with caution, for several reasons. The validity of any physical examination test should be established by a definitive standard, such as arthroscopy of the shoulder. Some studies have used magnetic resonance imaging (MRI) as the standard for diagnosis when evaluating the results of the physical examination for SLAP lesions. Although MRI has reported accuracies as high as 95% for SLAP lesions, that has not uniformly been our clinical experience. We have not studied the accuracy of MRI scanning for SLAP lesions in our clinical setting, but our experience has been that abnormalities of the superior labrum are difficult to distinguish from normal variants using MRI.[7] Because MRI tends to overdiagnose SLAP lesions, utilizing MRI criteria for establishing the accuracy of a clinical test for SLAP lesions will tend to produce better results for that test than if arthroscopy is the standard for making the diagnosis.

The results of the studies of examination tests for SLAP lesions also depend on the experience of the person who is performing the examination and on the number of examiners. It is preferable that one person performs the examination, but the inter- and intraobserver reliability of most of the reported tests has not been reported. The only studies that mention interobserver reliability for tests for SLAP lesions are the two studies by Kim et al[63,64] on the biceps load tests I and II. They mention that the kappa value for agreement between the two observers for the first test was 0.846 and for the second 0.815, which, according to the criteria of Landis and Koch[65] (fair: 0.21–0.40, moderate: 0.41–0.61; substantial: 0.61–0.8; excellent: 0.81–1), falls into the excellent range for interobserver agreement.

Another critical factor in interpreting the results of tests for SLAP lesions is the patient population studied (**Table 6–7**). For example, our study of SLAP lesions

TABLE 6–7 Review of Reported Diagnostic Accuracy for SLAP Lesions

Tests	Study	Lesion	Sensitivity	Specificity	PPV	NPV	DV
Compression rotation test	Snyder et al (1990)[12]	SLAP	22.0				
	Holovacs et al (2000)[93]	Glenoid labral tear	80.0	19.0			86
	McFarland et al (2002)[28]	SLAP	24.0	76.0	9	90	71
Anterior slide test	Kibler (1995)[79]	Superior Labral tear	78.0	92.0	84	87	
	McFarland et al (2002)[28]	SLAP	8.0	84.0	5	90	77
Active compression test	O'Brien et al (1998)[83]	Superior labral tear	100.0	99.0	95	100	99
	Morgan et al (1998)[16]	Anterior type II SLAP	88.0	42.0	42	88	57
		Posterior type II SLAP	32.0	13.0	17	27	20
		Combined type II SLAP	85.0	41.0	42	85	56
	McFarland et al (2002)[28]	SLAP	47.0	55.0	10	91	54
	Stenson and Templin (2002)[82]	SLAP	67.0	41.0	60		
	Guanche and Jones (2003)[94]	SLAP	54.0	47.0	57	45	
	Holovacs et al (2000)[93]		69.0	50.0			
	Parentis et al (2002)[62]	SLAP (type II)	65.0				
Biceps load test I	Kim et al (1999)[64]	SLAP (type II)	90.9	96.9	83	98	
Biceps load test II	Kim et al (2001)[85]	SLAP	90.0	92.0		95	
Crank test	Liu et al (1996)[80]	Glenoid labral tear	91.0	93.0	94	90	
	Mimori et al (1999)[81]	SLAP	83.0	100.0			

DV, diagnostic value; NPV, negative predictive value; PPV, positive predictive value; SLAP, superior labrum anterior and posterior.

includes a wide variety of patient groups with a variety of diagnoses.[52] This is in contrast to the study of Burkhart et al,[57] which includes primarily patients with shoulder symptoms associated with involvement in overhead sports. Including patients who do not have a history of overhead sports may tend to make the examinations appear less accurate, but including only the target group in the study may tend to overstate the accuracy and usefulness of the examination.

Using more than one test upon examination may increase the accuracy of the exam for SLAP lesions, but that has not been convincingly established. In our study[28] of only three physical examination tests for SLAP lesions, there was no added accuracy for combining the results of more than one test; however, further study is needed so that the best combination of findings can establish the diagnostic accuracy for SLAP lesions.

■ Specific Tests for the Biceps

Observation

Patients who complain of anterior shoulder pain should have the sides compared for asymmetry of the proximal shoulder and the acromioclavicular (AC) joint. Patients with a torn biceps tendon will have a typical swelling the middle of the arm called a "Popeye" sign due to the balling up of the tendon and muscle of the long head of the biceps (**Fig. 6–11**). The patient should be asked about a history of trauma, however, because this deformity should not occur without trauma. Progressive swelling without trauma should be evaluated with a careful history, examination, and appropriate radiographs. In our practice we have seen a patient who presented without trauma and with swelling at the proximal biceps tendon area that proved to be a soft tissue sarcoma (**Fig. 6–19**). In addition, synovial cysts can occur along the biceps tendon, which can appear either with or without pain.

Ludington Sign

The Ludington test was first described in 1923 as a way to increase the ability to detect full tears of the proximal tear of the biceps tendon.[66] In this test the patient is standing (**Fig. 6–20**) and is asked to place both hands on the head and to intertwine the fingers. This allows the arms to be supported by the hands on the head and allows the biceps to relax. The patient then is asked to relax and contract the biceps tendon. The examiner stands behind the patient and palpates the proximal biceps tendon to see if tension is found in the tendon with muscle contraction. If there is no tension in the tendon, then the proximal biceps tendon may be torn.

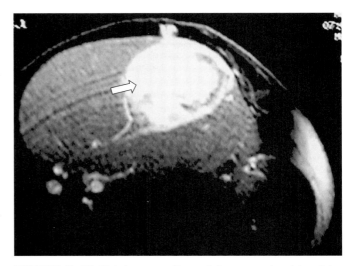

FIGURE 6–19 Painless swelling of the arm should not be assumed to be a tear of the long head of the biceps tendon because soft tissue sarcomas can occur in the arm. An axial image of a soft tissue sarcoma in the biceps muscle is shown (arrow) (axial and sagittal views).

This test is largely unnecessary in patients who have a ruptured proximal biceps tendon. In most instances the defect can be accentuated by merely asking the patient to tighten the biceps tendon with the elbow flexed and with the arm in front of the body (**Fig. 6–21**). There have been no studies of the Ludington test and its clinical usefulness.

Biceps Tenderness

Some consider the presence of tenderness along the proximal biceps tendon a necessary criterion for the diagnosis of biceps tendinitis or associated pathologies.

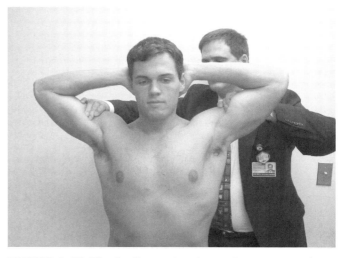

FIGURE 6–20 The Ludington test is another way to palpate for a torn long head of the biceps muscle.

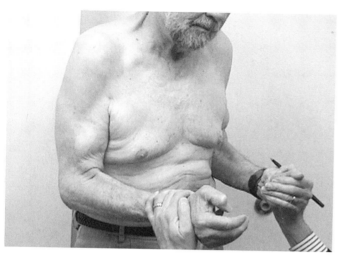

FIGURE 6–21 A tear of the long head of the biceps tendon can be detected by resisting elbow flexion of both arms and then palpating the muscle belly bilaterally.

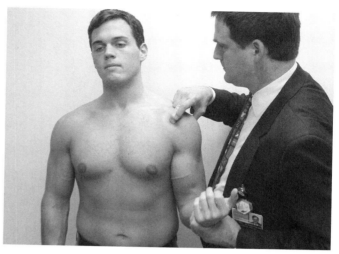

FIGURE 6–22 The long head of the biceps tendon can be palpated by externally rotating the arm 30 degrees, flexing and extending the elbow, and feeling for tendon movement anteriorly under the examiner's finger.

Crenshaw and Kilgore,[67] in their retrospective study of patients who underwent a biceps tenodesis at the Campbell Clinic, found that 88 of 89 patients had tenderness of the biceps at the intertubercular groove.

It is recognized by many physicians, however, that palpation of the intertubercular groove and proximal biceps tendon is not as easy as one might expect. There are many structures that converge at the upper end of the intertubercular groove, including the fasciculus obliquus from the anterior edge of the supraspinatus, the superior edge of the subscapularis tendon, the coracohumeral ligament, and portions of the superior glenohumeral ligament.[68-70] Also, in large or obese individuals it is difficult to identify reliably the intertubercular groove or the biceps tendon.

A second issue is the best position of the arm for palpating the bicipital groove. With the arm in an internally rotated position, the biceps tendon is beneath the conjointed tendon and near the anterior joint line. Palpation with the arm in this position will be unable to distinguish the bicipital groove from other structures. Matsen and Kirby[71] suggested that the bicipital groove is pointed directly anteriorly when the arm is in 10 degrees of internal rotation; however, we feel that with the biceps tendon in this position it is difficult to distinguish it from the anterior joint line. We suggest that the arm be externally rotated at least 30 degrees to remove it from the anterior joint line. Then, with the arm in this position, the elbow should be flexed and extended with one hand, while the tendon is palpated with the other (**Fig. 6–22**).

We studied the relationship of biceps tenderness to the presence of partial tears of the biceps tendon (unpublished data). In our cohort of 855 patients, 42 had partial biceps tears (5%). Biceps tenderness was found in 50% of the patients with a partial biceps tendon tear. The specificity

and sensitivity of tenderness of the biceps tendon for partial biceps tendon tears were 54 and 53%, respectively. The likelihood ratio for biceps tenderness making the diagnosis of partial biceps tearing was 1.52, indicating that biceps tenderness alone is not helpful in confirming the diagnosis of partial tears of the biceps tendon.

Despite these precautions, Burkhart et al[57] studied biceps tenderness as a sign for the varieties of type II SLAP lesions of the shoulder. They found that the incidence of tenderness varied according to the type, with tenderness more typical in anterior or combined type II lesions. In their study the sensitivity of biceps tenderness was 100% for anterior lesions, 74% for combined lesions, and 32% for posterior lesions; however, in their study the specificity of local tenderness for any of the lesions was less than 47%. This means that local tenderness along the biceps will make the diagnosis in only half of the patients, but when it is present, it can be specific.

> Local tenderness over the biceps tendon is not a sensitive or specific test for biceps tendon pathology.

Supination Sign of Yergason

In 1931 Yergason[72] described a test for biceps synovitis or of "wear and tear" of the biceps tendon. The test was performed with the elbow flexed 90 degrees and the forearm pronated. The examiner then should hold the subject at the wrist and resist active supination of the forearm. It was considered a positive test if the patient localized pain to the bicipital groove (**Fig. 6–23**). He suggested that this sign would be negative in cases of partial- or full-thickness tears of the rotator cuff.

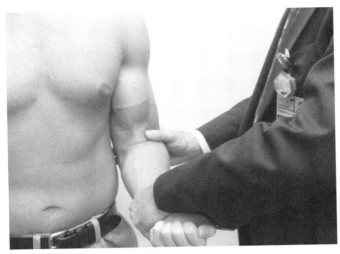

FIGURE 6–23 The Yergason's test is resisted supination of the forearm.

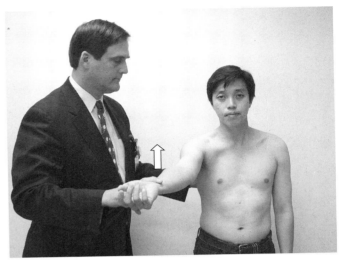

FIGURE 6–24 Speed's test is positive when pain is produced by resisted arm elevation.

The clinical usefulness of Yergason's test was studied by Holtby and Razmjou,[73] who evaluated a cohort of 50 patients with biceps tendon pathology. These pathologies included partial- and full-thickness tears of the biceps tendon. The authors found that Yergason's test had a sensitivity of 43%, a specificity of 79%, and an overall accuracy of 63%. The likelihood ratio was 2.05, which indicates that it is not a reliable test for making the diagnosis of biceps pathology.

Some authors have suggested that Yergason's test is helpful in the diagnosis of SLAP lesions; however, only one study by Parentis et al[62] used Yergason's test in the evaluation of a cohort of patients with shoulder pain and SLAP lesions. They found that in patients with type II SLAP lesions, Yergason's test had a sensitivity of 93%, but a specificity of only 13%.

Our personal experience with this test is that it rarely causes pain at the shoulder, regardless of the presence of biceps pathology or SLAP lesions. We no longer use this test.

Speed's Test

The history of Speed's test may never be entirely known, but Bennett[68] suggests that J. Spencer Speed of the Campbell Clinic made the association between biceps tendinitis and shoulder pain based on Speed's own personal experience. Crenshaw and Kilgore[67] also attributed this test to Speed in 1966, but to our knowledge Dr. Speed never described the test in the literature himself. Speed would apparently experience anterior shoulder pain when performing a straight leg examination on his patients, which he did with his forearm supinated, his elbow extended, and his arm forward flexed. He attributed the pain to biceps tendon synovitis.

Crenshaw and Kilgore[67] suggested that Speed's test is performed by having the patient elevate the extremity in flexion against resistance with the elbow extended and the forearm supinated (**Fig. 6–24**). The degree of horizontal extension was not specified, but the test has typically been performed with the arm directly in front of the shoulder or with slight horizontal extension (10 degrees). The test is positive if pain is localized to the bicipital groove.

There have been three studies evaluating the clinical usefulness of Speed's test (**Table 6–8**). The first study was performed by Bennett.[68] He studied prospectively 45 patients undergoing arthroscopy of the shoulder with a Speed's test. He considered pathology that would produce a positive test to include SLAP lesions, full tears of the biceps tendon, or partial biceps tendon tears visible at the time of arthroscopy of the shoulder. At the time of arthroscopy, Bennett would pull the

TABLE 6–8 Diagnostic Value of the Speed's Test in Three Different Studies (Percentages)

	Specificity	Sensitivity	NPV	PPV	Accuracy
Bennett[68]	13.8	90	83	23	NA
Holtby and Razmjou[73]	75	32	58	50	56
JHU cohort[a]	67	50	96	8	66

[a]The Johns Hopkins University Shoulder Database.

TABLE 6–9 Diagnostic Values of Clinical Tests in Patients with a Partial Biceps Tendon Tear (*N* = 40)

Clinical Tests	Sensitivity	Specificity	PPV	NPV	AC	LR
Biceps palpation	0.53	0.54	0.06	0.95	0.54	1.13
Speed test	0.50	0.67	0.08	0.96	0.66	1.51
Neer sign	0.64	0.41	0.05	0.96	0.43	1.09
Hawkins sign	0.55	0.38	0.05	0.94	0.39	0.89
Crank test	0.34	0.77	0.11	0.93	0.74	1.49
Belly press	0.17	0.92	0.24	0.88	0.82	2.01
Active compression palm down	0.68	0.46	0.08	0.95	0.47	1.24
Active compression palm up	0.40	0.57	0.06	0.93	0.56	0.93
Lift-off test	0.28	0.89	0.15	0.95	0.85	2.61
Kibler test	0.23	0.84	0.09	0.94	0.80	1.40

Source: Data from The Johns Hopkins University Shoulder Database.
AC, overall accuracy; LR, likelihood ratio; NPV, negative predictive value; PPV, positive predictive value.

biceps tendon intra-articularly to try to visualize lesions that might be in the portion of the tendon in the bicipital groove.

In his cohort of patients Speed's test was positive in 40 patients, but biceps pathology was seen in only 10 patients. The specificity of Speed's test was 14%, the sensitivity 90%, the positive predictive value 23%, and the negative predictive value 83%. Bennett noted that there were many associated pathologies that could produce a positive test; these included Bankart lesions, impingement, a tight capsule, partial subscapularis tendon tears, and spurs on the coracoacromial ligament. In his assessment, the low specificity of Speed's test and low positive predictive value limited its usefulness.

A study by Holtby and Razmjou[73] evaluated Speed's test in a cohort of 50 patients undergoing shoulder surgery for bicipital tendinosis, subluxated or dislocated biceps tendons, partial or complete rupture of the biceps tendon, or SLAP lesions type II or IV. They found that Speed's test had a sensitivity of 32%, a specificity of 75%, and an overall accuracy of 56% for detecting biceps pathology or types II and IV SLAP lesions. The likelihood ratio was 1.28, which indicates that this test is not useful for the diagnosis of biceps tendon conditions or for SLAP lesions.

We examined the usefulness of Speed's test for making the diagnosis of partial tears of the biceps tendon, which was present in 42 of our cohort of 855 patients who had undergone shoulder arthroscopy (**Table 6–9**). Our study (unpublished data) found that the specificity and sensitivity of Speed's test in detecting partial biceps tears were 67% and 50%, respectively. The overall accuracy was 66%, and the likelihood ratio was 1.52. These results are similar to those of Holtby and Razmjou and indicate that Speed's test is not reliable for making the diagnosis of biceps tendon pathology.

We also examined the usefulness of Speed's test in making the diagnosis of SLAP tears. In our study of type II SLAP lesions, we found that Speed's test had a sensitivity of 28%, a specificity of 72%, a positive predictive value of 12%, a negative predictive value of

91%, and an overall diagnostic accuracy of 68% for SLAP lesions. This compares favorably to the results of Bennett,[68] so a positive Speed's test cannot be interpreted as ruling in a SLAP lesion. These findings reinforce the complexity of interpreting clinical tests of the shoulder where multiple pathologies exist or where the symptoms overlap.

Gilchrist Sign

The Gilchrist sign[21] was described by Gilchrist in 1936 as a diagnostic test for bicipital tendon dislocations.[74] In this test the patient is standing and is asked to extend the arms to an overhead extension and marked external rotation, if possible while holding a 5-pound weight in each hand (**Fig. 6–25**). The examiner can stand in front of or behind the patient, and the patient is asked to lower his or outstretched arm to the side in the coronal plane. When the arm reaches an angle of 110 to 90 degrees, a

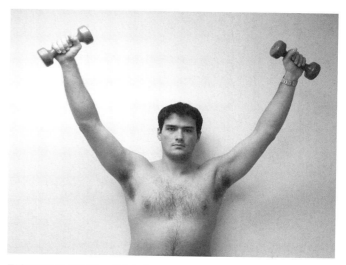

FIGURE 6–25 The Gilchrist sign is pain produced in the anterior shoulder when the patient is asked to elevate hand weights over several repetitions.

snap may be audible in the shoulder, and pain is felt in the region of the bicipital groove. This snap also may be felt by the examiner's fingers placed over the belly of the biceps and the tendon of the long head.

The Gilchrist sign has never been studied, and its clinical usefulness has not been established. The need to keep hand weights in the office is one disadvantage of this test.

Lippman Test

This test was described by Lippman[17] in 1943 to make the diagnosis of bicipital tendinosis or peri-tendinitis. This test is performed with the patient sitting or standing and with the examiner holding the arm of the patient flexed to 90 degrees. The examiner palpates the biceps tendon in the bicipital groove 6 to 8 cm below the glenohumeral joint and attempts to move it back and forth (**Fig. 6–26**). This test is positive if a sharp pain is felt by the patient in the biceps tendon where it is being flipped back and forth.

There are no studies of this test, and its clinical usefulness has never been studied. We have not found it easy to reliably palpate the biceps tendon or to be able to say that we are moving the tendon in that area as suggested.

Lateral Slide Test

In 1966 Crenshaw and Kilgore[67] described a test for biceps tendinitis that is similar in concept to the Lippman test. This is performed by attempting to hold the biceps tendon below the bicipital groove, then attempting to move it with one's fingers. Crenshaw and Kilgore described this test as flipping the tendon back

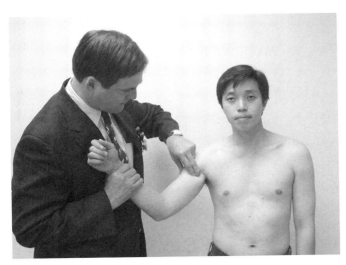

FIGURE 6–26 The Lippman test is palpation of the biceps tendon and involves flipping the long head of the biceps tendon beneath the examiner's finger.

and forth above its junction with the muscle belly. A positive result was pain localized to the bicipital groove.

The authors did not report what percentage of their patients had a positive test, and to our knowledge this test has not been studied or utilized in any study since that time. There is no indication that this test is a valuable examination technique.

Abbot Test for Biceps Instability

Instability of the biceps has become increasingly appreciated due to the ability to observe the biceps tendon arthroscopically. The test for biceps instability was initially described by Abbot et al in 1939.[75] This test for biceps instability involves first elevating the arm to full abduction and external rotation. The arm is then brought down to the side with progressive internal rotation. A positive test is a click or pop presumably due to the biceps tendon subluxating out of the groove. A variation of this test is to elevate the arm 90 degrees, then internally and externally rotate the arm. The patient or the examiner should feel a click or a clunk as the biceps tendon subluxates out of the bicipital groove.[51]

There are several concerns with this test. The first is that its validity has never been established by an anatomic or biomechanical study. There is currently no study that substantiates that the biceps tendon subluxates when the arm is placed in this position and rotated. There are no studies that demonstrate what structures would have to be torn to allow symptomatic subluxation to occur.

Second, one must keep in mind that there are many things in the shoulder that could be producing a click with the arm in this position, so it is difficult to ascribe a click to a subluxating biceps tendon. Third, biceps subluxations and dislocations are almost always associated with some form of rotator cuff pathology (particularly upper subscapularis tendon tears), so the symptoms of pain or of a click with an unstable biceps could be due in part to the cuff pathology.[49]

Last, there has been no reported study examining the validity or accuracy of this test in a large population. This test should currently be considered nonspecific and not diagnostic of any one pathology.

Biceps Entrapment Sign

A recently described entity of the biceps tendon is entrapment of the biceps tendon in the shoulder joint with elevation of the arm. Boileau et al[76] described this condition of the biceps tendon, which they called "hourglass biceps." This condition occurs when the bicep tendon develops an area of swelling in the bicipital groove, which gives it a fusiform shape. This abnormality of the biceps tendon can be seen only with the arthroscope when elevating the arm and viewing the joint through a posterior portal. With nearly full elevation the biceps tendon will be seen to fold into the joint, and a swollen or thickened area may be observed.

Werner et al[70] suggested that this entity can be suspected upon physical examination if the patient has a limitation of 10 to 20 degrees short of full elevation of the shoulder in flexion. This loss of motion is best demonstrated with the patient supine. Both active and passive motion should be restricted. Any attempt to increase the motion should result in increased shoulder pain. The authors suggest that this entity can appear like a frozen or stiff shoulder. The definitive diagnosis of "hourglass biceps" entrapment had to be made with arthroscopy.

Boileau et al[76] reported on 21 patients with biceps entrapment; 11 were involved in manual professions with some degree of overhead activity (e.g., painter, mason, carpenter). All of the patients had full-thickness rotator cuff tears. During arthroscopy all patients had hypertrophy and incarceration and buckling of the intra-articular portion of the long head of the biceps during passive elevation.

Other positive physical findings in this cohort of patients included a biceps tenderness in 15 patients (71%), a positive Speed's test in 10 patients (48%), and a positive Jobe's test for supraspinatus weakness in 17 patients (81%). The major characteristic of this patient population was the loss of terminal flexion of around 10 to 20 degrees of elevation.

There was no control group in this descriptive study by Boileau et al, so it is difficult to evaluate the specificity or sensitivity of this physical finding for making the diagnosis of hourglass biceps tendon. Further study is warranted of this finding and relatively recently reported entity.

Lift-off Test

The lift-off test was described by Gerber and Krushell[77] and was considered to be a sign of subscapularis tearing. However, Yamaguchi and Bindra[41] found that increased pain in the front of the shoulder with internal rotation up the back and with a positive lift-off test might indicate that the patient had biceps tendon pathology.

This test (**Fig. 6–27**) is performed by maximally internally rotating the patient's hand up his or her back; the patient then lifts the hand off the back. This test can be modified by asking the patient to hold his or her hand up the back at the level of the belt or buttocks. The patient is then asked to lift the hand off the back and hold it there. If the patient cannot hold it, then a partial- or full-thickness tear of the subscapularis should be considered. Because many patients with biceps tendon subluxations have partial- or full-thickness tears of the subscapularis, a

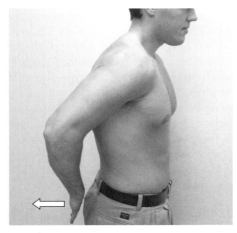

FIGURE 6–27 The lift-off test can be used to detect pathology of the long head of the biceps tendon, but it is more helpful for detecting tears of the subscapularis tendon.

positive test may indicate not only subscapularis but also biceps tendon pathology.

Although it is common to see patients with increased pain in the shoulder with internal rotation up the back, this observation is very nonspecific and could indicate a variety of diagnoses. The spectrum of entities that could cause pain with the arm up the back includes a stiff shoulder, supraspinatus tendon tears, subscapularis tendon tears, and arthritis of any cause. In our study of partial tears of the biceps tendon, however, we found that the lift-off test was sensitive in 27% and specific in 89%, and had an overall accuracy of 86%. The likelihood ratio is 2.53, which indicates that the liftoff test is not a good test for making the diagnosis of partial tears of the biceps tendon.

As a result, we do not feel that either increased pain up the back with internal rotation or a positive lift-off test is diagnostic for biceps tendon pathology. There have been no other studies to our knowledge that have examined the validity or accuracy of either of these observations for biceps tendon pathology.

Injection of the Biceps Tendon

Differential injections of various structures around the shoulder can be beneficial when attempting to make the diagnosis, especially of AC joint pathologies and rotator cuff disease. Injections into the biceps tendon for diagnostic or therapeutic reasons have not received widespread use for several reasons. First, the biceps tendon is intra-articular until it reaches the bicipital groove, where it is covered by the transverse ligament. This space is quite tight, and it is difficult to get a needle into it.

Second, locating the bicipital groove is not easy by palpation, particularly in muscular or heavy individuals. Third, if a patient has a rotator cuff tear and the biceps tendon or joint is exposed, theoretically any injection into the subacromial space will reach the biceps and bicipital groove. If a patient with a rotator cuff tear has relief of anterior shoulder pain with an injection, then it is impossible to know whether the pain was from the cuff tear or the biceps tendon.

Some have suggested that differential injections into the subacromial space and the shoulder joint can distinguish between biceps tendon pain and other etiologies of the pain.[41,78] Neviaser[78] suggested that if no pain relief is obtained from injecting the subacromial space with local anesthetic, then the joint should be injected. He commented that if the pain went away, presumably the anesthetic decreased the pain of bicipital tenosynovitis.

This approach of routinely injecting the long head of the biceps tendon has not been popular for several reasons. When injecting the bicipital groove area, it is difficult to know if the biceps has been accurately injected. In addition,, injections of the shoulder joint are equally difficult for both the experienced and inexperienced practitioner, and it is frequently difficult to know if the anesthetic has inadvertently entered the joint, the subacromial bursa, or other structures. Yamaguchi and Bindra[41] found that the accuracy of the injection can be improved with the use of ultrasound. Finally, an intra-articular injection into the shoulder joint could provide anesthesia for any number of shoulder pathologies, not just biceps pathologies. Intra-articular injections are nonspecific and do not reliably identify any single pathological process.

Technique
When injecting the biceps tendon, the patient can be sitting or supine. We prefer the supine position because the patient will be more relaxed and the arm can be extended slightly to bring the proximal shoulder more anterior (**Fig. 6–28**). The arm is then externally rotated

20 to 30 degrees to bring the biceps tendon away from the anterior shoulder. An assistant holds the patient by the elbow as the forearm is flexed and extended. The examiner then palpates the tendon and bicipital groove to feel the tendon as it slides in the groove.

The injection is done with sterile technique, and in some larger individuals a spinal needle may be needed to reach the bicipital groove area. We typically inject as the needle is inserted to provide anesthesia to the surrounding tissues. The needle is then inserted into the bicipital groove, and its location is confirmed by feeling the biceps tendon moving beneath the needle. Care is taken not to inject into the tendon itself. Once the anesthetic has had a chance to take effect, if the patient still has pain, we recommend injection of the subacromial space.

■ Specific Tests for SLAP Lesions

Compression Rotation Sign

This test was first described in 1990 by Snyder et al.[12] With the patient supine, the arm is abducted 90 degrees, and an axial load is applied to the proximal humerus, which compresses it into the glenoid (**Fig. 6–29**). The arm is then rotated around similar to the method used when performing a McMurray's test in the knee. The compression rotation sign is based on the idea that a labral fragment may get caught or trapped in the joint, much like a McMurray's test. There have been few studies that examine the clinical usefulness of this test.[28] Our study[28] of this test demonstrated that for type I SLAP lesions, it is 22% sensitive and 75% specific. For type II SLAP lesions, the test is 19% sensitive and 75% specific (**Table 6–10**). Although it is possible that the labrum is torn enough to produce symptoms of catching or

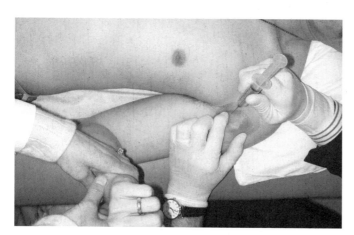

FIGURE 6–28 When injecting the long head of the biceps tendon, the tendon can be found by externally rotating the arm and then flexing and extending the elbow.

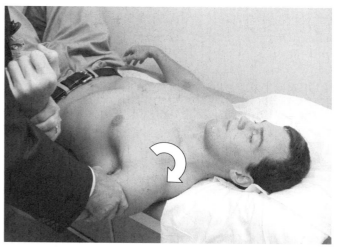

FIGURE 6–29 The compression rotation test for SLAP lesions involves compression of the humerus into the glenoid and then circular rotation of the arm.

and then an anterior apprehension maneuver is performed. When the patient becomes apprehensive, external rotation is stopped. The patient is then asked to actively flex the forearm at the elbow by bringing the hand toward his or her face. Upon resistance by the examiner, the patient is asked if the feeling of instability is improved, unchanged, or worsened. If the feeling of instability or apprehension is improved, then there is no SLAP lesion. If the pain is unimproved or worsened, then there is the suspicion of a SLAP lesion. The researchers note that the forearm should be supinated during the test and that the examiner should be at the same level of the patient by sitting in a chair.

In their analysis of this test, Kim et al compared the results of the biceps load test with other tests used for detecting biceps pathology. For the biceps load test, they found a sensitivity of 91%, a specificity of 97%, a positive predictive value of 83%, and a negative predictive value of 98% for combined SLAP lesions in shoulders with recurrent unilateral anterior dislocations. They emphasized that their results were based on a study of only patients with anterior shoulder instability.

It should be noted that in their study there was no control group and no mention of which examiners were performing the test. However, they did test the interobserver reliability and found that the examiners had a kappa of 0.846, which is in the good to excellent range. In addition, this test takes some coordination and cooperation on the part of the physician and the patient.

We have limited clinical experience with this test. To our knowledge there are no independent studies that support the findings of the originators of this test.

Biceps Load Test II

This test, described by Kim and co-workers,[85] is a variation of the biceps load test I designed for isolated SLAP lesions independent of shoulder instability. The rationale for the test is that resisted flexion of the arm with the forearm in a supinated position places stress on the proximal biceps anchor.

The second version of the biceps load test differs from the first in two ways: the arm position for the test and the definition of a positive test. In test II, the patient is supine, but the arm is abducted to 120 degrees of elevation. The arm is then externally rotated to its maximal extent, and the elbow is flexed 90 degrees and the forearm supinated (**Fig. 6–36**). The patient is asked to flex the elbow toward the head while the examiner resists that motion. A positive test is the presence of pain with the test or increased pain over baseline with the test. A negative test is the absence of pain or a lack of increase in the baseline pain. Kim et al studied 127 patients, and all of them underwent diagnostic arthroscopy. They found that for SLAP lesions the test had a sensitivity of 90%, a

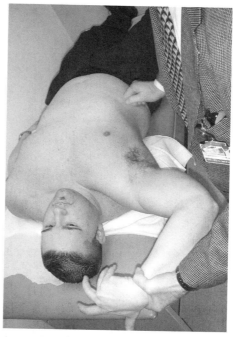

FIGURE 6–36 The biceps load II test adds resisted forearm supination to the biceps load I test.

specificity of 97%, a positive predictive value of 92%, and a negative predictive value of 96%. We have limited clinical experience with this test. There are no other independent studies evaluating its accuracy.

Pain Provocation Test

This test was described by Mimori et al[81] and is similar to the biceps load test described by Kim et al.[64] The patient is placed in a sitting position, and the arm is elevated to 90 to 100 degrees of abduction (**Fig. 6–37**). The examiner stands behind the patient and holds the arm with one hand while stabilizing the shoulder with the other. The arm is then externally rotated to its maximum until the patient reports pain. The test should be performed with the forearm in supination and in pronation. The authors say that this position is similar to an anterior apprehension position. A positive test is when the pain is present only with the forearm in the pronated position or if it is worse than the pain with the arm in the supinated position.

Mimori et al's study included 32 patients who experienced pain with overhead sports activities, such as baseball ($N = 30$), volleyball ($N = 1$), and football ($N = 1$). None of the patients had overt instability of the shoulder, and all had negative relocation tests for anterior shoulder instability. Only 15 of their patients underwent arthroscopic evaluation, and the results of MRI-arthrography were used to calculate the final results. The researchers found that the test had a sensitivity of 100%, a specificity of 90%, and an accuracy of 97%.

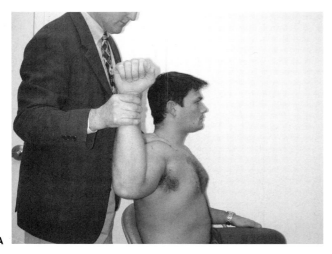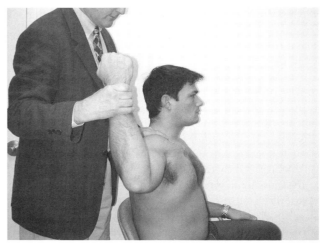

FIGURE 6–37 (A,B) The pain provocation test is positive when pain is produced in the shoulder with rotation of the forearm with the arm abducted 90 degrees.

There are no other studies of this test available in the literature. The results are influenced in part by patient selection and by the confidence of the authors in the accuracy of MRI-arthrography. Further study is needed before this test can be recommended.

"SLAPrehension" Test

This test was described in 1998 by Berg and Ciullo[61] and is almost identical to the active compression test described by O'Brien et al[83] in the same year. The patient is asked to flex the arm to 90 degrees and adduct the arm across the body at an unspecified angle (**Fig. 6–38**). The patient is to

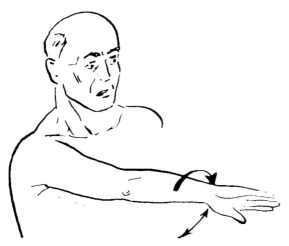

FIGURE 6–38 The "SLAPrehension test" is a variation of the active compression test and is positive if it produces pain in the anterior shoulder along the biceps tendon. (Adapted with permission from Berg EE, Ciullo JV. A clinical test for superior glenoid labral or SLAP lesions. Clin J Sport Med 1998;8(2): 121–123.)

hold the elbow in full extension and with the thumb pointed down. The examiner then resists an upward motion of the arm. If there is a SLAP lesion, then the patient should report pain into the bicipital groove area anteriorly. The test is then repeated with the forearm supinated, and the pain should decrease in intensity. If it does not increase, then the test is negative or indeterminate.

The authors suggested that the reason the pain diminished with the arm supinated was that the labrum fragment was not entrapped between the humeral head and the superior glenoid. They performed a retrospective study of 66 patients who at the time of arthroscopy were found to have SLAP lesions. Using the classification of Snyder,[12] there were 10 type I, 50 type II, 3 type III, and 3 type IV lesions. The test identified only 50% of the type I lesions (sensitivity of 50%) but 87.5% of the type II–IV-lesions.

The authors did not perform a thorough statistical analysis of this test and did not include patients who did not have SLAP lesions. They suggested that further study of this test was warranted, and we would agree. In our experience it is difficult to localize pain to the bicipital groove in patients with anterior shoulder pain. In addition, many patients with SLAP lesions report pain deep in the shoulder and not to the anterior aspect of the shoulder. This variation of the active compression test does not appear to have any advantages over that test and has not received widespread use among clinicians.

Relocation (Jobe) Test

The relocation test was first described by Dr. Frank Jobe and colleagues[86] in the late 1980s for evaluating shoulder pain in the overhead athlete. The test was performed with the patient supine, and the examiner placed the passive affected arm into abduction and

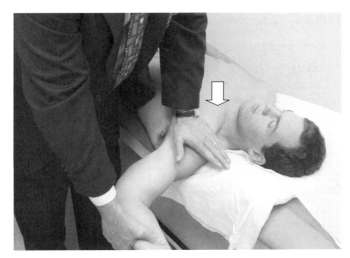

FIGURE 6–39 The relocation test may be positive in patients with SLAP lesions.

external rotation. The position of the arm was essentially a supine apprehension sign. According to Jobe et al, in the thrower with occult instability and stretching of the anterior capsule and ligaments, this position should produce impingement pain into the deltoid region. They felt this was due to the rotator cuff impinging upon the acromion. The examiner would then stabilize the humeral head by pushing posteriorly on the humeral head, which would relieve the impingement pain (Fig. 6–39). If the pain went away with stabilizing the humeral head, the patient was felt to have occult anteroinferior instability; if conservative measures failed, the patient would benefit from an anterior capsular shift.

Several years later, in the early 1990s, Dr. Chris Jobe[87] noticed that many of the throwers had posterior shoulder pain and also SLAP lesions. With the relocation test, the pain seen posteriorly in these athletes would often be relieved by stabilizing the humeral head with a posteriorly directed force. Jobe postulated that this pain was due to contact of the proximal humerus to the posterior and superior labrum, which Walch et al[55] had termed "internal impingement." Jobe believed that anteroinferior instability was responsible for this internal impingement, and when the head was stabilized, the contact would be relieved along with the pain.

This relief of contact of the rotator cuff to the posterior and superior labrum with a relocation maneuver can be demonstrated arthroscopically (see Chapter 5); however, not all patients who have pain when the arm is in abduction and external rotation experience pain relief with stabilization of the humeral head. Jobe never specified what it meant if the pain was not improved with this maneuver.

Burkhart et al[57] utilized the relocation test (Fig. 6–39) to evaluate their cohort of patients with one of three kinds of type II SLAP lesions. A positive test was the elimination of posterosuperior shoulder pain when the head was stabilized, and all of their patients had the diagnosis of a SLAP lesion confirmed with arthroscopy. The authors found that the relocation maneuver had the highest sensitivity for posterior type II SLAP lesions (85%), followed by combined type II SLAP lesions (59%) and type II anterior lesions (4%) (Table 6–11). The specificity of the relocation test for type II SLAP lesions varied from 68% (posterior lesions) to 54% (combined lesions) and 27% (anterior lesions). In their study of the relocation maneuver for SLAP lesions, 31% of the patients had rotator cuff tears that might have confounded the findings.

Further study of the accuracy of this test for the three variants of SLAP lesion is warranted. We have no clinical experience with this test in terms of its usefulness for one type of type II SLAP lesion over another type of SLAP lesion. Burkhart et al's study would suggest that the relocation test should be part of the evaluation of any patient who is suspected of having a SLAP lesion. Further study is warranted, and it will require large numbers of patients with these varieties of type II SLAP lesions to substantiate the usefulness of this test for the detection of SLAP lesions.

Mayo Shear Test

The Mayo shear test to date has only been presented by Dr. S. O'Driscoll (personal communication, 2000) at professional meetings and has not previously been described in the literature as a clinical study. The clinical exam is performed with the patient standing or sitting and the examiner behind the patient. The patient then elevates the arm and reports the location of the pain (Fig. 6–40). The patient should localize the pain to the

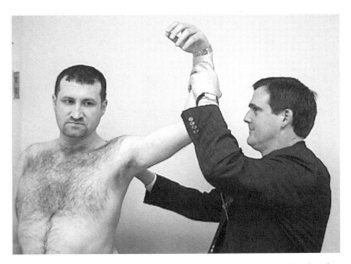

FIGURE 6–40 The Mayo shear test produces pain in the posterior shoulder when the arm is moved up and down in elevation with an anterior directed force on the shoulder.

posterior and superior shoulder with elevation and depression of the arm.

This test has not been statistically studied, but our experience has been that it may have promise in the detection particularly of type II combined or posterior lesions. This sentiment is echoed by Dr. Ben Kibler (personal communication, 2005). It also can cause pain in patients who have tight shoulders, so it should be interpreted with caution.

Savoie Test

This test was described by Savoie et al[88] and is designed to diagnose a specific injury complex called SLAC lesions (*s*uperior *l*abrum, *a*nterior *c*uff), which includes patients with SLAP lesions and partial-thickness supraspinatus tendon tears. This test is performed with the patient seated and the examiner standing to the side (**Fig. 6–41**). The arm is elevated to 90 degrees and the arm externally rotated. The examiner places his or her hand with the thumb in the back and the fingers in the front. An anteriorly directed force is applied by the thumb pushing the shoulder first straight anteriorly and then anteriorly/superiorly. A positive test is when there are one of three findings: (1) there is a clunk associated with some translation; (2) there is a clunk, and the humeral head stays subluxated out of the joint; or (3) there is pain only with the maneuver.

In his study of 40 patients with SLAC lesions, Savoie et al found this test positive in 35 of 40 patients (88%). In this same cohort they found that the anterior slide test (Kibler) was positive in 37 (93%), the active compression test was positive in 35 (88%), and the Whipple test for partial cuff tears was positive in 40 (100%).

To our knowledge there have been no independent studies of the validity or accuracy of the Savoie test. In our limited clinical experience, this test can be difficult

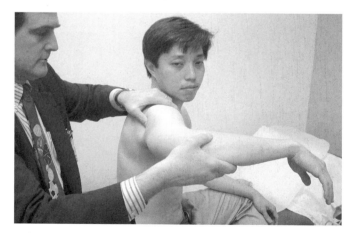

FIGURE 6–41 The Savoie test is another technique for creating shear on the shoulder with the arm in various positions.

TABLE 6–12 Analysis of Results in Patients Undergoing Three Tests (*N* = 294)

Positive Results	Control Group* (n = 266)	SLAP Group[†] (n = 28)	Significance (p Value)
None	114 (43%)	12 (43%)	>.05
One	104 (39%)	12 (43%)[‡]	>.05
Two	35 (13%)	4 (14%)[§]	>.05
Three	13 (5%)	0	NA

*266/299 in control group (299 patients with no lesions and 88 patients with type I SLAP lesions).

[†]28/34 in SLAP group (34 type II lesions, 1 type III lesion, and 4 type IV lesions).

[‡]Ten patients with SLAP lesions showed positive tests only in active compression test, and two showed positive compression rotation tests. No patient with a SLAP lesion showed a positive result only in the anterior slide test.

[§]Three patients with SLAP lesions showed positive results in both the compression rotation and active compression tests. One patient with a SLAP lesion showed positive results in both the compression rotation and anterior slide tests. NA, not applicable; SLAP, superior labrum anterior and posterior.

to perform in the patient who has pain with elevation to 90 degrees or with external rotation of the shoulder in this position. Also, pain with this maneuver may be nonspecific for SLAP lesions, and it should be interpreted with caution.

Combined Tests for SLAP Lesions

There are few studies that evaluate the usefulness of more than one test in the diagnosis of SLAP lesions. In our study of the compression rotation test, the active compression test, and the anterior slide test, we found that it was unusual for a patient with a SLAP lesion to have all three tests positive (**Table 6–12**).[28] The incidence of one, two, or three tests positive was nearly the same for patients with SLAP lesions as for patients who had no SLAP lesions.

This study was limited by the use of only three physical examinations designed specifically for SLAP lesions; however, we performed a similar study using a variety of physical examination tests (**Table 6–11**). We again found that no one test or combination of tests typically used for evaluating the painful shoulder would accurately diagnose a SLAP lesion.[52]

As a result, there is no study that demonstrates that one combination of tests increases the accuracy of the examination for SLAP lesions.

■ Arthroscopy and SLAP–Biceps Lesions

There is increasing evidence that the gold standard for making the diagnosis of SLAP lesions is an arthroscopic evaluation of the shoulder. Although many signs upon physical examination may be sensitive for SLAP lesions, their specificity is low, which means that they will miss a large percentage of SLAP lesions. In addition, these physical examination tests are difficult to interpret because they can produce pain in a variety of locations in the shoulder.

In our practice, we do not operate on a patient because we feel that he or she has a SLAP lesion upon examination; rather, we do so when the the patient has failed nonoperative treatment. The archetypical patient who is suspicious for a SLAP lesion is an overhead athlete who has posterior and superior shoulder pain. This pain in the posterior and superior shoulder can be reproduced with any maneuver where the arm is abducted and externally rotated. The battery of tests described earlier will probably be more accurate in studies limited to these individuals.

The diagnosis of isolated biceps pathology continues to be controversial, and there are no tests that accurately predict biceps pathology. We do not place any faith in Speed's and Yergason's tests, and the diagnosis of biceps pathology remains an arthroscopic one. The patient at risk for biceps pathology typically has rotator cuff disease, and we feel that one should not be considered without the other. There is little support for operating on the biceps tendon based on physical examination alone.

REFERENCES

1. Codman, E., *The Shoulder: Rupture of the Supraspinatus Tendon and Other Lesions in or about the Subacromial Bursa.* 1934, Boston: Thomas Todd.
2. Meyer, A., *Spontaneous dislocation and destruction of the tendon of the long head of the biceps brachii.* Arch Surg, 1921. **17**:p.493–506.
3. Meyer, A., *Spontaneous dislocation of the tendon of the long head of biceps brachii.* Arch Surg, 1926. **13**:p.109–119.
4. Habermeyer, P., P. Magosch, M. Pritsch, M.T. Scheibel, and S. Lichtenberg, *Anterosuperior impingement of the shoulder as a result of pulley lesions: A prospective arthroscopic study.* J Shoulder Elbow Surg, 2004. **13**(1):p.5–12.
5. Vangsness, C.T., Jr., S.S. Jorgenson, T. Watson, and D.L. Johnson, *The origin of the long head of the biceps from the scapula and glenoid labrum. An anatomical study of 100 shoulders.* J Bone Joint Surg Br, 1994. **76**(6):p.951–954.
6. Ilahi, O.A., *Anatomical variants in the anterosuperior aspect of the glenoid labrum.* J Bone Joint Surg Am, 2004. **86-A**(2):p.432–3; author reply 433.
7. Rao, A.G., T.K. Kim, E. Chronopoulos, and E.G. McFarland, *Anatomical variants in the anterosuperior aspect of the glenoid labrum: a statistical analysis of seventy-three cases.* J Bone Joint Surg Am, 2003. **85-A**(4):p.653–9.
8. Nove-Josserand, L. and G. Walch, *Long biceps tendon*, in *Shoulder Surgery*, N. Wulker, M. Mansat, and F.H. Fu, Editors. 2001, Martin Dunitz: London. p.243–259.
9. Neer, C.S., 2nd, *Impingement lesions.* Clin Orthop Relat Res, 1983(173):p.70–7.
10. Neer, C.S., L.U. Bigliani, and R.J. Hawkins, *Rupture of the long head of biceps related to subacromial impingement.* Orthop trans, 1977. **1**:p.111.
11. Hitchcock, H.H. and C.O. Bechtol, *Painfull shoulder: Observations on the role of the tendon of the long head of biceps brachii and it's causation.* J Bone Joint Surg Am, 1948. **30**:p.263–273.
12. Snyder, S.J., R.P. Karzel, W. Del Pizzo, R.D. Ferkel, and M.J. Friedman, *SLAP lesions of the shoulder.* Arthroscopy, 1990. **6**(4):p.274–9.
13. Burkhart, S.S. and D.L. Fox, *SLAP lesions in association with complete tears of the long head of the biceps tendon: a report of two cases.* Arthroscopy, 1992. **8**(1):p.31–5.
14. Andrews, J.R., W.G. Carson, Jr., and W.D. McLeod, *Glenoid labrum tears related to the long head of the biceps.* Am J Sports Med, 1985. **13**(5): p.337–41.
15. Maffet, M.W., G.M. Gartsman, and B. Moseley, *Superior labrum-biceps tendon complex lesions of the shoulder.* Am J Sports Med, 1995. **23**(1): p.93–8.
16. Morgan, C.D., S.S. Burkhart, M. Palmeri, and M. Gillespie, *Type II SLAP lesions: three subtypes and their relationships to superior instability and rotator cuff tears.* Arthroscopy, 1998. **14**(6):p.553–65.
17. Lippman, R.K., *Frozen shoulder; Periarthritis; Bicipital tendinitis.* Arch Surg, 1943. **7**:p.283–296.
18. Warner, J.J. and P.J. McMahon, *The role of the long head of the biceps brachii in superior stability of the glenohumeral joint.* J Bone Joint Surg Am, 1995. **77**(3):p.366–72.
19. Itoi, E., S.R. Newman, D.K. Kuechle, B.F. Morrey, and K.N. An, *Dynamic anterior stabilisers of the shoulder with the arm in abduction.* J Bone Joint Surg Br, 1994. **76**(5):p.834–6.
20. Rodosky, M.W., C.D. Harner, and F.H. Fu, *The role of the long head of the biceps muscle and superior glenoid labrum in anterior stability of the shoulder.* Am J Sports Med, 1994. **22**(1):p.121–30.
21. Itoi, E., D.K. Kuechle, S.R. Newman, B.F. Morrey, and K.N. An, *Stabilising function of the biceps in stable and unstable shoulders.* J Bone Joint Surg Br, 1993. **75**(4):p.546–50.
22. Pradhan, R.L., E. Itoi, Y. Hatakeyama, M. Urayama, and K. Sato, *Superior labral strain during the throwing motion. A cadaveric study.* Am J Sports Med, 2001. **29**(4):p.488–92.
23. Levy, A.S., B.T. Kelly, S.A. Lintner, D.C. Osbahr, and K.P. Speer, *Function of the long head of the biceps at the shoulder: electromyographic analysis.* J Shoulder Elbow Surg, 2001. **10**(3):p.250–5.
24. Yamaguchi, K., K.D. Riew, L.M. Galatz, J.A. Syme, and R.J. Neviaser, *Biceps activity during shoulder motion: an electromyographic analysis.* Clin Orthop, 1997(336):p.122–9.
25. Jobe, C.M., M.M. Pink, F.W. Jobe, and B. Shaffer, *Anterior Shoulder Instability, Impingement, and Rotator Cuff Tear*, in *Operative Techniques in Upper Extremity Sports Injuries*, F.W. Jobe, Editor. 1996, Mosby: St. Louis.p.164–272.
26. Werner, S.L., T.J. Gill, T.A. Murray, T.D. Cook, and R.J. Hawkins, *Relationships between throwing mechanics and shoulder distraction in professional baseball pitchers.* Am J Sports Med, 2001. **29**(3): p.354–8.
27. Bey, M.J., G.J. Elders, L.J. Huston, J.E. Kuhn, R.B. Blasier, and L.J. Soslowsky, *The mechanism of creation of superior labrum, anterior, and posterior lesions in a dynamic biomechanical model of the shoulder: the role of inferior subluxation.* J Shoulder Elbow Surg, 1998. **7**(4): p.397–401.
28. McFarland, E.G., T.K. Kim, and R.M. Savino, *Clinical assessment of three common tests for superior labral anterior-posterior lesions.* Am J Sports Med, 2002. **30**(6):p.810–5.
29. Burkhart, S.S., C.D. Morgan, and W.B. Kibler, *The disabled throwing shoulder: spectrum of pathology Part I: pathoanatomy and biomechanics.* Arthroscopy, 2003. **19**(4):p.404–20.
30. Burkhart, S.S., C.D. Morgan, and W.B. Kibler, *The disabled throwing shoulder: spectrum of pathology. Part II: evaluation and treatment of SLAP lesions in throwers.* Arthroscopy, 2003. **19**(5):p.531–9.
31. Burkhart, S.S., C.D. Morgan, and W.B. Kibler, *The disabled throwing shoulder: spectrum of pathology Part III: The SICK scapula, scapular dyskinesis, the kinetic chain, and rehabilitation.* Arthroscopy, 2003. **19**(6):p.641–61.
32. Schulz, C.U., H. Anetzberger, M. Maier, M. Pfahler, and H.J. Refior, *The sublabral foramen: Does it affect stress distribution on the anterior glenoid?* J Shoulder Elbow Surg, 2004. **13**(1):p.35–38.
33. Pagnani, M.J., X.H. Deng, R.F. Warren, P.A. Torzilli, and D.W. Altchek, *Effect of lesions of the superior portion of the glenoid labrum on*

glenohumeral translation. J Bone Joint Surg Am, 1995. **77**(7): p.1003–10.

34. McMahon, P.J., A. Burkart, V. Musahl, and R.E. Debski, *Glenohumeral translations are increased after a type II superior labrum anterior-posterior lesion: A cadaveric study of severity of passive stabilizer injury.* J Shoulder Elbow Surg, 2004. **13**(1):p.39–44.

35. Burkhart, S.S. and C.D. Morgan, *The peel-back mechanism: its role in producing and extending posterior type II SLAP lesions and its effect on SLAP repair rehabilitation.* Arthroscopy, 1998. **14**(6):p.637–40.

36. McFarland, E.G., Hsu CY, Neira C, O'Neil O., *Internal impingement of the shoulder: A clinical and arthroscopic analysis.* J Shoulder Elbow Surg, 1999. **8**(5):p.458–60.

37. Kessel, L. and M. Watson, *The painful arc syndrome. Clinical classification as a guide to management.* J Bone Joint Surg Br, 1977. **59**(2): p.166–72.

38. Gill, T.J., E. McIrvin, S.D. Mair, and R.J. Hawkins, *Results of biceps tenotomy for treatment of pathology of the long head of the biceps brachii.* J Shoulder Elbow Surg, 2001. **10**(3):p.247–9.

39. Osbahr, D.C., A.B. Diamond, and K.P. Speer, *The cosmetic appearance of the biceps muscle after long-head tenotomy versus tenodesis.* Arthroscopy, 2002. **18**(5):p.483–7.

40. West, R.V., M. Koenig, and R.J. Neviaser. *Functional Symptomatology following biceps tenodesis compared to biceps tenotomy or rupture.* in *Open Meeting of American Shoulder and Elbow Surgeons.* 2/8/2003. New Orleans, Louisiana.

41. Yamaguchi, K. and R. Bindra, *Disorders of Biceps Tendon,* in *Disorders of the Shoulders: Diagnosis and Management,* J.P. Iannotti and G.R. Williams, Editors. 1999, Lippincott Williams: Philadelphia. p.159–190.

42. Walch, G., P. Boileau, E. Noel, J.P. Liotard, and H. Dejour, *[Surgical treatment of painful shoulders caused by lesions of the rotator cuff and biceps: Treatment as a function of lesions. Reflections on Neer's concept].* Rev Rhum Mal Osteoartic, 1991. **58**(4):p.247–57.

43. Neer, C.S., 2nd, *Anterior acromioplasty for the chronic impingement syndrome in the shoulder: a preliminary report.* J Bone Joint Surg Am, 1972. **54**(1):p.41–50.

44. Neer, C.S., 2nd and R.P. Welsh, *The shoulder in sports.* Orthop Clin North Am, 1977. **8**(3):p.583–91.

45. Becker, D.A. and R.H. Cofield, *Tenodesis of the long head of the biceps brachii for chronic bicipital tendinitis. Long-term results.* J Bone Joint Surg Am, 1989. **71**(3):p.376–81.

46. Soifer, T.B., H.J. Levy, F.M. Soifer, F. Kleinbart, V. Vigorita, and E. Bryk, *Neurohistology of the subacromial space.* Arthroscopy, 1996. **12**(2):p.182–6.

47. Valadie, A.L., 3rd, C.M. Jobe, M.M. Pink, E.F. Ekman, and F.W. Jobe, *Anatomy of provocative tests for impingement syndrome of the shoulder.* J Shoulder Elbow Surg, 2000. **9**(1):p.36–46.

48. Burns, W.C., 2nd and T.L. Whipple, *Anatomic relationships in the shoulder impingement syndrome.* Clin Orthop, 1993(294):p.96–102.

49. Walch, G., L. Nove-Josserand, P. Boileau, and C. Levigne, *Subluxations and dislocations of the tendon of the long head of the biceps.* J Shoulder Elbow Surg, 1998. **7**(2):p.100–8.

50. O'Donoghue, D.H., *Subluxing biceps tendon in the athlete.* Clin Orthop, 1982(164):p.26–9.

51. O'Donoghue, D.H., *Injuries of the shoulder girdle,* in *Treatment of Injuries to Athletes,* D.H. O'Donoghue, Editor. 1976, Saunders: Philadelphia. p.142–243.

52. Kim, T.K., W.S. Queale, A.J. Cosgarea, and E.G. McFarland, *Clinical features of the different types of SLAP lesions: an analysis of one hundred and thirty-nine cases. Superior labrum anterior posterior.* J Bone Joint Surg Am, 2003. **85-A**(1):p.66–71.

53. Davidson, P.A., N.S. Elattrache, C.M. Jobe, and F.W. Jobe, *Rotator cuff and posterior-superior glenoid labrum injury associated with increased glenohumeral motion: a new site of impingement.* J Shoulder Elbow Surg, 1995. **4**(5):p.384–90.

54. Jobe, C., *Superior glenoid impingement.* Orthop Clin North Am, 1997. **28**(2):p.137–143.

55. Walch, G., P. Boileau, E. Noel, and S.T. Donnel, *Impingement of the deep surface of the supraspinatus tendon on the posterosuperior glenoid rim: An arthroscopic study.* J Shoulder Elbow Surg, 1992. **1**(5):p.238–245.

56. Burkhart, S.S. and C. Morgan, *SLAP lesions in the overhead athlete.* Orthop Clin North Am, 2001. **32**(3):p.431–41, viii.

57. Burkhart, S.S., C.D. Morgan, and W.B. Kibler, *Shoulder injuries in overhead athletes. The "dead arm" revisited.* Clin Sports Med, 2000. **19**(1):p.125–58.

58. Kim, T.K. and E.G. McFarland, *Internal impingement of the shoulder in flexion.* Clin Orthop Relat Res, 2004(421):p.112–9.

59. Clavert, P., F. Bonnomet, J.F. Kempf, P. Boutemy, M. Braun, and J.L. Kahn, *Contribution to the study of the pathogenesis of type II superior labrum anterior-posterior lesions: A cadaver model of a fall on the outstretched hand.* J Shoulder Elbow Surg, 2004. **13**(1):p.45–50.

60. Stenson, W.B., S.E. Snyder, R.P. Karzel, M.P. Banas, and S.E. Rahal, *Long-term clinical follow-up of isolated SLAP lesions of the shoulder.* Arch Am Acad Orthop Surg, 1997. **1**(1):p.61–64.

61. Berg, E.E. and J.V. Ciullo, *A clinical test for superior glenoid labral or 'SLAP' lesions.* Clin J Sport Med, 1998. **8**(2):p.121–3.

62. Parentis, M.A., K.J. Mohr, and N.S. el Attrache, *Disorders of the superior labrum: review and treatment guidelines.* Clin Orthop, 2002(400): p.77–87.

63. Kim, S.H., K.I. Ha, J.H. Ahn, and H.J. Choi, *Biceps load test II: A clinical test for SLAP lesions of the shoulder.* Arthroscopy, 2001. **17**(2): p.160–4.

64. Kim, S.H., K.I. Ha, and K.Y. Han, *Biceps load test: a clinical test for superior labrum anterior and posterior lesions in shoulders with recurrent anterior dislocations.* Am J Sports Med, 1999. **27**(3):p.300–3.

65. Landis, J.R. and G.G. Koch, *An application of hierarchial kappa-type statistics in the assessment of majority agreement among multiple observers.* Biometrics, 1977. **33**(2):p.363–374.

66. Ludington, N.A., *Rupture of the long head of the biceps flexor cubiti muscle.* Ann Surg, 1923. **77**:p.358–363.

67. Crenshaw, A.H. and W.E. Kilgore, *Surgical treatment of bicipital tenosynovitis.* J Bone Joint Surg Am, 1966. **48**(8):p.1496–502.

68. Bennett, W.F., *Specificity of the Speed's test: arthroscopic technique for evaluating the biceps tendon at the level of the bicipital groove.* Arthroscopy, 1998. **14**(8):p.789–96.

69. Walch, G., L. Nove-Josserand, and C. Levinge, *Tears of the supraspinatus tendon associated with "hidden" lesions of the rotator interval.* J Shoulder Elbow Surg, 1992. **74**:p.353–360.

70. Werner, A., T. Mueller, D. Boehm, and F. Gohlke, *The stabilizing sling for the long head of the biceps tendon in the rotator cuff interval. A histoanatomic study.* Am J Sports Med, 2000. **28**(1):p.28–31.

71. Matsen, F.A., 3rd and R.M. Kirby, *Office evaluation and management of shoulder pain.* Orthop Clin North Am, 1982. **13**(3):p.453–75.

72. Yergason, R.M., *Supination sign.* J Bone Joint Surg Am, 1931. **13**(Jan):p.160.

73. Holtby, R. and H. Razmjou, *Accuracy of the Speed's and Yergason's tests in detecting biceps pathology and SLAP lesions: comparison with arthroscopic findings.* Arthroscopy, 2004. **20**(3):p.231–6.

74. Gilchrist, E.L., *Dislocation and elongation of the long head of the biceps brachii.* Ann of Surg, 1936. **104**(1):p.118–138.

75. Abbot, L.C. and J.B.d.M. Saunders, *Acute traumatic dislocation of the tendon of long head of biceps brachii. A report of six cases with operative findings.* Surgery, 1939. **6**:p.817–840.

76. Boileau, P., P.M. Ahrens, and A.M. Hatzidakis, *Entrapment of the long head of the biceps tendon: the hourglass biceps—a cause of pain and locking of the shoulder.* J Shoulder Elbow Surg, 2004. **13**(3): p.249–57.

77. Gerber, C. and R.J. Krushell, *Isolated rupture of the subscapularis muscle.* J Bone Joint Surg Br, 1991. **73**:p.389–394.

78. Neviaser, T.J., *The role of the biceps tendon in the impingement syndrome.* Orthop Clin North Am, 1987. **18**(3):p.383–6.

79. Kibler, W.B., *Specificity and sensitivity of the anterior slide test in throwing athletes with superior labral tears.* Arthroscopy, 1995. **11**(3):p.296–300.

80. Liu, S.H., M.H. Henry, and S.L. Nuccion, *A prospective evaluation of a new physical examination in predicting glenoid labral tears.* Am J Sports Med, 1996. **24**(6):p.721–5.

81. Mimori, K., T. Muneta, T. Nakagawa, and K. Shinomiya, *A new pain provocation test for superior labral tears of the shoulder.* Am J Sports Med, 1999. **27**(2):p.137–42.

82. Stenson, W.B. and K. Templin, *The crank test, the O'Brien test, and routine magnetic resonnance imaging scans in the diagnosis of labral tears.* Am J Sports Med, 2002. **30**(6):p.806–9.

83. O'Brien, S.J., Pagnani MJ, Fealy S, McGlynn SR, Wilson JB., *The active compression test: a new and effective test for diagnosing labral tears and acromioclavicular Joint Abnormality.* Am J Sports Med, 1998. **26**(5):p.610–613.

84. Chronopoulos, E., T.K. Kim, H.B. Park, D. Ashenbrenner, and E.G. McFarland, *Diagnostic value of physical tests for isolated chronic acromioclavicular lesions.* Am J Sports Med, 2004. **32**(3):p.655–61.

85. Kim, S.H., K.I. Ha, H.S. Kim, and S.W. Kim, *Electromyographic activity of the biceps brachii muscle in shoulders with anterior instability.* Arthroscopy, 2001. **17**(8):p.864–8.

86. Jobe, F.W., R.S. Kvitne, and C.E. Giangarra, *Shoulder pain in the overhead or throwing athletes. The relationship of anterior instability and rotator cuff impingement.* Orthop Rev, 1989. **18**:p.963–975.

87. Jobe, C.M., *Posterior superior glenoid impingement: expanded spectrum.* Arthroscopy, 1995. **11**(5):p.530–6.

88. Savoie, F.H., 3rd, L.D. Field, and S. Atchinson, *Anterior superior instability with rotator cuff tearing: SLAC lesion.* Orthop Clin North Am, 2001. **32**(3):p.457–61, ix.

89. Snyder, S.J., M.P. Banas, and R.P. Karzel, *An analysis of 140 injuries to the superior glenoid labrum.* J Shoulder Elbow Surg, 1995. **4**(4):p.243–8.

90. Tomonobu, H., K. Masaaki, S. Kihumi, O. Kenji, F. Sunao, K. Akihiko, A. Mituhiro, U. Masamichi, and I. Seiichi, *The incidence of gleno-humeral joint abnormalities concomiant to rotator cuff tears.* J Shoulder Elbow Surg, 1999. **8**(4):p.383.

91. Handelberg, F., S. Willems, M. Shahabpour, J.P. Huskin, and J. Kuta, *SLAP lesions: a retrospective multicenter study.* Arthroscopy, 1998. **14**(8):p.856–62.

92. Altman, D.G., *Practical Statistics for Medical Research.* 1991, London: Chapman & Hall.

93. Holovacs, T.F., D.C. Osbahr, H. Singh, and K.P. Speer, *The sensitivity and specificity of the physical examination to detect glenoid labrum tears.*, in *Meeting of the American Shoulder and Elbow Society.* 2000: Orlando, FL.

94. Guanche, C.A. and D.C. Jones, *Clinical testing for tears of the glenoid labrum.* Arthroscopy, 2003. **19**(5):p.517–23.

7

The Acromioclavicular and Sternoclavicular Joints

This chapter discusses the examination of the acromioclavicular (AC) and sternoclavicular (SC) joints. Although AC joint conditions are more commonly seen in patients, conditions of the SC joint continue to be some of the more vexing problems in the shoulder to treat. Even though they are infrequent, injuries to both ends of the clavicle at the AC joint and SC joint can occur, so the examiner should be able to see the SC joint as part of the AC examination.

■ Examination of the Acromioclavicular Joint

AC Examination

The AC joint may be one of the few joints in the shoulder where an examiner can get his or her hands on the joint and where the tests upon examination are fairly accurate and reliable. Although this makes the joint easier to examine and to treat, there are some AC joint conditions that require further study before definitive statements can be made about the accuracy and reliability of examination for those entities. The most common conditions of the AC joint include idiopathic osteoarthritis, posttraumatic arthritis, AC separations, and osteolysis.[1] Most of these can be reliably diagnosed with a history, physical examination, and radiographs. In patients with a history of trauma, AC separations and posttraumatic arthritis are the most common. In patients with insidious onset of pain without trauma, the most frequent diagnosis will be idiopathic osteoarthritis or osteolysis.

Osteolysis is a condition of increased bone turnover due to stress at the distal clavicle, but its presentation is similar to primary or secondary osteoarthritis. It is most common in weight lifters and active individuals who perform exercises known to stress the AC joint and to cause pain, specifically push-ups, bench presses, and dips. Other conditions that can cause this condition are hyperparathyroidism, rheumatoid arthritis, and other forms of systemic arthritis.[2-7]

The examination of the AC joint should involve comparing both sides; this may be one of the most helpful tools in making the diagnosis (**Fig. 7–1**). Asymmetry of the AC joints can be a helpful finding upon examination but does not necessarily correlate with symptoms in all cases. It is important to do a complete examination because other conditions may mimic AC joint problems.

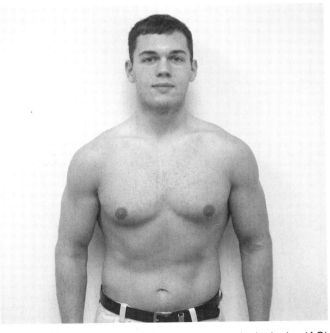

FIGURE 7–1 The examination of the acromioclavicular (AC) joint, comparing both sides.

It is also possible that AC joint problems can mimic other shoulder pathologies. Patients with severe AC joint pain may have significant inflammation and pain of the whole shoulder region, with or without loss of range of motion and function.[8] Patients may be unable to lift their arms over shoulder level, and they may report dysfunction with other activities.

AC joint disease can also mimic other shoulder pathologies by presenting with a pain distribution similar to rotator cuff problems and by producing pain with maneuvers traditionally felt to be diagnostic of impingement. In our study of patients with isolated AC joint problems, 57% had a positive Neer sign, 47% a positive Hawkins sign, 50% a painful arc, 24% a positive Speed's test, and 35% a drop arm sign.[9] In their study of patients with isolated AC joint problems, Maritz and Oosthuizen[10] found that 59% had a painful arc sign, 86% a positive Speed's test, 57% neck tenderness, and 91% a positive Jobe's test. (see chapter 4)

There are three major entities that can mimic AC joint problems. The first is cervical spine disease, which frequently radiates down the trapezius into the superior shoulder. The second entity, which can have symptoms similar to AC joint problems, is a superior labrum anterior and posterior (SLAP) lesion. Berg and Ciullo[11] reported on SLAP lesions that were missed and discovered only after the distal clavicle excision did not relieve the patient's pain. The third most common entity that can mimic AC joint problems is rotator cuff disease.

In addition, more than one diagnosis can occur at one time, and the most common condition seen to coexist with AC joint problems is rotator cuff disease.[1,12–16] In our cohort of 737 patients who underwent surgery between 1992 and 2001, there were 42 cases of isolated distal clavicle resection, but there were 105 cases of distal clavicle excision with acromioplasties and rotator cuff repairs. This indicates that AC joint problems frequently coexist with rotator cuff problems, which require surgery. When operating on younger patients with AC joint problems, Berg and Ciullo[16] recommended arthroscopy of the shoulder to avoid missing other entities such as SLAP lesions that might be masked or coexist with AC joint pathologies. We agree with these recommendations and routinely perform diagnostic arthroscopy of the shoulder in patients who are having what seem to be isolated AC joint problems.

The other reason to do a complete examination is to verify the findings of AC joint pathology seen in imaging modalities and to determine if they are part of the clinical presentation. In our practice, many patients present to the office with plain radiographs or magnetic resonance imaging (MRI) scans that demonstrate arthritis of the AC joint. Patients often confuse AC arthritis with glenohumeral arthritis and seek consultation with the orthopedic surgeon because they have arthritis in their shoulder. Patients and practitioners often do not realize that AC joint arthritis is nearly a normal condition with aging of the individual.

The incidence of asymptomatic idiopathic arthritis of the AC has been shown to increase linearly with age. This has been verified in studies using plain radiographs, MRIs, and cadaveric studies.[17,18] Cadaveric studies show degenerative changes of the AC joint in the fourth decade, with increasing frequency with each successive decade.[19] Petersson[20] performed dissections of the acromioclavicular joint in 85 cadavers (168 AC joints) of all ages. He found increased severity of degenerative changes with age and suggested that this was a consequence of regression of the acromioclavicular disk. Bonsell et al[18] studied radiographs of 84 asymptomatic individuals between 40 and 83 years of age and found significant relationship between specific radiological degenerative changes and age. In this study, 45% individuals overall had radiological evidence of AC degenerative disease.

Recent MRI studies demonstrate that degenerative changes begin in the AC joint in the third decade and can affect up to 93% of shoulders over the fourth decade.[17] A vast majority of these degenerative acromioclavicular joints are not symptomatic, and they do not warrant treatment. In a study on 50 shoulders by Stein et al,[17] the prevalence of AC joint arthritis with MRI in asymptomatic patients was 68% in the 30-and-under age group and 93% in the over-30 age group. In one study of asymptomatic volunteers, MRI findings indicative of AC joint arthritis were present in 75% of shoulders.[21]

Observation

One of the most helpful hints for the presence of AC joint problems is to compare the two shoulders for asymmetry of the AC joints. There is a wide range of normal variation in the degree of prominence of the AC joint in patients; this is probably because of the high degree of asymptomatic arthritis in the AC joint. Asymmetry is not diagnostic of any one condition, but it should direct the examiner to inquire about pathology or pain in the AC joint.

Other causes of swelling of the AC joint region can be due to trauma, tumors, infections, or synovial cysts. Malignant tumors of the distal clavicle are unusual, but the authors are reminded of a case of a metastatic breast cancer to the distal clavicle in their practice, which was the cause of swelling and pain. The diagnosis was made by a history of increasing pain and increasing swelling near the AC joint with no trauma in a patient with a history of breast cancer. Plain radiographs revealed the tumor and imminent pathological fracture. Although this presentation is uncommon, it demonstrates that the AC joint region is not immune to conditions that can affect other joints.

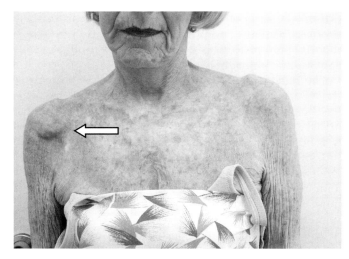

FIGURE 7–2 Synovial cyst near the AC joint (arrow).

Sepsis of the AC joint can produce symptoms of pain and swelling, but usually the patient has or eventually develops other symptoms of a septic arthritis such as a fever, redness, and warmth. It can be due to hematogenous seeding of the joint, but this is more common in immunosuppressed individuals, such as those patients who are leukopenic due to chemotherapeutic agents or human immunodeficiency virus (HIV) disease. Sepsis can be iatrogenic after AC joint injections or after surgical procedures.

Synovial cysts can appear near the AC joint, and the patient typically will have a painless swelling that is insidious. These cysts sometimes regress in size, and they can be quite small or very large (**Figs. 7–2, 7–3**). They can be associated with isolated AC joint arthritis, rotator cuff tears, rheumatoid arthritis, or other conditions about the shoulder.[12,22,23] Some authors have suggested transilluminating the cysts with a light to establish the diagnosis, because cysts should transilluminate, and more

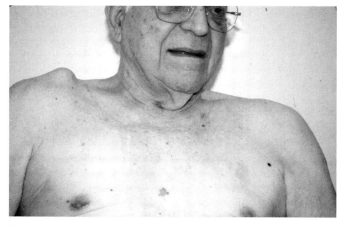

FIGURE 7–3 Clinical presentation of a synovial cyst over the AC joint.

solid masses will not. This is not diagnostic, however, and in patients where the diagnosis is uncertain, either aspiration of the cyst or MRI of the shoulder and AC joint may confirm the diagnosis.

Ecchymosis, swelling, and pain after trauma are common in this region, and the differential diagnosis is quite long. The major differential diagnosis is between fractures and AC separations. AC separations have been classified as three types by Allman[24] and modified by Rockwood[25] as six types (**Fig. 7–4**). Almost each of these types can be mimicked by a distal clavicle fracture, so observation and examination should be accompanied by radiographic evaluation. Grade I injuries typically have only swelling and no deformity (**Fig. 7–5**). Grade II injuries usually have swelling and a mild deformity, but this diagnosis must be confirmed with radiographs that demonstrate a step-off between the AC joint and the acromion (**Fig. 7–6**).

Grade III injuries have displacement of the clavicle superiorly with a characteristic deformity (**Fig. 7–7**). Sometimes this displacement can be difficult to evaluate acutely due to swelling and in patients who are large or heavy. In addition, patients often present hunched over due to pain with the involved extremity lower than the other side. This often makes the diagnosis uncertain, and other injuries should be ruled out. Grade IV injuries are displacement of the clavicle posteriorly into the trapezius fascia. These injuries are less common, but axillary radiographs can confirm the displacement (**Fig. 7–8**). Grade V injuries are where the clavicle displaces significantly superiorly and may tent the skin (**Fig. 7–9**). They are difficult to distinguish from grade III lesions acutely and warrant further evaluation once the pain and swelling have diminished. Radiographs can help with determining the degree of displacement, but often the clinical appearance is the more important determinant of treatment. Last, grade VI lesions are subcoracoid dislocations of the clavicle, and these are extremely rare. A review of the literature demonstrates only a handful of cases of grade VI lesions, but these patients may present with a wide variety of symptoms due to compression of the brachial plexus by the displaced clavicle. Patients with trauma, deformity of the shoulder, and neurovascular findings should be carefully and thoroughly evaluated for these lesions.

Fractures of the distal clavicle can mimic or coexist with AC joint problems. As a result, radiographs are indicated in most cases of deformity of the AC joint. Distal clavicle fractures are classified according the location and displacement (**Figs. 7–10, 7–11, 7–12**). Type I fractures can appear like grade I or II AC separations. Type II clavicle fractures can appear like grade III or IV AC separation. The clinical appearance of type II A and type II B distal clavicle is the same, and they cannot be distinguished by physical examination. Type III distal

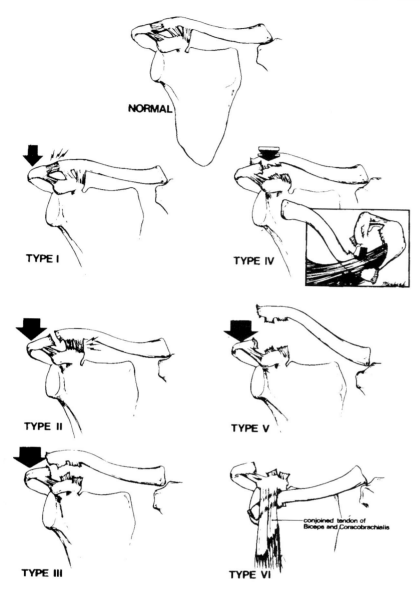

FIGURE 7–4 Types of AC joint separation. (Adapted with permission from Rockwood CA Jr. Subluxations and dislocations about the shoulder: injuries to acromioclavicular separations. In: Rockwood CA Jr, Green DP, eds. Fractures. Philadelphia: JB Lippincott; 1984:860–910.)

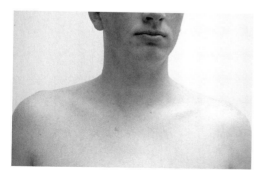

FIGURE 7–5 Clinical presentation of a grade I AC separation (right side) can be very subtle.

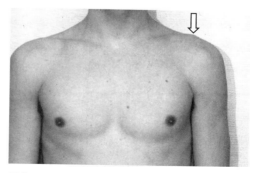

FIGURE 7–6 Clinical presentation of a grade II AC joint separation (arrow).

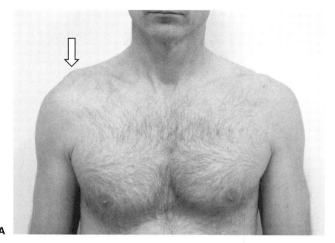
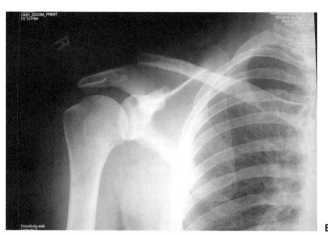

A

B

FIGURE 7–7 Clinical and radiological presentation of a grade III AC joint separation (arrow).

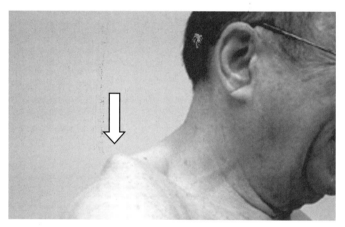

FIGURE 7–8 Clinical presentation of a grade IV AC joint separation.

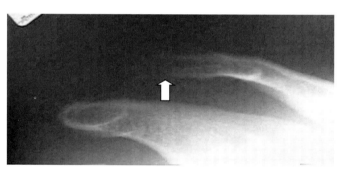

FIGURE 7–9 Radiograph of a grade V AC joint separation showing elevation of the distal clavicle (arrow).

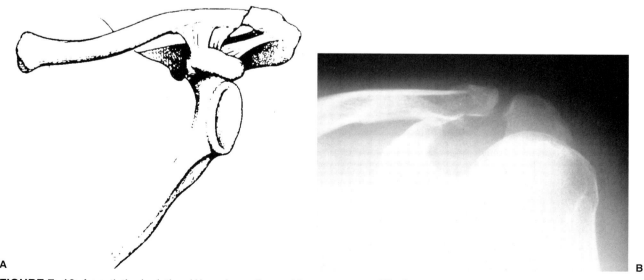

A

B

FIGURE 7–10 An artist's depiction (A) and a radiographic appearance (B) of a type I distal clavicle fracture.

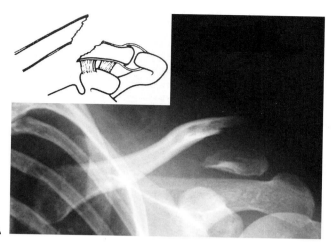

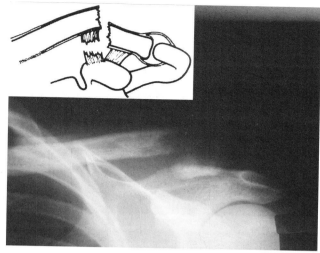

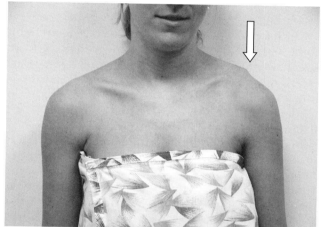

FIGURE 7–11 Type IIa **(A)** and IIb **(B)** distal clavicle fractures can appear similar on clinical examination **(C)**. (Adapted with permission from Craig EV Fractures of the clavicle. In: Rockwood CA Jr, Matsen FA, eds. The Shoulder, Vol. 1. Philadelphia: WB Saunders; 1998:428–482.)

clavicle fracture typically appears like grade II or III AC separation (**Fig. 7–12**).

Pain Distribution and Local Tenderness

One of the major hints that a patient may have AC joint pathology is the distribution of pain. Whereas rotator cuff symptoms typically radiate into the deltoid and proximal arm, the pain of the AC joint is usually located over the joint and radiates into the trapezius (**Fig. 7–13**). Afflictions of the AC joint should be considered in the differential diagnosis of trapezius and neck pain.

Gerber et al[26] performed a simple but elegant study to demonstrate the difference in pain distributions by injecting saline selectively into either the AC joint or the subacromial space. The injection into the AC joint produced pain into the trapezius in 80% of patients (12 of 15), and injections into the subacromial space produced pain into the deltoid region in 100% (8 of 8 patients). Gerber and colleagues concluded that the

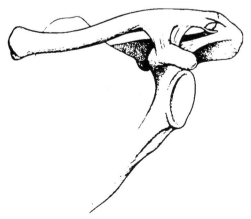

FIGURE 7–12 Type III distal clavicle fracture where the fracture enters the AC joint. (Adapted with permission from Craig EV. Fractures of the Clavicle. In: Rockwood CA Jr, Matsen FA, eds. The Shoulder, Vol. 1. Philadelphia: WB Saunders; 1998:428–482.)

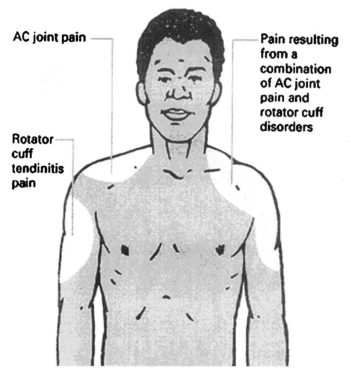

FIGURE 7–13 Pathology of the AC joint and rotator cuff creates different pain patterns. (Adapted with permission from McFarland EG, Hobbs WR. The active shoulder: AC joint pain and injury. Your Patient & Fitness 1998;12 (4):23–27.)

pain pattern alone is a reliable observation to support the diagnosis of AC joint pathology; however, they noted that patients reported pain in a variety of locations after irritation of the AC joint (**Table 7–1**). This indicates that other pain patterns can be present due to AC joint irritation. One limitation of their study was that the pain distribution of AC joint pathology could not be compared with that of SLAP lesions, which can mimic AC joint problems.[11,27]

TABLE 7–1 Localization of Pain after Irritation of the Acromioclavicular Joint (N = 15)

Local pain	15 (100%)
Supraspinatus fossa	12 (80%)
Upper trapezius muscle	12 (80%)
Lateral clavicle	12 (80%)
Anterolateral deltoid region	9 (60%)
Medial aspect of upper arm	4 (27%)
Thumb	4 (27%)
Sternocleidomastoid muscle	3 (20%)
Posterolateral acromion	2 (13%)
Radial forearm	1 (7%)
Infraspinatus fossa	0
Triceps region	0
Posterior deltoid region	0

Source: Adapted with permission from Gerber C, Galantay RV, Hersche O. The pattern of pain produced by irritation of the acromioclavicular joint and the subacromial space. J Shoulder Elbow Surg 1998;7(4):352–355.

TABLE 7–2 Pain on Clinical Testing after Irritation of the Acromioclavicular Joint

Findings	Symptoms and Subjects: Number (%)		
	Increased	Unchanged	Relieved
Local pressure	15 (100%)	2 (13%)	1 (7%)
Coracoid pressure	13 (87%)	9 (60%)	6 (40%)
Forced abduction	6 (40%)	13 (87%)	1 (7%)
Cross-body adduction	2 (13%)	12 (80%)	
Movement of neck	3 (20%)	11 (73%)	
Resisted exterior rotation	3 (20%)	6 (40%)	
Resisted interior rotation	3 (20%)	12 (80%)	
Palm-up test	3 (20%)	11 (73%)	
Supraspinatus test	3 (20%)		

Source: Adapted with permission from Gerber C, Galantay RV, Hersche O. The pattern of pain produced by irritation of the acromioclavicular joint and the subacromial space. J Shoulder Elbow Surg 1998;7(4):352–355.

Local tenderness at the AC joint is considered by many to be the sine qua non of AC joint pathology. In their study after irritating the AC joint with saline, Gerber et al[26] examined the AC joint and found that the only physical finding that was consistent in 100% was AC joint tenderness (**Table 7–2**). Maritz and Oosthuizen[10] found that local tenderness had a sensitivity of 96%.

In their study of AC joint pathology and the best way to make the diagnosis of AC conditions, Walton et al[28] found that local tenderness was 96% sensitive but only 10% specific. Their study underscores that sometimes it is difficult to determine if the patient's tenderness is located at the AC joint, proximal rotator cuff, biceps tendon, or coracoid. This is presumably due to the close proximity of these structures, and it can be compounded when these other conditions are present.

The high incidence of asymptomatic degeneration of the AC joint with age almost requires that the joint be tender to establish that it is the source of pain. The distinction between a symptomatic and asymptomatic AC joint is important to avoid unnecessary treatment directed at the AC joint, including surgery. In this circumstance where it is unclear if the AC joint is the source of pain for the patient, selective injection of different structures can be helpful in determining the location of the pain.[1,29–32] The use of injections is discussed later in this chapter.

One-Finger Test

One technique useful for establishing the location of pain in the shoulder is to ask the patient to point one finger at the source or location of the pain (**Fig. 7–14**). Typically, patients with isolated AC joint pathology will point directly at the AC joint at the top of the shoulder. This test is less useful in patients with associated pathologies, especially biceps tendon problems, because they will point to the anterior aspect of the AC joint near the coracoid or biceps tendon. In that case, other tests should be utilized

TABLE 7–4 Diagnostic Values of Combined Tests

Test	Sensitivity % of N	Specificity % of N	PPV % of N	NPV % of N	Overall Accuracy* % of N
Positive in all 3 tests	25 (4 of 16)	97 (290 of 299)	31 (4 of 13)	96 (290 of 302)	93 (294 of 315)
Positive in 2 or more than 2 of the tests	81 (13 of 16)	89 (266 of 299)	28 (13 of 46)	99 (266 of 269)	89 (279 of 315)
Positive in 1 or more than 1 of the tests	100 (16 of 16)	74 (221 of 299)	17 (16 of 94)	100 (221 of 221)	75 (237 of 315)

Source: Adapted with permission from Chronopoulos E, Kim TK, Park HB, Ashenbrenner D, McFarland EG. Diagnostic value of physical tests for isolated chronic acromioclavicular lesions. Am J Sports Med 2004;32(3):655–661.

*Three hundred fifteen patients (16 in the AC lesion group, 299 in the no AC lesion group) who underwent all three tests (cross-body adduction stress test, AC-resisted extension test, and active compression test) were included in this analysis.

AC, acromioclavicular; NPV, negative predictive; PPV, positive predictive value.

Combination of Tests for More Accurate Diagnosis

There are two studies that evaluate the increased diagnostic accuracy if upon physical examination more than one test is considered when making the diagnosis of AC joint pathology. We found that when using the crossed arm adduction stress test, the active compression test, and the arm extension test, if all three were positive, the overall accuracy was 93%, but the sensitivity was only 25% (**Table 7–4**). One limitation of our study was that the patients were included only if they had AC joint tenderness, and the presence or absence of AC joint tenderness was not addressed as either a diagnostic sign or a prognostic sign for the results of surgery.

A second study by Walton et al[28] used physical examination and imaging modalities to determine which combination provided the highest accuracy for the diagnosis of isolated AC joint pathology. They studied 42 subjects who had pain within an area bounded by the midclavicle and deltoid insertion. Their results demonstrate that the highly sensitive tests, such as AC joint tenderness and MRI scans, had low specificity and highly specific tests, such as O'Brien's test and X-rays, had low sensitivity for AC joint pain; however, a combination of positive AC compression test and positive bone scan can predict AC joint damage as the cause of shoulder pain with a high degree of confidence (**Table 7–5**).[28]

TABLE 7–5 Sensitivity and Specificity for Clinical and Imaging Diagnostic Tests

Test	Sensitivity (%)	Specificity (%)
Paxinos test	82	50
AC tenderness	96	10
O'Brien's	16	90
X-rays	41	90
MRI	85	50
Bone scan	82	70

Source: Adapted with permission from Walton J, Mahajan S, Paxinos A, et al. Diagnostic values of tests for acromioclavicular joint pain. J Bone Joint Surg Am 2004;86-A(4):807–812.

AC, acromioclavicular; MRI, magnetic resonance imaging.

Clinical Summary: Acromioclavicular Joint

Based on these studies, the most important findings for confirming the diagnosis of AC joint problems are the ability of the patient to localize the pain to the AC joint area, local tenderness to the AC joint, and a positive result to an injection test. Other tests upon examination are used to support the diagnosis made by these factors. The examination we have found to be most helpful for confirming AC joint problems is local tenderness of the AC joint. When performing other tests meant to provoke AC joint pain, it is important that the patient localize the pain to the AC joint and not to other areas of the shoulder. We routinely utilize a combination of the arm extension test, the O'Brien's test, and the crossed arm adduction stress test; if all three of these tests are positive, then the diagnosis of AC pathology is confirmed in more than 90% of cases.

■ Sternoclavicular Joint

The sternoclavicular joint is not a frequently injured joint in the body, and its evaluation seems straightforward in most instances. Most conditions of the SC joint fortunately can be treated effectively nonoperatively because the surgical results of treatment seem to fall short of those of other joints in the body. The relative low frequency of injury is balanced by the difficulty in treating this joint. The examination of the SC joint presents fewer challenges to the provider than does the treatment.

History and Examination

A history of trauma is an important element in the evaluation of the SC joint. In adults fractures, subluxations, and dislocations of the SC joint are the most frequent injuries. In adolescents, because the physis is one of the last in the body to close, a physeal fracture with a periosteal sleeve type of disruption is most common. The

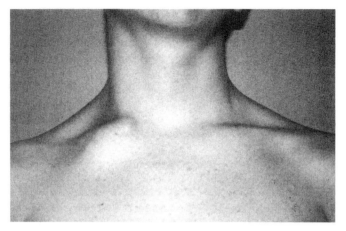

FIGURE 7–21 In adolescents with open physis, a fracture through the growth plate can produce a deformity similar to an anterior sternoclavicular dislocation. (Adapted with permission from O'Neill PJ, Cosgarea AJ, McFarland EG. Unusual double clavicle fracture in a lacrosse player. Clin J Sport Med 2000;10:69–71.)

most common displacement of these fractures and instabilities is anterior (**Fig. 7–21**), and a prominence will be seen on the chest.

Posterior displacements of the proximal clavicle may be difficult to see in patients due to swelling, and they should be suspected with pain and swelling in this area with no obvious displacements. Because posteriorly displaced proximal clavicles can compress the great vessels or structures in the posterior neck, patients with acute SC joint trauma should be asked about dysphagia and be observed for distension of the veins in the neck or affected arm and difficulty speaking, breathing, or swallowing.

In patients with no trauma and swelling about the SC joint, the most common diagnosis is degenerative arthritis.[42] Tumors and benign conditions, however, such as osteitis condensans, Freiberg's avascular necrosis, and sternoclavicular hyperostosis can also cause swelling of the proximal end of the clavicle near the SC joint. These conditions are quite rare, but they typically present with pain and swelling of the proximal clavicle and SC joint. Infections of the SC are typically accompanied by pain, swelling, warmth, erythema, and tenderness. The SC joint can be readily evaluated by undressing the patient and comparing both sides. Unless the patient is large or there is significant hematoma, the joint can be visualized easily. If the patient has popping or subluxations of the joint sometimes, they can demonstrate the maneuvers that produce the symptoms. Crepitus can be detected by placing the hand over the joint as the patient moves the extremity.

Range of motion of the shoulder should be tested to determine if the SC condition has affected shoulder movements and also because motion can accentuate deformities of the joint. In patients with chronic instability or those who have had previous surgery to the SC joint, motion of the shoulder complex can also demonstrate how much translation of the proximal clavicle occurs in both anteroposterior and inferosuperior directions. Reductions of acute sternoclavicular instabilities, especially posterior instabilities, should not be attempted in the office or outpatient setting. When the patient is not in pain, the examiner can grasp the proximal clavicle and translate it in these directions. When the patient is experiencing pain, however, it is sometimes necessary to anesthetize the area with local anesthetic prior to attempting any translations.

Voluntary Sternoclavicular Subluxations

One of the most uncommon conditions seen at the SC joint is voluntary subluxations of the joint. This is typically seen in adolescents who have generalized ligamentous laxity who discover that they can subluxate the joint with movement of the shoulder.[43,44] In some instances this subluxation occurs after an injury, but this is the least common presentation of this condition.

This subluxation is uniformly characterized by displacement of the proximal clavicle anteriorly. Like demonstrable or voluntary subluxations of the glenohumeral joint, these subluxations may become sore if they occur too often or if they occur with the repetitive motions of sports. We have seen it be symptomatic in patients involved in swimming or weight lifting.

The desired treatment for this condition is nonoperative with activity modification, cryotherapy, medication, and, rarely, cortisone shots. Surgical treatment has a high failure rate, and at least one study suggests that patients do worse with surgery than without it.[44]

REFERENCES

1. Shaffer, B.S., *Painful conditions of the acromioclavicular joint.* J Am Acad Orthop Surg, 1999. **7**(3):p.176–88.
2. Preusen, S.E., K. Pierce, T.C. Demos, and L.M. Lomasney, *Radiologic case study. Stress-induced osteolysis of the distal clavicle.* Orthopedics, 2003. **26**(2):p.136, 214–6.
3. Flatow, E.L., X.A. Duralde, G.P. Nicholson, R.G. Pollock, and L.U. Bigliani, *Arthroscopic resection of the distal clavicle with a superior approach.* J Shoulder Elbow Surg, 1995. **4**(1 Pt 1):p.41–50.
4. Petersson, C.J., *The acromioclavicular joint in rheumatoid arthritis.* Clin Orthop Relat Res, 1987(223):p.86–93.
5. Grey, T., *Osteomyelitis of the clavicle.* Br J Surg, 1945. **32**:p.466–467.
6. Levine, A.H., M.J. Pais, and E.E. Schwartz, *Posttraumatic osteolysis of the distal clavicle with emphasis on early radiologic changes.* AJR Am J Roentgenol, 1976. **127**(5):p.781–4.
7. Nathanson, L. and M. Slobodkin, *Acromioclavicular changes in primary and secondary hyperparathyroidism.* Radiology, 1950. **55**(1):p.31–5.

8. Moseley, H.F., *Athletic injuries to the shoulder region.* Am J Surg, 1959. **98**:p.401–22.

9. Chronopoulos, E., T.K. Kim, H.B. Park, D. Ashenbrenner, and E.G. McFarland, *Diagnostic value of physical tests for isolated chronic acromioclavicular lesions.* Am J Sports Med, 2004. **32**(3):p.655–61.

10. Maritz, N.G.J. and P.J. Oosthuizen, *Diagnostic criteria for acromioclavicular joint pathology.* J Bone Joint Surg Br, 2002. **84**(Supp 1):p.78–a.

11. Berg, E.E. and J.V. Ciullo, *A clinical test for superior glenoid labral or 'SLAP' lesions.* Clin J Sport Med, 1998. **8**(2):p.121–3.

12. Craig, E.V., *The acromioclavicular joint cyst. An unusual presentation of a rotator cuff tear.* Clin Orthop, 1986(202):p.189–92.

13. Neer, C.S., 2nd, *Anterior acromioplasty for the chronic impingement syndrome in the shoulder: a preliminary report.* J Bone Joint Surg Am, 1972. **54**(1):p.41–50.

14. Neer, C.S., 2nd, *Impingement lesions.* Clin Orthop, 1983(173): p. 70–7.

15. Stuart, M.J., A.J. Azevedo, and R.H. Cofield, *Anterior acromioplasty for treatment of the shoulder impingement syndrome.* Clin Orthop, 1990 (260):p.195–200.

16. Berg, E.E. and J.V. Ciullo, *The SLAP lesion: a cause of failure after distal clavicle resection.* Arthroscopy, 1997. **13**(1):p.85–9.

17. Stein, B.E., J.M. Wiater, H.C. Pfaff, L.U. Bigliani, and W.N. Levine, *Detection of acromioclavicular joint pathology in asymptomatic shoulders with magnetic resonance imaging.* J Shoulder Elbow Surg, 2001. **10**(3): p.204–8.

18. Bonsell, S., A.W.t. Pearsall, R.J. Heitman, C.A. Helms, N.M. Major, and K.P. Speer, *The relationship of age, gender, and degenerative changes observed on radiographs of the shoulder in asymptomatic individuals.* J Bone Joint Surg Br, 2000. **82**(8):p.1135–9.

19. DePalma, A., J. White, and G. Callery, *Degenerative lesions of the shoulder joint at various age groups which are compatible with good function, in Instructional Course Lectures. The American Academy of Orthopaedic Surgeons,* J. Edwards, Editor. 1950: Ann Arbor.p.168–80.

20. Petersson, C.J., *Degeneration of the acromioclavicular joint. A morphological study.* Acta Orthop Scand, 1983. **54**(3):p.434–8.

21. Needell, S.D., M.B. Zlatkin, J.S. Sher, B.J. Murphy, and J.W. Uribe, *MR imaging of the rotator cuff: peritendinous and bone abnormalities in an asymptomatic population.* AJR Am J Roentgenol, 1996. **166**(4):p.863–7.

22. Groh, G.I., T.M. Badwey, and C.A. Rockwood, Jr., *Treatment of cysts of the acromioclavicular joint with shoulder hemiarthroplasty.* J Bone Joint Surg, 1993. **75**(12):p.1790–4.

23. Postacchini, F., D. Perugia, and S. Gumina, *Acromioclavicular joint cyst associated with rotator cuff tear. A report of three cases.* Clin Orthop, 1993(294):p.111–3.

24. Allman, F.L., Jr., *Fractures and ligamentous injuries of the clavicle and its articulation.* J Bone Joint Surg Am, 1967. **49**(4):p.774–84.

25. Rockwood, C.A.J., *Subluxations and dislocations about the shoulder. Injuries to acromioclavicular separations, in Fractures,* R.C.A. Jr. and G.D.P., Editors. 1984, Lippincott J.B.: Philadelphia.p.860–910.

26. Gerber, C., R.V. Galantay, and O. Hersche, *The pattern of pain produced by irritation of the acromioclavicular joint and the subacromial space.* J Shoulder Elbow Surg, 1998. **7**(4):p.352–5.

27. O'Brien, S.J., M.J. Pagnani, S. Fealy, S.R. McGlynn, and J.B. Wilson, *The active compression test: a new and effective test for diagnosing labral tears and acromioclavicular joint abnormality.* Am J Sports Med, 1998. **26**(5):p.610–3.

28. Walton, J., S. Mahajan, A. Paxinos, J. Marshall, C. Bryant, R. Shnier, R. Quinn, and G.A. Murrell, *Diagnostic values of tests for acromioclavicular joint pain.* J Bone Joint Surg Am, 2004. **86-A**(4):p.807–12.

29. Bogduk, N. and A. Marsland, *The cervical zygapophysial joints as a source of neck pain.* Spine, 1988. **13**(6):p.610–617.

30. Kellgren, J.H., *On the distribution of pain arising from deep somatic structures with charts of segmental pain areas.* Clin Sci, 1939. **4**:p.35–45.

31. Kellgren, J.H., *Observations on pain arising from muscle.* Clin Sci, 1938. **3**:p.175–90.

32. Inman, V.T. and J.B. Saunders, *Referred pain from skeletal structures.* J Nerve Ment Dis, 1944. **99**:p.660–7.

33. McLaughlin, H.L., *On the frozen shoulder.* Bull. Hosp. Joint Dis. Orthop. Inst., 1951. **12**:p.383–393.

34. Jacob, A.K. and P.I. Sallay, *Therapeutic efficacy of corticosteroid injections in the acromioclavicular joint.* Biomed Sci Instrum, 1997. **34**: p.380–5.

35. Blazar, P.E., J.P. Iannotti, and G.R. Williams, *Anteroposterior instability of the distal clavicle after distal clavicle resection.* Clin Orthop, 1998(348):p.114–20.

36. Bigliani, L.U., G.P. Nicholson, and E.L. Flatow, *Arthroscopic resection of the distal clavicle.* Orthop Clin North Am, 1993. **24**(1): p. 133–41.

37. Worcester, J.N., Jr. and D.P. Green, *Osteoarthritis of the acromioclavicular joint.* Clin Orthop Relat Res, 1968. **58**:p.69–73.

38. Neer, C.S., 2nd, *Shoulder reconstruction.* 1990, W.B. Saunders: Philadelphia.p.433–36.

39. Salter, E.G., Jr., R.J. Nasca, and B.S. Shelley, *Anatomical observations on the acromioclavicular joint and supporting ligaments.* Am J Sports Med, 1987. **15**(3):p.199–206.

40. Hollingworth, G.R., R.M. Ellis, and T.S. Hattersley, *Comparison of injection techniques for shoulder pain: results of a double blind, randomised study.* Br Med J (Clin Res Ed), 1983. **287**(6402):p.1339–41.

41. Partington, P.F. and G.H. Broome, *Diagnostic injection around the shoulder: hit and miss? A cadaveric study of injection accuracy.* J Shoulder Elbow Surg, 1998. **7**(2):p.147–50.

42. Hamilton-Wood, C., P. Hollingworth, P. Dieppe, C. Ackroyd, and I. Watt, *The painful swollen sterno-clavicular joint.* Br J Radiol, 1985. **58**(694):p.941–5.

43. Rockwood, C.A., Jr. and J.M. Odor, *Spontaneous atraumatic anterior subluxation of the sternoclavicular joint.* J Bone Joint Surg Am, 1989. **71**(9):p.1280–8.

44. Sadr, B. and M. Swann, *Spontaneous dislocation of the sterno-clavicular joint.* Acta Orthop Scand, 1979. **50**(3):p.269–74.

Appendix

Statistical Terms and Analysis

One of the goals of this book has been to examine the usefulness of shoulder examinations upon making the diagnosis of various shoulder conditions. As clinicians who do not use statistical terms everyday, the language utilized by statisticians is sometimes confusing. This appendix describes the statistics used in this book so that the provider (whether trainer, therapist, surgeon, physician, or chiropractor) can understand the terms.

Prevalence The prevalence of a condition is the number of individuals in a population who have the disease at a given time. The prevalence is expressed as the number of people with the disease divided by the number of people in the group studied at that time. For example, if we study with ultrasound the shoulders of everyone in the country on a given day, there will be a certain number of cases present. The number of cases related to the total number of subjects is the prevalence.

The prevalence of a disorder can affect the results of studies that evaluate the effectiveness of examination of the shoulder or any other test in a population. The prevalence does not affect the sensitivity and specificity of a test per se. It will affect how often you get false-positives and false-negatives, however, which can affect the predictive values and post-test probabilities discussed below.

Validity The validity of a test is its ability to measure what it claims to measure. This "face validity" is essentially the measure of truthfulness and believability of a test. For example, a muscle is tested by an examiner who exclaims that the test that is being used is the best for this particular muscle. However, further study indicates that the muscle tested is next to another muscle, and that the test is really measuring the muscle next to the one intended.

In this case, the test is not valid. It does not measure what it claims to measure . Many tests used in physical examination of the shoulder lack adequate study to know if they are valid or not. Many of the tests were described many years ago on the basis of observations of clinicians who did not have the knowledge we have now of the anatomy, physiology, and pathologies of the shoulder complex.

When determining the validity of a test, it is important that the standard used also is credible and truthful. For example, to determine if a particular test really determines cartilage fraying, you decide to use magnetic resonance imaging (MRI) as the standard to validate the test it. In this case, you must prove that the MRI is an adequate standard. If the standard chosen does not have validity and is not established, then the validity of the test can be questioned. This is called criterion validity, which means that a new tool or instrument is consistent with and has similar results to other measures.

There are other forms of validity that make subtle distinctions between the new test and other standards. Content validity is whether the items of the test represent the variables or symptoms that constitute the condition being studied. It is possible that the test may represent only a subset of the symptoms or variables of a condition, which may affect the validity of the test. There is also construct validity, which means that the components of the test measure items that are true for the condition being studied.

It is possible that some measures will not be free of some error. However, a test or physical examination that is described should be able to measure what it says it will measure, and the test should be designed to minimize error.

In some cases it may not be possible to determine a test's validity with current knowledge. Although the validity may not have been tested and may not be discoverable, it is possible that the test still has some value in the decision-making process.

Sensitivity The sensitivity of a test is the proportion of patients testing positive out of all patients with the disease. It is also a measure of the probability that an individual with the disease will test positive for the disease. Sensitivity measures the "true-positive" rate, in that the denominator is individuals who are known to definitely have the condition by some other standard. The sensitivity of a test is its ability to obtain a positive result when the condition or disease entity is present in an individual as determined by the standard. In other words, it is the ability of the test to be positive when the condition is present.

A high sensitivity means that the test has a good ability to pick out the individuals who have the condition. As sensitivity increases, the test correctly identifies those who have the disorder, and fewer of the individuals who have the condition are missed. As sensitivity decreases, the test is less able to identify those who have the condition.

Specificity The specificity is the proportion of patients testing negative for a condition among those patients without the condition. In other words, specificity measures the "true-negative" rate, as measured against a standard. It is a measure of the probability that a subject without the disease will have a negative test result. It is also a measure of the chance that a patient will test negative for the condition who actually does not have the condition. A high specificity means that the test identifies reliably those without the condition.

Positive predictive value The positive predictive value (PPV) of a test is the probability that an individual with a positive test will actually have the disease. PPV differs from sensitivity in that sensitivity has a different denominator; PPV measures positives in a population of individuals with and without the condition, whereas sensitivity is restricted to those who have the disease. A PPV is the positive rate when the denominator includes those who are true-positives and false-positives A high PPV means that a positive test will have a high chance of identifying an individual with the disorder.

Negative predictive value Negative predictive value (NPV) of a test is the probability that an individual who tested negative does not have the disease. NPV differs from sensitivity in that the calculation of NPV has in the denominator those individuals who tested negative, including true-negatives and false-negatives. A high NPV means that a negative test has a high chance of identifying an individual who does not have the disorder.

Relationship of prevalence to predictive values The prevalence of a condition in a population can affect the predictive values. If the condition has a low prevalence, the positive predictive value can look unacceptably low even if the test has a high sensitivity. This is because when calculating the predictive values, the false-negatives and -positives are in the denominator. If the prevalence is very low, then a few false-negatives or -positives can have a larger impact on the predictive values, even when the test may have good sensitivity and specificity.

Accuracy Accuracy is the proportion of correctly categorized individuals (both true-positives and true-negatives) divided by all the subjects in the study. This denominator includes all true- and false-positives and all true- and false-negatives. The accuracy is not very useful because the prevalence must be 50% for this statistic to be helpful. If the prevalence is low, then a test will tend to identify most negatives as negatives, which will give it a high accuracy regardless of whether it successfully identifies any cases.

Likelihood ratio The likelihood ratio (LR) is an important statistical value that has not been used by many clinical studies, but it is a very valuable measure for clinicians who want to know the probability that the test will identify someone with a given condition. A likelihood ratio is a measure of the odds that a test will identify a person with the condition being studied over the odds that it will incorrectly identify an individual who does not have the condition. In other words, for a positive test, how much more likely is it o be a true case rather than a false-positive? Thus, if the LR is 10, the test is 10 times more likely to be a true-positive than a false-positive. If an individual tests positive for a labrum lesion, and the test has a LR of 10, then the individual has a 10-fold increase in odds that they actually have a labrum tear.

A likelihood ratio of 10 is felt to be a clinically significant increase in probability that a test will be positive. A test with a likelihood ratio over 10 is considered a strong and significant indicator that the test will be predictive that the condition is present. A test with a likelihood ratio of 5 to 10 indicates a moderate increase in post-test probability, and an LR of 2 to 5 indicates a small increase in post-test probability.

Reliability Reliability is the ability of a test to obtain the same result if it is repeated. This test–re-test concept can determine if a test can give the same results either between individuals or if one individual is performing the test. There are two types of reliability. The first is when one examiner repeats the test either the same day or at a later date. This is called intraexaminer reliability. The second type of reliability is when two individuals perform the test at nearly the same time. This is called intertester reliability. These measures of the usefulness of a test are particularly important if the test is subjective or does not have distinct criteria for its application.

When performing reliability with one examiner, the results can be reported in several ways. If the examiner repeats a test within a short period of time, the percentage of times the test results were the same can be reported. For example, if a test of a labrum tear is performed by the same individual on the same subject 6 hours apart, the results can be compared for both positive and negative responses. If the examinations were in agreement with one another 80% of the time, then one would then say that the intratester agreement of the test was 80%. The higher the reliability, the greater the chance that the test will have the same results.

When performing intertester reliability, the results can be reported in a similar fashion. If two individuals examine the same subject within a few minutes or hours, then the number of times they obtained the same results can be reported. If the intertester agreement was 80%, then it would indicate that they had the same results 80% of the time.

However, there are limitations to the statistical analysis, which merely mentions the percentage of times two or more examiners agree. The amount of variation that exists between two observers can be determined statistically with a test known as a kappa coefficient.

Kappa coefficients The kappa coefficient is a way of measuring how much two or more observers agree upon a certain measurement. The reason to use kappa values over "percent agreement" is that kappa statistics account for the fact that some agreement between observers will be due to chance alone. For example, in a population with a lot of negatives, two observers have a greater chance of agreement based on chance alone.

For example, if two examiners read radiographs and then determine the type of fracture present according to a classification system, the kappa coefficient is a way of determining how much the observers of the fractures agree upon the types of fractures. The test reports the agreement using a scale, where 1.0 means that the examiners agreed upon the classification 100% of the time. There are several ways to perform this calculation, but a common classification of the results with this test is by Landis and Koch. According to their recommendations, a kappa value of 0.0 to 0.2 represents poor agreement between observers, 0.21 to 0.4 fair agreement, 0.41 to 0.6 moderate agreement, 0.61 to 0.8 substantial, and 0.81 to 1.0 perfect agreement.

Post-test probability A further tool for interpreting diagnostic tests includes the post-test probability. This statistic is not commonly used in studies of clinical tests but is being used more and more for clinical studies. This number tells the actual probability of a subject having or not having the diseases given a positive or negative result, respectively. The post-test probability is calculated by multiplying the likelihood ratio (see above) by the pretest probability (i.e., the prevalence of the disease). Because post-test probabilities include the prevalence, they are not as informative in case control studies where the prevalence is artificially set by the design of the study.

Descriptive statistics Descriptive statistics are the most basic statistical techniques to describe data and populations. The most commonly used descriptive statistics are the mean, median, and standard deviation. The mean is the sum of all the values in a distribution divided by the sample size, and the standard deviation is the square root of the mean of the differences between each data point and the mean. When describing a normal (bell-shaped) distribution, the mean lies at the center, or median position, of the distribution, and each standard deviation encompasses a known percent of the data. In cases in which the data are distinctly not normal, the median becomes a better estimate of the center of the distribution than the mean.

Confidence interval A confidence interval is a range of values that has a high probability of containing the parameter being estimated, such as the mean or a relative risk. The 95% confidence interval is constructed in such a way that 95% of such intervals will contain the parameter. Similarly, 99% of 99% confidence intervals contain that parameter. The level of confidence is only justified to the extent that bias is absent from the study.

Measures of significance Tests of significance are used to evaluate the results we observe to decide whether they are sufficiently beyond the expected range of results to be regarded as "significant." In statistical terms, the goal of the test is to reject the null hypothesis that the result can be explained by chance alone. To do so, we set a significance level (also known as p value) at which we will reject the null hypothesis, that is, a level at which we feel confident the observed differences cannot be explained by chance alone. In practice, most investigators used a $p = .05$ significance level. In other words, they feel confident that their results cannot be explained by chance alone when this result had a 1 in 20 or less probability of occurring. Tests of significance using these basic principles are used to evaluate several types of results. The most common are summarized in **Table A–1**.

Correlation Sometimes, the goal of an analysis is not to measure how different two distributions are, but rather how they are related. The most common method used to evaluate the strength of a relationship between two variables is to examine their correlation. Correlation is generally assessed using the Pearson correlation coefficient. Pearson correlation coefficients can range from −1.00 (a perfectly negative relationship) to +1.00 (a perfectly positive relationship). A coefficient of 0 indicates complete independence. Because correlation is an assessment of the degree of linear relationship between two continuous variables, variables that may have a strong nonlinear (e.g., U-shaped) relationship may yield coefficients close to 0.

Utility The utility of a test is a measure of whether the patient is truly better off as a result of the test. A test

TABLE A–1 Results from Commonly Used Significance Tests

Type of Result	Commonly used Significance Test
Difference between two proportions; all cells have > 5 cases	Chi-square
Difference between two proportions; some cells have < 5 cases	Fisher's exact
Difference between the means of two normal distributions	t-test
Difference between single normal populations at two time points	Paired t-test
Difference between the means of two non-normal distributions	Wilcoxon rank
Difference between the means of more than two distributions	ANOVA*

ANOVA, analysis of variance.

could have a high sensitivity, specificity, and good likelihood ratios and still have low utility if it is very invasive or poses other risks or inconvenience to the patient.

SUGGESTED READINGS

Bhandari M, et al. User's guide to the surgical literature: how to use an article about a diagnostic test. J Bone Joint Surg Am 2003;85-A (6):1133–1140

Carmines EG, Zeller RA. Reliability and Validity Assessment:Quantitative Applications in the Social Sciences. Newbury Park, CA: Sage; 1979

Daniel WW. Biostatistics: A Foundation for Analysis in the Health Sciences, 7th ed. New York: Wiley; 1999

DeVellis RF. Scale Development: Theory and Applications. Newbury Park, CA: Sage; 1991

Ebell M, Barry H. Evidence-based Medicine. Michigan: Office of Medical Education Research and Development, College of Human Medicine, Michigan State University; 1999

Galen RS, Gambino S. Beyond Normality. New York: Wiley; 1975

Gordis L. Epidemiology. Philadelphia: WB Saunders; 2000

Greenfield ML, Kuhn JE, Wojtys EM. A statistics primer: validity and reliability. Am J Sports Med 1998;26(3):483–485

Jaeschke R, Guyatt GH, Sackett D. How to use an article about a diagnostic test: are the results of the study valid? JAMA 1994;271:289–291

Landis J, Koch GG. An application of hierarchical kappa-type statistics in the assessment of majority agreement among multiple observers. Biometrics 1977;33(2):363–374

Litwin MS. How to Measure Survey Reliability and Validity, vol. 7. Newbury Park: Sage; 1995

Nicoll D, McPhee SJ. Pignone. M. Pocket Guide to Diagnostic Tests, 4th ed. New York: McGraw-Hill/Appleton & Lange; 2003

Sackett DL HR. Guyatt GH, Tugwell P. Clinical epidemiology: A Basic Science for Clinical Medicine, 2nd ed. Boston: 1991

Sackett DL SS. Richardson WS, Rosenberg W, Haynes RB. Evidence-based Medicine: How to Practise and Teach EBM, 2nd ed. Edinburgh: Churchill Livingstone; 2000

Szklo M, Nieto FJ. Epidemiology: Beyond the Basics. New York: Aspen; 1999

Weiss N. Clinical Epidemiology: The Study of the Outcome of Illness, 2nd ed. New York: Oxford University Press; 1996

Index

Page numbers followed by an italic *f* or *t* indicate the entry on that page is in a figure or table.

A

Abbot test, for biceps instability, 230
Abdominal compression test
  in biceps pathology, 229*t*
  resisted, 119, 119*f*
  of subscapularis muscle, 118–119, 118*f*–119*f*
Abduction. *See also specific tests*
  combined tests of, 74, 74*f*
  dynamometer values in, 96, 96*t*
  elevation in, 16–17, 17*f*, 26, 57
    measurement of, 26–28, 27*f*–28*f*
  normal range of, 16*t*
  passive, range of, 189–190
Abductor digiti minimi muscle, innervation of, 12*f*
Abductor pollicis brevis muscle, innervation of, 12*f*
Abductor pollicis longus muscle, innervation of, 11*f*
Abrasion sign, in rotator cuff disease, 140, 140*f*
Accuracy, definition of, 259
Acromioclavicular (AC) joint, 244–255
  active compression test (O'Brien test) of, 252, 252*f*
  age and, 245, 250
  anteroposterior instability of, 253–254
  arthritis of, 8, 10*f*, 244–245
  asymmetry of, 8–10, 9*f*–10*f*, 244, 244*f*, 245
  asymptomatic *versus* symptomatic, 250
  cross-body adduction stress test of, 251, 251*f*
  cysts of, 8, 9*f*, 246, 246*f*
    clinical presentation of, 246, 246*f*
    diagnosis of, 246
    transillumination of, 246
  disorders/injuries of. *See also specific types*
    versus cervical spine disease, 245
    coexisting conditions with, 245
    common, 244
    differential diagnosis of, 246, 249

    glenohumeral motion in, 41*t*
    mechanisms of, 6*t*
    mimicking other conditions, 245
    muscle atrophy in, 8*t*
    pain provocation tests of, 249–250, 250*t*
    radiography of, 245
    versus rotator cuff disease, 245
    scapular dyskinesia with, 61
    side-to-side comparisons in, 8–10, 9*f*–10*f*, 244, 244*f*, 245
    versus SLAP lesions, 245
    sports-related, 5*t*, 244
    tests for, 250–255
      combined, 255, 255*t*
      diagnostic values of, 251*t*, 255*t*
      sensitivity and specificity of, 251*t*, 255*t*
  examination of, 244–249
  injection test of, 249–250, 254
    accuracy of, 254
    challenges in, 254
    technique for, 254, 254*f*
  local tenderness in, evaluation of, 249–255
  normal variation in, 245
  observation of, 8, 9*f*–10*f*, 245–249
  one-finger test of, 250–251, 251*f*
  osteolysis of, 244
  pain in, 2, 244
    activities aggravating, 5*t*
    distribution of, 2, 3*f*, 249–255, 250*f*
    localization of, 249–255, 250*t*, 251*f*
    patterns of, 5*t*
  Paxinos test of, 253, 253*f*
  resisted arm extension test of, 252–253, 252*f*
  separation of, 8, 9*f*, 244, 246
    versus clavicle fracture, 246–249, 248*f*–249*f*
    clinical presentation of, 246, 247*f*–248*f*

grade I, 246, 247*f*
grade II, 246, 247*f*
grade III, 246, 247*f*–248*f*
grade IV, 246, 247*f*–248*f*
grade V, 246, 247*f*–248*f*
grade VI, 246, 247*f*
radiographic features of, 246, 248*f*
sepsis of, 246
stability function of, 170
swelling of, causes of, 245
Acromion
anterior spur of, 130, 130*f*
in rotator cuff impingement, 129–131,
129*f*–130*f*
shapes of, 130–131, 130*f*
slope of, 131
stability function of, 170
Active compression test
for acromioclavicular disorders, 252, 252*f*
diagnostic values of, 251*t*, 252
sensitivity and specificity of, 251*t*, 252, 255*t*
for biceps pathology, 229*t*
for SLAP lesions, 224*t*, 235–236, 235*f*–236*f*
diagnostic accuracy of, 225*t*, 233*t*, 236
patient interpretation in, 236
sensitivity and specificity of, 224*t*–225*t*, 236
Active range of motion, 22
Active rotation, 42
with arm at 90 degrees, 44–45, 45*f*–46*f*
with arm at side, 42–43, 43*f*–44*f*
Activities of daily living
in range of motion assessment, 50, 50*t*, 71–72, 72*f*
in strength testing, 98
Adduction. *See also specific tests*
cross-body, 17, 18*f*, 73–75, 74*f*, 143*t*, 251, 251*f*
dynamometer values in, 96, 96*t*
horizontal, 17, 18*f*
Adductor pollicis muscle, innervation of, 12*f*
Adhesive capsulitis, 71
Age
and acromioclavicular joint, 245, 250
and biceps tendon tears, 216
and laxity, 184, 185*t*
in patient history, 1*t*
and range of motion, 20–21
and rotator cuff disease, 126–127, 127*t*,
157–158, 157*t*
and SLAP lesions, 224
and strength testing, 91
American Academy of Orthopaedic Surgeons (AAOS),
range of motion measures of, 16–17, 16*t*
American Medical Association (AMA), range of motion
measures of, 15–16, 16*t*
Analysis of variance (ANOVA), 260*t*
Anconeus muscle
actions of, 11*t*
innervation of, 11*t*
Andrews' anterior instability test, 196, 196*f*
Anesthesia, general, and laxity, 184, 184*t*
Anginal pain, 2, 3*f*

ANOVA (analysis of variance), 260*t*
Anterior capsule, stability function of, 169
Anterior dislocation, sports-related, 5*t*
Anterior drawer test, 182–184, 183*f*
as instability test, 190
Anterior glide test, for SLAP lesions, 224*t*,
233–234, 233*f*
diagnostic values of, 224*t*–225*t*, 233*t*, 234
Anterior instability, 190–198
Andrews' test for, 196, 196*f*
anterior drawer test for, 190
apprehension test for, 190–192, 190*f*–191*f*
augmentation test for, 194–195
combined tests for, 198
crank test for, 195, 195*f*
diagnostic values of tests for, 192*t*
fulcrum test for, 195, 195*f*
prone test for, 196
release test for, 197–198, 197*f*
relocation test for, 192–194, 193*f*
sensitivity and specificity of tests for, 192*t*
standing Rowe test for, 195, 196*f*
surprise test for, 198
in throwing athlete (APIT lesion), 165
Anterior internal impingement, 136,
196–197, 196*f*
Anterior labrum, stability function of, 169
Anterior laxity
drawer test of, 182–184, 183*f*
load and shift test of, 185–186, 186*f*
measurement of, 182–187
Protzman test of, 187, 187*f*
Anterior pseudolaxity, 219
Anterior subluxation
demonstrable or voluntary, 206, 206*f*
test for, 80–81, 81*f*
Anteroinferior labrum, detachment of, 163, 163*f*
Anteroposterior instability, of acromioclavicular
joint, 253–254
Anteroposterior laxity
drawer tests of, 182–184, 182*f*–183*f*
load and shift test of, 185–186, 185*f*–186*f*
measurement of, 182–187
Protzman test of, 187, 187*f*
push-pull test of, 186–187, 187*f*
tests for, use in posterior instability, 203
Anteroposterior laxity, measurement of, 182–187
Anteroposterior radiograph, 13, 13*f*
of subacromial impingement, 129–130, 129*f*
Anterosuperior capsule, stability functions of, 170
APIT (anteroposterior instability in the throwing athlete)
lesion, 165
Apley scratch test, 72, 72*f*–73*f*
Apoptosis, in rotator cuff disease, 127
Apprehension test
for anterior instability, 190–192, 190*f*–191*f*
accuracy of, 191–192, 191*t*
augmentation variation of, 194–195
crank variation of, 195, 195*f*
diagnostic values of, 192*t*

Apprehension test (*Continued*)
    fulcrum variation of, 195, 195*f*
    pain *versus*, 192
    reliability of, 192
    sensitivity and specificity of, 192, 192*t*
    for demonstrable or voluntary subluxation, 205
    for posterior instability, 199–201, 200*f*–201*f*
    for SLAP lesions, 224*t*
    validity of, 186*t*
Archery injuries, 5*t*
Arc of motion, total, in overhead athletes, 35–37
Arm(s). *See also specific tests*
    adduction of, horizontal or cross-body, 17, 18*f*, 73–75,
        74*f*, 143*t*, 251, 251*f*
    elevation of
        in abduction, 16–17, 17*f*, 26–28, 27*f*–28*f*
        in flexion, 16–17, 17*f*, 26, 28, 28*f*, 57
        measurement of, 26–28
    extension of
        horizontal, 17
        at side, behind body, 16
    rotation of
        external, 16–17
        internal, 16–18
        lateral, 17
        medial, 17
Arthritis
    acromioclavicular joint, 244–245
    glenohumeral motion in, 41*t*
    mechanisms of, 6*t*
    muscle atrophy in, 8*t*
    pain in
        activities aggravating, 5*t*
        patterns of, 5*t*
    shrug sign test in, 80, 80*t*
    sternoclavicular joint, 256
Arthrography
    of internal impingement, 134, 134*f*, 135
    of rotator cuff tears, 126–127, 127*t*
Arthrometer, 167
Arthroscopic suturing, of ligaments, 164
Arthroscopy
    in instability, 164
    in internal impingement, 133–134, 133*f*, 135
    of SLAP-biceps lesions, 240–241
Asymmetry
    of acromioclavicular joint, 8–10, 9*f*–10*f*,
        244, 244*f*, 245
    observation of, 8–10, 9*f*–10*f*, 244, 244*f*
    of scapula, 10, 10*f*
        in scoliosis, 81, 81*f*
    in total arc of motion, in overhead athletes, 35–37
Atrophy, muscular. *See also specific muscles*
    observation of, 7–8, 8*f*
    shoulder pathologies associated with, 8*t*
Augmentation test, for anterior instability, 194–195
    validity of, 186*t*
Axillary nerve
    distribution of, 108, 108*f*
    injection studies of, 110, 113

    muscles innervated by, 11*f*, 11*t*, 108, 120
    palsy of, 108, 108*f*, 110
        deltoid lag sign in, 110, 111*f*, 155–156
        versus rotator cuff injury, 110
        scaphoid sign in, 110, 110*f*
Axillary radiograph, 13, 13*f*

B
Babinski's reflex, 13
Bankart lesion, 163, 163*f*, 216
    bony, 167–168
Baseball players
    biceps tendon function in, 217–218
    glenohumeral motion in, 41–42
    infraspinatus atrophy in, 114
    injuries in, 5*t*. *See also specific types*
    latissimus dorsi syndrome in, 102, 102*f*
    posterior shoulder tightness test in, 75
    rotational injuries in, 29–37
        active *versus* passive motion in, 35
        biomechanical study of, 34
        bone alterations in, 35
    rotational range of motion in, 30*t*
    rotator cuff disease in, biomechanics of, 128, 128*f*
    scapular dyskinesia in, 61
    strength testing in, dynamometer for, 97
    total arc of motion in, 35–37
    triceps tendinitis in, 121
Belly press test
    in biceps pathology, 229*t*
    resisted, 119, 119*f*
    of subscapularis muscle, 118–119, 118*f*–119*f*
Bench press injuries, 5, 5*t*, 105–106, 244
Biceps brachii muscle
    actions of, 11*t*, 121
    anatomy of, 120–121, 120*f*, 213–214, 213*f*
    EMG studies of, 90
    innervation of, 11*t*, 12*f*, 121
    long head of, 120, 213, 213*f*
    short head of, 120, 120*f*, 213, 213*f*
Biceps entrapment sign, 230–231
Biceps load test I, 236–237, 236*f*
    diagnostic values of, 225*t*, 237
Biceps load test II, 237, 237*f*
    diagnostic values of, 225*t*, 237
Biceps tendon, 213–241
    anatomy of, 120–121, 213–214, 213*f*
    arthroscopy of, 240–241
    attachment anatomy of, 120–121, 120*f*, 214–215, 214*f*–215*f*
    entrapment sign in, 230–231
    function of, 217–218
        dynamic, 218
        as spacer, 217
        stabilizing, 217–218
        static, 217–218
    Gilchrist sign in, 229–230, 229*f*
    injections of, 231–232
        technique for, 232, 232*f*
    instability of, 221–222
        Abbot test for, 230

lateral slide test of, 230
lift-off test of, 231, 231*f*
Lippman test of, 230, 230*f*
Ludington test of, 226, 226*f*
observation of, 8, 9*f*, 226
palpation of, 227, 227*f*, 229*t*
pulley system of, 213–214
and rotator cuff disease, 220–221, 221*f*
and shoulder instability, 218–220
and shoulder pain, 220–221, 221*f*
soft tissue sarcoma of, 226, 226*f*
Speed's test of, 228–229, 228*f*
supination sign of Yergason in, 227–228, 228*f*
synovial cysts of, 226
tears of, 8, 9*f*, 121, 216
   age and, 216
   bulge or lump with, 216, 216*f*
   evaluation for, 226–232
   location of, 216
   "Popeye arm" in, 121, 216, 216*f*, 226
   with superior labrum tears, 216–217.
      See also Superior labrum injury, anterior to
      posterior (SLAP)
tenderness of, testing for, 226–227, 227*f*
tests for, 225–232
   diagnostic values of, 228*t*–229*t*
Biceps tenodesis, 220
Biceps tenotomy, 220
Bicipital groove pain, in SLAP lesion evaluation,
   233–234, 234*t*
Biodex, for strength testing, 97
Biomechanics, clinically relevant, 22–26
Blackburn position, for supraspinatus testing, 112, 112*f*
Blix's curve, 89, 89*f*
Bone laxity, 167, 167*f*
Bone scan, of acromioclavicular joint, 255, 255*t*
Bone-to-bone end feel, 49
Bony Bankart lesion, 167–168
Brachialis muscle
   actions of, 11*t*
   innervation of, 11*t*, 12*f*
Brachioradialis muscle, innervation of, 11*f*
Breast cancer, metastatic to clavicle, 245
Buford complex, 215, 216*f*
Bursitis, subscapular, 82, 82*f*

C

Capsular contraction, in overhead athletes, 34–35
Capsular failure, in instability, 163
Capsular feel, 49
Capsular ligaments, stability functions of, 169–170, 169*t*
Capsular shift, for instability, 163–164
Cervical levels, reflex testing at, 10–13, 13*f*
Cervical spine disorders
   versus acromioclavicular disorders, 245
   pain in, 2, 3*f*
Chest pain, 2, 3*f*
Chi-square, 260*t*
Chock block, labrum as, 167, 167*f*
Circle concept, of stability, 169–170, 170*f*

Clavicle
  distal
    excision of, and AC joint instability, 253
    fracture of, 246–249
      versus acromioclavicular separation, 247–249
      type I, 246, 248*f*
      type II, 246
      type II A, 246, 249*f*
      type II B, 246, 249*f*
      type III, 246–249, 249*f*
    malignant tumors of, 245
   pain medial to, 2, 3*f*
   proximal, disorders of, 256
Clinically significant motions, in range of motion
      assessment, 49–50, 50*f*, 50*t*, 51*f*, 71–72, 72*f*
Clunk test, for SLAP lesions, 233, 233*f*
Codman, hammock position of, 78–79, 79*f*
Codman's paradox, 77, 77*f*
Combined abduction test, 74, 74*f*
Combing hair, range of motion for, 50*t*
Compression, concavity, 168, 168*f*
Compression forces
  in rotator cuff disease, 127–128
  in shoulder stability, 168–169, 168*f*
Compression rotation sign
  diagnostic accuracy of, 225*t*, 232–233, 233*t*
  in SLAP lesions, 224*t*, 232–233, 232*f*
Computed tomography (CT), 14
Concavity compression, 168, 168*f*
Confidence interval, 260
Construct validity, 258
Content validity, 258
Coracoacromial ligament
  in pulley system, 213–214
  stability function of, 170
Coracoantecubital distance test, 73. *See also* Cross-body
      adduction
Coracobrachialis muscle
  actions of, 11*t*
  innervation of, 11*t*, 12*f*
Coracohumeral ligament, 162*f*
  stability functions of, 169–170, 169*t*
Coracoid impingement, 131–133, 131*f*
  biceps tendon in, 221, 221*f*
  functional, 133
  iatrogenic, 131–133
  idiopathic, 132
  pain in, 131–132
  posterior glenoid osteotomies and, 132–133
  posttraumatic, 132–133
  testing for, 147–148, 147*f*
  Trillat procedure and, 131–132
Coracoid impingement sign, 147–148, 147*f*
Coracoid stress fracture, sports-related, 5*t*
Correlation, 260
Corticosteroids, subacromial injection of, 149–150
Cortisone injection, in subscapular bursitis, 82, 82*f*
Crank test
  for anterior instability, 195, 195*f*
  for biceps pathology, 229*t*

Crank test (*Continued*)
  for SLAP lesions, 234–235, 234*f*
    diagnostic values of, 224*t*–225*t*, 235
Crepitus
  in rotator cuff disease, 140, 140*f*
  in scapular motion, 81
  in sternoclavicular pathology, 256
Cross-body adduction, 17, 18*f*
Cross-body adduction test
  of acromioclavicular joint, 251, 251*f*, 251*t*
    diagnostic values of, 251, 251*t*
    sensitivity and specificity of, 251,
      251*t*, 255*t*
  of mobility/flexibility, 73–75, 74*f*
  of rotator cuff, 143*t*
Cybex II, for strength testing, 92–93, 97
Cysts
  of acromioclavicular joint, 8, 9*f*, 246, 246*f*
  of biceps tendon, 226
Cyriax system, 49
Cytokines, in shoulder pain, 128–129

D
Dawbarn's sign, 141
"Dead arm" syndrome, 163
Deltoid lag sign, 110, 111*f*, 155–156, 155*f*
Deltoid muscle
  actions of, 11*t*, 108
  anatomy of, 90, 107–108, 108*f*
  anterior, 108, 108*f*
    testing of, 108–109, 109*f*
      optimal position for, 93*t*
  atrophy of
    conditions associated with, 8*t*
    scaphoid sign in, 8, 9*f*, 110, 110*f*
    side-to-side comparisons in, 8, 9*f*, 110
    swollen appearance in, 110, 110*f*
  innervation of, 11*f*, 11*t*, 108, 108*f*
  middle, 108, 108*f*
    testing of, 109, 109*f*
      optimal position for, 93*t*
  posterior, 108, 108*f*
    testing of, 109–110, 109*f*
      optimal position for, 93*t*
  in rotator cuff disease, 138, 138*f*–139*f*
  strength testing of, 107–110, 109*f*
Demonstrable scapular dyskinesia, 67, 67*f*
Demonstrable scapular winging, 67, 67*f*
Demonstrable subluxation, 198, 198*f*, 205–207
  anterior, 206, 206*f*
  evaluation of, 205
  inferior, 206–207, 206*f*
  posterior, 205–206, 206*f*
  sternoclavicular, 256
Dermatomes, 10, 12*f*
Descriptive statistics, 260
Digital inclinometers, 20, 20*f*
Dislocation(s), 162. *See also* Instability
  anterior, sports-related, 5*t*
  biceps tendon, 221–222

  inferior, 203–204
  sternoclavicular, 255–256
Distal clavicle
  excision of, and AC joint instability, 253
  fracture of, 246–249
    versus acromioclavicular separation, 247–249
    type I, 246, 248*f*
    type II, 246
    type II A, 246, 249*f*
    type II B, 246, 249*f*
    type III, 246–249, 249*f*
  malignant tumors of, 245
Diurnal variations, in strength testing, 91–92
Dominance of extremity, 1–2, 1*t*
  and glenohumeral motion, 39, 39*t*–40*t*
  and laxity measurements, 184
  and range of motion, 21, 29, 30*t*–33*t*, 34–36
  and strength testing, 91
Dorsal scapular nerve, muscles innervated
    by, 11*t*, 104
Downward rotation, scapular, 55, 56*f*
Drawer test(s)
  anterior, 182–184, 183*f*
    as instability test, 190
  posterior, 182–184, 182*f*, 203
Drooping, in tennis shoulder, 63, 63*f*
Drop arm sign
  in acromioclavicular disorders, 251*t*
  definition of, 151
  in rotator cuff disease, 151–152, 151*f*
    accuracy of, 142*t*–144*t*
    diagnostic values of, 143*t*
    sensitivity and specificity of, 142*t*–144*t*, 151–152
Drop sign, 120, 154–155, 155*f*
Dynamometer(s), 94–97
  disadvantages of, 97
  duration of force/fatigue with, 96–97
  handheld, 95–97, 95*f*
  isokinetic, 95, 95*f*, 97–98
  placement of, 96, 96*t*
  reference values for, 96, 96*t*
  reliability of, 95–96, 95*t*
  spring scale, 95–96, 95*f*, 95*t*
  strain gauge, 95, 95*f*
  tests positions for, 96, 96*t*
Dysphagia, in sternoclavicular pathology, 256

E
Eating, range of motion for, 50*t*
Eccentric phase, 55
Ehlers-Danlos syndrome, 205
Elbow, hyperextension of, 207, 207*f*
Electrical shock, and posterior instability, 198
Electromagnetic devices, for motion studies, 23–25,
    23*f*–25*f*
Electromyography, 89–90
  intramuscular fine-wire, 89
  optimal muscle testing position determined by, 92, 93*t*
  quantitative, 89–90
  surface, 89–90

Elevation. *See also specific tests*
 in abduction, 16–17, 17*f*, 26, 57
  measurement of, 26–28, 27*f*–28*f*
 in flexion, 16–17, 17*f*, 26, 57
  measurement of, 26, 28, 28*f*
 measurement of, 26–28
  positions or maneuvers hampering, 27–28,
   27*f*–28*f*
 radiographic studies of, 22–25
 scapular motion in, 57
  biomechanics of, 53–58
  versus glenohumeral motion, 51–52
 in scapular plane, 17, 17*f*, 27*f*, 52
Ellman classification, of partial rotator
   cuff tears, 133, 133*t*
Embolism, finger, 13
"Empty can" position, 152–153, 152*f*
 for supraspinatus testing, 112–113, 112*f*–113*f*
Empty feel, 49
End feel, 43*f*, 48–49
 bone-to-bone, 49
 capsular, 49
 Cyriax's classification of, 49
 empty, 49
 Maitland's scheme for, 48–49, 49*t*
 spasm, 49
 springy block, 49
 tissue approximation, 49
Entrapment sign, biceps, 230–231
E³ program, 90
Etiology, 1
Extension, 16. *See also specific tests*
 dynamometer values in, 96, 96*t*
 horizontal, 17
 normal range of, 16*t*
Extensor carpi radialis brevis muscle,
   innervation of, 11*f*
Extensor carpi radialis longus muscle,
   innervation of, 11*f*
Extensor digiti minimi muscle, innervation of, 11*f*
Extensor digitorum muscle, innervation of, 11*f*
Extensor indicis muscle, innervation of, 11*f*
Extensor pollicis brevis muscle, innervation of, 11*f*
Extensor pollicis longus muscle, innervation of, 11*f*
External rotation, 16–17, 16*t*. *See also specific tests*
 active
  with arm at 90 degrees, 45, 46*f*
  with arm at side, 43, 44*f*
 with arm at 90 degrees, 16*t*, 44–45, 45*f*–46*f*
 with arm at side, 42–43, 43*f*–44*f*
 functional positions for, 50, 51*f*
 in lateral decubitus position, 47, 47*f*
 normal range of, 16*t*
 180 degree rule, 36
 in overhead athletes, 29–37, 41–42
 passive
  with arm at 90 degrees, 45, 45*f*
  with arm at side, 42–43, 43*f*
 scapular, 55*t*, 56, 57*f*
External rotation lag sign, 154, 154*f*

F
Face validity, 258
Fall(s)
 mechanism of injuries in, 4, 5*t*–6*t*
 superior labrum injury in, 222–223, 223*t*
Feagin test, for inferior laxity, 204, 204*f*
Fibroblasts, in rotator cuff disease, 127
Fine-wire electromyography, 89
Fingers, examination of, 13
Fisher's exact, 260*t*
Flexibility, 71–81
 Apley scratch test of, 72, 72*f*–73*f*
 combined abduction test of, 74, 74*f*
 crossed-arm test of, 73–74, 74*f*
 hammock position of Codman in, 78–79, 79*f*
 horizontal flexion test of, 73, 73*f*
 locked quadrant position in, 78, 78*f*
 pectoralis minor muscle contracture test of, 76–77,
   76*f*–77*f*
 pivotal position/area in, 78–80, 79*f*
 posterior shoulder tightness test of, 74–76, 74*f*–75*f*
 quadrant position and test in, 77, 77*f*–78*f*
 reverse scapulothoracic rhythm in, 81
 shrug sign in, 80, 80*f*, 80*t*
 subluxation test of, 80–81, 81*f*
 subscapularis muscle tightness test of, 76
 zero position of Saha in, 78, 79*f*
Flexion. *See also specific tests*
 contact of rotator cuff in, 136–138, 136*f*
 dynamometer values in, 96, 96*t*
 elevation in, 16–17, 17*f*, 26, 57
  measurement of, 26, 28, 28*f*
 forward, 17, 17*f*
 horizontal, test of, 73, 73*f*
 normal range of, 16*t*
 weighted scapular test of, 65
Flexor carpi radialis muscle, innervation of, 12*f*
Flexor carpi ulnaris muscle, innervation of, 12*f*
Flexor digiti minimi brevis muscle, innervation of, 12*f*
Flexor digitorum profundus muscle, innervation of, 12*f*
Flexor digitorum superficialis muscle, innervation of, 12*f*
Flexor pollicis brevis muscle, innervation of, 12*f*
Flexor pollicis longus muscle, innervation of, 12*f*
Flip sign, scapular, 64–65, 65*f*
Football injuries, 5*t*
 posterior instability in, 198, 199*f*
Force-length relationship, in muscle strength, 89, 89*f*
Forward flexion, 17, 17*f*
Fracture(s)
 coracoid stress, sports-related, 5*t*
 of distal clavicle, 246–249
  versus acromioclavicular separation, 247–249
  type I, 246, 248*f*
  type II, 246
  type II A, 246, 249*f*
  type II B, 246, 249*f*
  type III, 246–249, 249*f*
 rib stress, sports-related, 5*t*
 sternoclavicular joint, 255–256
  physeal, 255–256, 256*f*

Freiberg's avascular necrosis, 256
Frozen shoulder, 71
  glenohumeral motion in, 41*t*
  shrug sign test in, 80, 80*t*
Fukada test, for posterior instability, 202, 202*f*
Fulcrum test, of anterior instability, 195, 195*f*
"Full can" position, 152–153, 152*f*
  for supraspinatus testing, 113, 113*f*
Functional motions, in range of motion assessment,
    49–50, 50*f*, 50*t*, 51*f*, 71–72, 72*f*

G

Gender
  and physical examination, 6–7, 6*f*–7*f*
  and range of motion, 21, 21*t*
  and strength testing, 91
General anesthesia, and laxity, 184, 184*t*
Generalized ligamentous laxity, 207–208, 207*f*–208*f*
Gilchrist sign, in biceps pathology, 229–230, 229*f*
Glenohumeral internal rotation deficit (GIRD), 29–37
  lateral decubitus examination for, 47, 47*f*
  scapular dyskinesia with, 61
Glenohumeral joint
  active rotation of, 42
  inflexibilities of, 72
  instability of, 162–166. *See also* Instability
  laxity of, 171–190. *See also* Laxity
  motion of, 37–42
    clinical studies of, 38–42, 38*t*–41*t*
    versus combined motions, 38–42, 38*t*–40*t*
    distribution of
      by age, 41, 41*t*
      by diagnosis, 41, 41*t*
    in dominant *versus* non-dominant shoulder, 39, 39*t*–40*t*
    goniometry of, 41
    hip abnormalities and, 68–69
    in lateral decubitus position, 47, 47*f*
    in overhead athletes, 41–42
    reliability of measurements of, 39–40
    versus scapular, in elevation, 51–52
    scapular motion in, 46–47, 46*f*
    versus scapulothoracic motion, 22–26, 23*t*, 25*t*, 37–39, 37*t*
    in standing *versus* supine position, 39–40, 40*t*
    visual observation of, 40–41
  passive rotation of, 42
    external
      with arm at 90 degrees, 45, 45*f*
      with arm at side, 42, 43*f*
    internal, with arm at 90 degrees, 43–44, 44*f*
Glenohumeral protectors, 90
Glenohumeral-scapulothoracic rotation, combined
  active, 42
    with arm at 90 degrees, 44, 45*f*
    with arm at side, 43, 44*f*
  passive, 42
    with arm at 90 degrees, 44–45, 45*f*
    with arm at side, 43, 43*f*
Glenoid
  biceps tendon attachment to, 214, 214*f*
  bony configuration of, 167

labrum attachment to, 214–215, 215*f*
  osseous defects of, 168, 168*f*
  retroversion of, 167
  stability functions of, 167–169
  surface of, integrity of, 167–168
Glenoid dysplasia, 167
Global coordinate system, for range of motion, 18, 18*f*
Golf injuries, 5*t*
Goniometers, handheld, 19
Goniometry
  versus clinically significant motions, 49–50
  of elevation in abduction, 26–28, 27*f*
  of elevation in flexion, 28, 28*f*
  of glenohumeral motion, 41
  reliability of, 50
  of scapular motion, 46–47
Gowns, for female patients, 6, 6*f*–7*f*
Greater tuberosity of humerus, supraspinatus tendon
    attachment on, 111–112, 112*f*

H

Hammock position of Codman, 78–79, 79*f*
Hand(s)
  examination of, 13
  placing behind head, range of motion for, 50*t*
  position, in Codman's paradox, 77, 77*f*
  up the back, internal rotation with, 48, 48*f*
Handheld dynamometers, 95–97, 95*f*
Handheld goniometers, 19
Hawkins classification, of humeral head translation
  based on clinical feel, 181–182, 181*f*
  based on millimeters, 179–180, 180*f*
Hawkins impingement sign, 144–145, 144*f*
  accuracy of, 142*t*–143*t*, 144–145, 144*t*
  in acromioclavicular disorders, 251*t*
  biceps tendon in, 220–221, 221*f*, 229*t*
  diagnostic values of, 143*t*, 144, 251*t*
  sensitivity and specificity of, 142*t*–143*t*, 144, 144*t*
Head posture, and scapular motion, 69–70, 69*f*
Hip movements, abnormal, and shoulder pathology,
    68–69
History, patient, 1, 1*t*, 7
Hoffmann's maneuver, 13, 13*f*
Horizontal adduction, 17, 18*f*
Horizontal extension, 17
Horizontal flexion test, 73, 73*f*
Hornblower's sign, 156–157, 156*f*
Humeral head
  bony configuration of, 167
  diameter of, 167
  retroversion of, 167
  translation of, 171–182
    anatomical restraints to, 169–170
    anteroposterior
      drawer tests of, 182–184, 182*f*–183*f*
      load and shift test of, 185–186, 185*f*–186*f*
      measurement of, 182–187
      Protzman test of, 187, 187*f*
      push-pull test of, 186–187, 187*f*
      total, 178, 178*t*

cadaveric studies *versus* physical findings of, 178, 178*t*
clinical feel of, 181–182, 181*f*
force for, 171, 178–179
Hawkins classifications of, 179–182,
    180*f*–181*f*
inferior
    hyperabduction test in, 189–190, 189*f*
    measurement of, 187–190
    sulcus sign in, 187–189, 188*f*, 203–204
    true (luxatio erecta), 188–189, 188*f*
labrum as chock block to, 167, 167*f*
literature review of, 172*t*–177*t*
in millimeters, 179–180, 179*f*
in percent head diameters, 180
quantitative measures of, 179–182
sulcus sign in, 179–180, 187–189, 188*f*
Humeral positioners (muscles), 90
Humeroscapular muscles, strength testing of, 120–122
Humerus
    greater tuberosity of, supraspinatus tendon attachment
        on, 111–112, 112*f*
    hyperangulation of, 29, 134, 164, 164*f*
    motion studies of, 22–26
    in overhead athlete, 29–37
    retroversion ("spun back") of, 35–36
    stability functions of, 167–169
Hyperabduction test, for inferior laxity, 189–190, 189*f*
Hyperangulation, of humerus, 29, 134, 164, 164*f*
Hyperlaxity, 207–208, 207*f*–208*f*
Hyperreflexia, 13
Hypertonicity, 13

I

Impingement
    in athletes, 134–136, 138
    biceps pathology and, 220–221, 221*f*
    coracoid, 131–133, 131*f*
        biceps tendon in, 221, 221*f*
        functional, 133
        iatrogenic, 131–133
        idiopathic, 132
        pain in, 131–132
        posterior glenoid osteotomies and, 132–133
        posttraumatic, 132–133
        testing for, 147–148, 147*f*
        Trillat procedure and, 131–132
    coracoid sign of, 147–148, 147*f*
    examination for, 138–151
        accuracy of tests in, 142–144, 142*t*–144*t*
        diagnostic values of tests in, 143, 143*t*
        sensitivity and specificity of tests in, 142*t*–144*t*
    glenohumeral motion in, 41*t*
    internal, 29, 133–136, 134*f*, 164, 165*f*
        anterior, 136, 196–197, 196*f*
        arthroscopic findings of, 133–135, 133*f*
        cadaveric studies of, 135, 135*f*–136*f*
        versus internal contact, 135
        in occult instability, 196–197, 196*f*
        osteophytes and, 135, 135*f*
        physical therapy for, 136

physiologic contact in, 135
radiographic studies of, 134–135, 134*f*
scapular dyskinesia and, 135
SLAP lesions with, 136, 223
stage I, 136
stage II, 136
stage III, 136
mechanism of injury in, 6*t*
Neer sign of, 80, 141–144, 142*f*
pain in
    activities aggravating, 5*t*
    patterns of, 5*t*
    versus posterior instability, 201, 201*f*
rotator cuff, 129–158
    and scapular motion, 70–71, 135
    types of, 129–138
scapular adaptation in, 66–67
secondary, 193
shrug sign test in, 80*t*
subacromial, 129–131
    acromial shape and, 130–131, 130*f*
    biceps tendon in, 221, 221*f*
    diagnostic injection in, 148–151, 150*f*
    radiographic studies of, 129–130, 129*f*–130*f*
    secondary, posterior shoulder tightness test in, 75
Inclinometers, 20
    digital, 20, 20*f*
    mechanical, 20, 20*f*
    scapular positioning with, 60–61
Inferior glenohumeral ligament, 162*f*
    in internal impingement, 134–135
    stability functions of, 169–170, 169*t*
Inferior instability, 203–204
    examination in, 203–204
    Feagin test for, 204, 204*f*
    history of, 203–204
    Rowe test for, 204, 204*f*
Inferior laxity
    Feagin test for, 204, 204*f*
    hyperabduction test in, 189–190, 189*f*
    measurement of, 187–190, 203–204
    sulcus sign in, 187–189, 188*f*, 203–204
    true (luxatio erecta), 188–189, 188*f*, 203
Inferior subluxation, demonstrable or voluntary,
    206–207, 206*f*
Infraspinatus lag signs, 116, 154–155, 154*f*–155*f*
Infraspinatus muscle
    actions of, 11*t*
    anatomy of, 114, 114*f*
    atrophy of, 114–115
        bilateral, 115, 115*f*
        conditions associated with, 8*t*
        etiology of, 114
        observation of, 8, 8*f*, 115, 115*f*
    innervation of, 11*f*, 11*t*, 114
    Patte test of, 145–146, 145*f*
    in rotator cuff disease, 139, 139*f*, 143*t*, 145–146, 146*f*, 153
    strength testing of, 114–116, 116*f*, 153
        optimal position for, 93*t*, 115–116
    tenderness of, palpation for, 139, 139*f*

Injection(s)
  acromioclavicular, 249–250, 254, 254*f*
  biceps tendon, 231–232, 232*f*
  subacromial, 148–151, 150*f*, 231–232, 249–250, 254
Instability (shoulder), 162–166
  anterior, 190–198
    Andrews' test for, 196, 196*f*
    anterior drawer test for, 190
    apprehension test for, 190–192, 190*f*–191*f*
    augmentation test for, 194–195
    combined tests for, 198
    crank test for, 195, 195*f*
    diagnostic values of tests for, 192*t*
    fulcrum test for, 195, 195*f*
    prone test for, 196
    release test for, 197–198, 197*f*
    relocation test for, 192–194, 193*f*
    sensitivity and specificity of tests for, 192*t*
    standing Rowe test for, 195, 196*f*
    surprise test for, 198
  in athletes, 29, 163–165
  biceps pathology and, 218–220
  biomechanics of, 167–170
  circle concept of, 169–170, 170*f*
  demonstrable or voluntary, 205–207
  diagnosis of, difficulties in, 162
  dislocation *versus* subluxation, 162
  glenohumeral motion in, 41*t*
  glenoid osseous defects in, 168, 168*f*
  history of concepts of, 162–165
  hyperlaxity and, 207–208, 207*f*–208*f*
  inferior, 203–204
    Feagin test for, 204, 204*f*
    Rowe test for, 204, 204*f*
  in internal impingement, 134–136
  labrum detachment in, 163, 163*f*
  versus laxity, 167–179
  mechanism of injury in, 6*t*
  muscle atrophy in, 8*t*
  nonstructural, 205
  occult, 163–167
    challenge of, 165–167
    glenohumeral motion in, 41*t*
    internal impingement sign for, 196–197, 196*f*
  pain in, 163–164
    activities aggravating, 5*t*
    patterns of, 5*t*
  posterior, 198–203
    apprehension test for, 199–201, 200*f*–201*f*
    demonstrable or voluntary, 198, 198*f*
    as football injury, 198, 199*f*
    in football injury, 198, 199*f*
    Fukada test for, 202, 202*f*
    glenohumeral motion in, 41*t*
    history of, 198–199
    jerk test for, 201–202, 201*f*
    pain in, *versus* impingement, 201, 201*f*
    physical examination of, 199, 199*f*
    posterior laxity tests used for, 203
    posterior subluxation (Miniaci) test for, 202, 202*f*

  push-pull test for, 202–203
  Rowe test for, 201, 201*f*, 203
  in seizure disorders, 198–199
  spectrum of, 205*t*
  sports-related, 5, 5*t*
  radiographic studies of, 179, 179*t*
  in rotator cuff disease, 163–164
  shrug sign test in, 80*t*
  SLAP lesions and, 218–220
  sulcus sign in, 179–180, 186*t*, 187–189, 188*f*, 203–204
  superior, 218–219
  testing related to, 207–208
  tests for, 190–207
    clinical, validity of, 186*t*
Instability, of acromioclavicular joint, anteroposterior, 253–254
Instability, of biceps tendon, 221–222
Instability, of sternoclavicular joint, 255–256
Internal contact
  versus internal impingement, 135
  of rotator cuff, in flexion, 136–138, 136*f*
Internal impingement, 29, 133–136, 134*f*, 164, 165*f*
  anterior, 136, 196–197, 196*f*
  arthroscopic findings of, 133–135, 133*f*
  cadaveric studies of, 135, 135*f*–136*f*
  versus internal contact, 135
  in occult instability, 196–197, 196*f*
  osteophytes and, 135, 135*f*
  physical therapy for, 136
  physiologic contact in, 135
  radiographic studies of, 134–135, 134*f*
  scapular dyskinesia and, 135
  SLAP lesions with, 136, 223
  stage I, 136
  stage II, 136
  stage III, 136
Internal impingement sign, for occult instability, 196–197, 196*f*
Internal rotation, 16, 16*t*, 17–18. *See also specific tests*
  with arm at 90 degrees, 16*t*, 43–44, 44*f*–45*f*
  functional positions for, 50, 50*f*
  glenohumeral deficit of, 29–37, 47, 47*f*, 61
  with hand up the back, 48, 48*f*
  in lateral decubitus position, 47, 47*f*
  normal range of, 16*t*
  180 degree rule for, 36
  in overhead athletes, 29–37, 41–42
  passive isolated glenohumeral, with arm at 90 degrees, 43–44, 44*f*
  in posterior instability, 199, 199*f*
  scapular, 55*t*, 56–58, 57*f*
Intertester reliability, 259–260
Intra-articular pressure, 168
Intraexaminer reliability, 259
Isokinetic dynamometers, 95, 95*f*, 97–98
Isokinetic strength testing, 97–98

J
Jerk test, for posterior instability, 201–202, 201*f*
Jigs, for laxity testing, 171

Jobe, Frank, 192–193
Jobe position/test
    diagnostic values of, 143*t*, 153
    for rotator cuff disease, 143*t*, 152–153, 152*f*
    for supraspinatus testing, 112–113, 112*f*–113*f*,
        152–153, 152*f*
Jobe relocation test
    for anterior instability, 192–194, 193*f*
        diagnostic values of, 192*t*, 193–194
        evaluation of, using different criteria for positive
            result, 194, 194*t*
        in rotator cuff disease, 193
        sensitivity and specificity of, 192*t*, 193–194
    for internal impingement/occult instability,
        196–197, 196*f*
    for SLAP lesions, 224*t*, 238–239, 239*f*
        diagnostic accuracy of, 224*t*, 239
        sensitivity and specificity of, 224*t*, 234*t*, 239
    validity of, 186*t*
Joint above/joint below assessment, 10

K
Kappa coefficients, 260
Kayaking injuries, 5*t*
Kennedy-Hawkins (Hawkins) sign, 144–145, 144*f*
    accuracy of, 142*t*–143*t*, 144–145, 144*t*
    in acromioclavicular disorders, 251*t*
    biceps tendon in, 220–221, 221*f*, 229*t*
    diagnostic values of, 143*t*, 144, 251*t*
    sensitivity and specificity of, 142*t*–143*t*, 144, 144*t*
Kibler, Ben, 68
Kibler's positions, for scapular positioning test, 59–60, 59*f*
Kibler test
    for biceps pathology, 229*t*
    diagnostic accuracy for, 229*t*, 233*t*, 234
    for SLAP lesions, 233–234, 233*f*
Kincom isokinetic dynamometers, 95, 95*f*, 97
Kinetic chain, 24, 67–71
King Kong's arm, 63, 63*f*
Knee, hyperextension of, 207, 208*f*
KT-1000 arthrometer, 167
Kyphosis, and scapular motion, 69–70, 69*f*

L
Labrum. *See also* Superior labrum
    attachment to superior glenoid, 214–215, 215*f*
    biceps tendon attachment to, 214–215, 214*f*
    as chock block, 167, 167*f*
    in concavity compression, 168–169, 168*f*
    detachment, in instability, 163, 163*f*
    stability functions of, 167–169, 167*f*, 169
Lag sign(s), 89, 154–157
    deltoid, 110, 111*f*, 155–156, 155*f*
    infraspinatus, 116, 154–155, 154*f*–155*f*
    subscapularis, 156, 156*f*
    supraspinatus, 154–155, 154*f*–155*f*
Lateral decubitus position, rotation measurements in,
    47, 47*f*
Lateral pectoral nerve, muscle innervated by, 11*t*, 105
Lateral rotation, scapular, 55

Lateral slide test
    biceps tendon, 230
    scapular, 58–60, 59*f*
        reliability of, 60
        specificity of, 60
        validity of, 60
Latissimus dorsi muscle, 90
    actions of, 11*t*, 101–102
    anatomy of, 101, 101*f*
    innervation of, 11*t*, 101
    strength testing of, 101–102, 102*f*
        optimal position for, 93*t*
    tenderness of, palpation for, 139–140, 140*f*
Latissimus dorsi syndrome, 102, 102*f*
Laxity, 171–190
    age and, 184, 185*t*
    anteroposterior
        drawer tests of, 182–184, 182*f*–183*f*
        load and shift test for, 185–186, 185*f*–186*f*
        measurement of, 182–187
        Protzman test of, 187, 187*f*
        push-pull test of, 186–187, 187*f*
        tests for, use in posterior instability, 203
    biceps pathology and, 218–220
    dominance of extremity and, 184
    generalized (hyperlaxity), 207–208, 207*f*–208*f*
    inferior
        Feagin test for, 204, 204*f*
        hyperabduction test in, 189–190, 189*f*
        measurement of, 187–189, 188*f*, 203–204
        sulcus sign in, 187–189, 188*f*, 203–204
        true (luxatio erecta), 188–189, 188*f*
    versus instability, 167–179
    in internal impingement, 134–136
    measurement of, 167
    normal, 167, 167*f*
    posterior, tests for, use in posterior instability, 203
    preoperative, under general anesthesia, 184, 184*t*
    SLAP lesions and, 218–220
    sulcus sign in, 179–180, 186*t*, 187–189, 188*f*, 203–204
    testing of, 171–179. *See also specific laxity types and tests*
        arm position in, 170–171, 171*f*
        cadaveric, 178, 178*t*
        clinical, 178–182
        for demonstrable or voluntary subluxation, 205
        end points in, 171
        excursion in, force for, 171
        in occult instability, 165–166
        quantitative measures in, 179–182
        radiographic, 179, 179*t*
        results of, review of literature on, 172*t*–177*t*
        translation in, 171–182
            cadaveric studies *versus* physical findings of,
                178, 178*t*
            clinical feel of, 181–182, 181*f*
            force for, 171, 178–179
            Hawkins classifications of, 179–182, 180*f*–181*f*
            in millimeters, 179–180, 179*f*
            in percent head diameters, 180
            total anteroposterior, 178, 178*t*

Laxity (*Continued*)
  validity of tests for, 186*t*
  venting of joint in, 171
  in zero or loose packed position, 170–171, 171*f*
Lennie test
  accuracy of, 60
  resting scapular position and, 52–53, 53*f*
Levator scapulae muscle
  actions of, 11*t*
  innervation of, 11*f*, 11*t*
Levine sign, 2, 3*f*
Lidocaine injection, for diagnosis of rotator cuff disease, 148–151, 150*f*
Lift-off test
  of biceps tendon, 231, 231*f*
    diagnostic values of, 229*t*, 231
  resisted, 118, 118*f*
  of subscapularis muscle, 117–119, 117*f*–118*f*, 153, 153*f*
Ligament(s)
  anatomy of, 162, 162*f*–163*f*
  laxity of, 167, 167*f*
    generalized (hyperlaxity), 207–208, 207*f*–208*f*
    testing of, 171–179
  stability functions of, 169–170, 169*t*, 170*f*
  surgical tightening of, 163–164
Likelihood ratio, definition of, 259
Lippman test, of biceps tendon, 230, 230*f*
Little League shoulder, 5*t*. *See also* Baseball players
Load and shift test
  for anteroposterior laxity, 185–186, 185*f*–186*f*
  for posterior instability, 203
  validity of, 186*t*
Locked quadrant position, 78, 78*f*
Long thoracic nerve
  muscle innervated by, 11*t*, 102
  palsy, and scapular winging, 58, 58*f*, 65–66, 82, 99, 99*f*
Loose packed position, 170–171, 171*f*
Lordosis, and scapular motion, 69–70
Lower extremities, and shoulder pathology, 67–69, 68*f*
Ludington test, of biceps tendon, 226, 226*f*
Lumbrical muscle, innervation of, 12*f*
Luxatio erecta, 188–189, 188*f*, 203

M
Maffet's classification, of SLAP lesions, 216, 217*f*
Magnetic resonance imaging (MRI), 14
  of acromioclavicular joint, 245, 255, 255*t*
  of impingement
    accuracy of, 142*t*
    internal, 134–135, 134*f*
  of rotator cuff tears, 126–127, 127*t*
  of SLAP lesions, 225
Maitland range of motion scheme, 48–49, 49*t*
Manual muscle testing (MMT), 93–94
  ceiling effect in, 94
  as clinical standard, 93
  disadvantages of, 93–94
  grading scales for, 93, 94*t*
  individual muscles *versus* muscle groups in, 94
  reliability of, 94–96, 95*t*

small differences in, difficulty detecting, 94
strength-function relationship in, 98
subjectivity of, 94
Maximal voluntary contraction (MVC), 90
Mayo shear test, for SLAP lesions, 239–240, 239*f*
Measures of significance, 260, 260*t*
Mechanical force, dynamometer measurement of, 94–97
Mechanical inclinometers, 20, 20*f*
Mechanism of injury, 4, 5*t*–6*t*.
    See also specific injuries
Medial pectoral nerve, muscle innervated by, 11*t*, 105–106
Medial shoulder blade, pain in, 2
Median nerve, muscles innervated by, 11*t*, 12*f*
Men
  physical examination of, 6, 6*f*
  range of motion in, 21, 21*t*
  strength testing in, 91
Middle glenohumeral ligament, 162*f*–163*f*
  stability functions of, 169–170, 169*t*
  variability of, 215, 215*f*–216*f*
Millimeters, translation of humeral head in, 179–180, 179*f*
Miniaci test, 202, 202*f*
Mobility, 71–81
  Apley scratch test of, 72, 72*f*–73*f*
  clinical measures of, 71
  combined abduction test of, 74, 74*f*
  crossed-arm test of, 73–74, 74*f*
  hammock position of Codman in, 78–79, 79*f*
  horizontal flexion test of, 73, 73*f*
  locked quadrant position in, 78, 78*f*
  measurements and tests of, 71–81
  pectoralis minor muscle contracture test of, 76–77, 76*f*–77*f*
  pivotal position/area in, 78–80, 79*f*
  posterior shoulder tightness test of, 74–76, 74*f*–75*f*
  quadrant position and test in, 77, 77*f*–78*f*
  reverse scapulothoracic rhythm in, 81
  shrug sign in, 80, 80*f*, 80*t*
  subluxation test of, 80–81, 81*f*
  subscapularis muscle tightness test of, 76
  zero position of Saha in, 78, 79*f*
Morgan's classification, of SLAP lesions, 217, 217*f*
Motivation, patient, in strength testing, 92
Muscle(s). *See also specific muscles*
  anterior view of, 88*f*
  as functional groups, 90
  posterior view of, 88*f*
Muscle activity, and shoulder motion, 25–26
Muscle testing, 10, 88–122. *See also* Range of motion; Strength testing
Muscular strength
  definition of, 88
  testing of, 88–122. *See also* Strength testing
Musculocutaneous nerve
  muscles innervated by, 11*t*, 12*f*, 121
  palsy of, 121
Musculoskeletal examination, 6–14, 6*t*
Myocardial infarction, pain in, 2

N

Nausea, with pain, 2
Neer impingement sign, 80, 141–144, 142f
  accuracy of, 142–144, 142t–144t
  in acromioclavicular disorders, 251t
  in biceps pathology, 229t
  contact in flexion and, 137
  diagnostic values of, 143, 143t, 224t–225t, 251t
  sensitivity and specificity of, 142t–143t, 144,
    144t, 224t
Negative predictive value (NPV), definition of, 259
Neurovascular examination, 10–13
Night, pain during, 4, 5t
90-degree external rotation, 16t, 44–45, 45f–46f
90-degree internal rotation, 16t, 43–44, 44f–45f
Nobuhara's zero position, 79–80, 79f

O

O'Brien test. *See also* active compression test
  for acromioclavicular disorders, 252, 252f
    diagnostic values of, 251t, 252
    sensitivity and specificity of, 251t, 252, 255t
  for biceps pathology, 229t
  for SLAP lesions, 224t, 235–236, 235f–236f
    diagnostic accuracy of, 225t, 233t, 236
    patient interpretation in, 236
    sensitivity and specificity of, 224t–225t, 234t, 236
Observation of patient, 6–10, 6f–9f
Occult instability, 163–167
  challenge of, 165–167
  glenohumeral motion in, 41t
  internal impingement sign for, 196–197, 196f
One-finger test, of acromioclavicular joint, 250–251, 251f
180 degree rule, for internal *versus* external rotation, 36
One-leg stability series, 68, 68f
Opponens digiti minimi muscle, innervation of, 12f
Osteitis condensans, 256
Osteoarthritis
  acromioclavicular joint, 244–245
  glenohumeral motion in, 41t
  mechanisms of, 6t
  muscle atrophy in, 8t
  pain in
    activities aggravating, 5t
    patterns of, 5t
  shrug sign test in, 80, 80t
  sternoclavicular joint, 256
Osteolysis, of acromioclavicular joint, 244
Osteophytes, in internal impingement, 135, 135f
Overhead athletes
  APIT lesion in, 165
  glenohumeral motion in, 41–42
  impingement in, 134–136, 138
  infraspinatus atrophy in, 114
  injuries in, 5t. *See also specific types*
  instability in, 163–166
  kinetic chain in, 67–69
    abnormal hip movements in, 68–69
    one-leg stability test of, 68, 68f
  latissimus dorsi syndrome in, 102, 102f

  pain in, 29, 164–166
  relocation sign in, 193
  return to sports by, after surgery, 166t
  rotational injuries in, 29–37, 30t–33t
    active *versus* passive motion in, 35
    180-degree rule for, 36
    osseous changes in, 35–36
  rotator cuff disease in, 128, 128f, 134–136,
    138, 163–164
  scapular motion in, 51
  serratus anterior fatigue in, 104
  strength testing in, 98
    dynamometer for, 97
  total arc of motion in, 35–37
  triceps tendinitis in, 121

P

Pain
  acromioclavicular joint, 2, 244
    activities aggravating, 5t
    distribution of, 2, 3f, 249–255, 250f
    localization of, 249–255, 250t, 251f
    patterns of, 5t
  activities aggravating, 4, 5t
  adaptation to, scapular dyskinesia as, 66–67
  anginal, 2, 3f
  versus apprehension sign, 192
  biceps pathology and, 220–221, 221f
  bicipital groove, in SLAP lesion evaluation,
    233–234, 234t
  chest or rib, 2, 3f
  in coracoid impingement, 131–132
  diffuse, differential diagnosis of, 4
  distribution of, 2–4, 3f
  improvement in, as indicator of etiology, 4
  in instability, 5t, 163–164
    posterior, *versus* impingement, 201, 201f
  medial shoulder blade, 2
  in multiple areas, 4
  nausea with, 2
  during night (sleep), 4, 5t
  in overhead athlete, 29, 164–165
  progressive, 4
  in range of motion measurement, 48–49, 49t
  referred, to shoulder, 2, 4f, 4t
  in rotator cuff disease, 2, 128–129, 137–138
    distribution of, 2, 3f, 138, 138f–139f
  scapular, localization of, 81–82, 82f
  in SLAP lesions, 5t, 224
  slower onset of, 2
  in strength testing, 92
  sudden onset of, 2
  thoracic, 2, 3f
  weakness secondary to, 2
  worsening of, patterns of, 4, 5t
Painful arc syndrome, 146–147, 146f
  in acromioclavicular disorders, 251t
  anterior, 146, 146t
  posterior, 146, 146t
  superior, 146–147, 146t

Painful arc syndrome (*Continued*)
  testing for
    accuracy of, 142*t*–144*t*, 147
      diagnostic values of, 143*t*, 147, 251*t*
      sensitivity and specificity of, 142*t*–144*t*, 147
    types of, 146, 146*t*
Pain provocation test
  for acromioclavicular pathology, 249–250, 250*t*
  for SLAP lesions, 237–238, 238*f*
    diagnostic values of, 224*t*, 237
Paired *t*-test, 260*t*
Palmar interosseous muscle, innervation of, 12*f*
Palmaris brevis muscle, innervation of, 12*f*
Palmaris longus muscle, innervation of, 12*f*
Palpation
  of biceps tendon, 227, 227*f*, 229*t*
  of infraspinatus muscle, 139, 139*f*
  of latissimus dorsi muscle, 139–140, 140*f*
  in rotator cuff disease
    for muscle defects, 139–140, 139*f*–140*f*
    for tendon defects, 140–141, 141*f*
  of scapula, 81–82
  of supraspinatus muscle, 139, 139*f*
  transdeltoid, 140–141
Passive range of abduction, 189–190
Passive range of motion, 22
Passive rotation, 42
  with arm at 90 degrees, 43–45, 44*f*–45*f*
  with arm at side, 42–43, 43*f*–44*f*
Patient history, 1, 1*t*, 7
Patient positioning. *See also specific tests*
  and range of motion, 21–22
  and strength testing, 92–93
Patte sign, 120, 145–146, 145*f*
Paxinos test, of acromioclavicular joint, 253, 253*f*
  sensitivity and specificity of, 255*t*
Pearl, Michael, 50, 50*f*–51*f*
Pectoralis major muscle, 90
  absence of, 105
  actions of, 11*t*, 105
  anatomy of, 105, 105*f*
  clavicular head of, 105, 105*f*
  innervation of, 11*t*, 105
  rupture of, 105–106, 106*f*
  sports injuries of, 105–106
  sternal head of, 105, 105*f*
  strength testing of, 105–106, 106*f*
Pectoralis major tendon tear, sports-related, 5, 5*t*
Pectoralis minor muscle
  absence of, 107
  actions of, 11*t*, 106–107
  anatomy of, 106, 107*f*
  contracture (tightness) test of, 76–77, 76*f*–77*f*
  innervation of, 11*t*, 106
  isolated testing of, unlikelihood of, 107
  strength testing of, 106–107, 107*f*
Pectoralis muscle. *See also* Pectoralis major muscle;
    Pectoralis minor muscle
  congenital absence of, 105, 107
    observation of, 7, 7*f*

rupture of, 105–106, 106*f*
  observation of, 8, 9*f*
  strength testing of, 105–107, 106*f*–107*f*
    optimal position for, 93*t*
Perineum care, range of motion for, 50*t*
Peripheral nerve(s)
  distribution of, 12*f*
  muscles innervated by, 11*f*, 11*t*, 12*f*
  testing of, 10
Physeal fracture, of sternoclavicular joint,
    255–256, 256*f*
Physical examination, 6–14, 6*t*. *See also specific disorders
    and tests*
Physical therapy, for internal impingement, 136
Pivotal area, 79–80, 79*f*
Pivotal position, 78–80, 79*f*
Plain radiographs, 14
  of acromioclavicular joint, 245, 255, 255*t*
"Pop," 1, 216
"Popeye arm," in biceps rupture, 121, 216, 216*f*, 226
Positioning, patient. *See also specific tests*
  and range of motion, 21–22
  and strength testing, 92–93
Positive predictive value (PPV), definition of, 259
Posterior capsular contracture, in overhead athletes,
    34–35
Posterior capsule, stability functions of, 169–170
Posterior drawer test, 182–184, 182*f*, 203
Posterior glenoid osteotomies, and coracoid
    impingement, 132–133
Posterior instability, 198–203
  apprehension test for, 199–201, 200*f*–201*f*
  demonstrable or voluntary, 198, 198*f*
  in football injury, 198, 199*f*
  Fukada test for, 202, 202*f*
  glenohumeral motion in, 41*t*
  history of, 198–199
  jerk test for, 201–202, 201*f*
  pain in, *versus* impingement, 201, 201*f*
  physical examination of, 199, 199*f*
  posterior laxity tests used for, 203
  posterior subluxation (Miniaci) test for, 202, 202*f*
  push-pull test for, 202–203
  Rowe test for, 201, 201*f*, 203
  in seizure disorders, 198–199
  spectrum of, 205*t*
  sports-related, 5, 5*t*
  in throwing athlete (APIT lesion), 165
Posterior laxity
  drawer test of, 182–184, 182*f*
  load and shift test of, 185–186, 186*f*
  measurement of, 182–187
  Protzman test of, 187, 187*f*
  push-pull test of, 186–187, 187*f*
  tests for, use in posterior instability, 203
Posterior shoulder flexibility test, 73, 73*f*
Posterior shoulder tightness test, 74–76, 74*f*–75*f*
Posterior subluxation
  demonstrable or voluntary, 205–206, 206*f*
  test for, 80–81, 81*f*, 202, 202*f*

Posterosuperior labrum, in internal impingement, 134–136
Post-test probability, 260
Posture, and scapular motion, 69–70, 69*f*
Power drivers (muscles), 90
Predictive value
    negative, definition of, 259
    positive, definition of, 259
    relationship of prevalence to, 259
Preoperative laxity, 184, 184*t*
Prevalence
    definition of, 258
    relationship to predictive values, 259
Pronator quadratus muscle, innervation of, 12*f*
Pronator teres muscle
    actions of, 11*t*
    innervation of, 11*t*, 12*f*
Prone instability test, 196
Protraction, scapular, 53–55, 54*f*–55*f*, 82, 82*f*
Protzman test, of anteroposterior laxity, 187, 187*f*
Proximal humeral apophysitis, sports-related, 5*t*
Pseudolaxity
    anterior, 219
    in superior labrum injury, 34, 219
Pulley system, of biceps tendon, 213–214
Push-pull test
    for posterior instability, 202–203
    for posterior laxity, 186–187, 187*f*

Q
Quadrant position, locked, 78, 78*f*
Quadrant position and test, 77, 77*f*–78*f*
Quantitative measures, of laxity, 179–182

R
Radial nerve, muscles innervated by, 11*f*, 11*t*
Radiography, 13–14, 13*f*
    of acromioclavicular joint, 245–246, 248*f*, 255, 255*t*
    deficiencies in motion studies, 23
    of instability/laxity, 179, 179*t*
    of internal impingement, 134–135, 134*f*
    of rotator cuff tears, 126–127, 127*t*
    of shoulder elevation, 22–25
    of subacromial impingement, 129–130, 129*f*–130*f*
Range of motion, 15–82
    active, 22
    for activities of daily living, 50, 50*t*, 71–72, 72*f*
    age and, 20–21
    dominance of extremity and, 21, 29, 30*t*–33*t*, 34–36
    electromagnetic studies of, 23–25, 23*f*–25*f*
    elevation, 26–29
    gender and, 21, 21*t*
    measurements of, 10
        AAOS guidelines for, 16–17, 16*t*
        AMA guidelines for, 15–16, 16*t*
        biomechanical considerations in, 22–26
        challenges in, 15
        end feel in, 43*f*
            Cyriax's classification of, 49
            factors affecting, 48–49
            Maitland's scheme for, 48–49, 49*t*
    functional, 49–50, 50*f*, 50*t*, 51*f*, 71–72, 72*f*
    global coordinate system for, 18, 18*f*
    handheld goniometers for, 19, 49–50
    inclinometers for, 20, 20*f*
    Maitland scheme of, 48–49, 49*t*
    nomenclature in, 15–17
    normative values in, 16, 16*t*
    reliability of, 19, 19*t*, 20
    techniques for, 19–20
    validity of, 18–19
    variables affecting, 17–18, 20–22
    visual estimation for, 19
    zero positions in, 15, 16*f*
    muscle activity and, 25–26
    in overhead athletes, 29–37, 30*t*–33*t*
    passive, 22
    patient positioning and, 21–22
    radiographic studies of, 22–25
    rotational, 29–48
    scapular, 51–71
    in sternoclavicular pathology, 256
Range of passive abduction (RPA), 189–190
Referred pain, 2, 4*f*, 4*t*, 220
Reflex testing, 10–13, 13*f*
Release test
    for anterior instability, 197–198, 197*f*
    validity of, 186*t*
Reliability
    definition of, 259–260
    intertester, 259–260
    intraexaminer, 259
    of range of motion measurements, 19, 19*t*, 20
    of strength testing systems, 93–98, 95*t*
Relocation test
    for anterior instability, 192–194, 193*f*
        diagnostic values of, 192*t*, 193–194
        evaluation of, using different criteria for positive
            result, 194, 194*t*
        in rotator cuff disease, 193
        sensitivity and specificity of, 192*t*, 193–194
    for internal impingement/occult instability,
        196–197, 196*f*
    for SLAP lesions, 224*t*, 238–239, 239*f*
        diagnostic accuracy of, 225*t*, 239
        sensitivity and specificity of, 224*t*–225*t*,
            234*t*, 239
    validity of, 186*t*
Rent sign, in rotator cuff disease, 140–141, 141*f*
Repetitive stress, 165
Resistance, in range of motion measurement,
    48–49, 49*t*
Resisted arm extension test, of acromioclavicular
    disorders, 252–253, 252*f*
    diagnostic values of, 251*t*, 253
Resisted belly press test, of subscapularis muscle,
    119, 119*f*
Resisted lift-off test, of subscapularis muscle,
    118, 118*f*
Retraction, scapular, 54–55, 54*f*
Reverse scapulothoracic rhythm, 81

Rhomboid major muscle
  actions of, 11*t*, 104
  anatomy of, 104, 104*f*
  innervation of, 11*f*, 11*t*, 104
  strength testing of, 104–105, 104*f*–105*f*
  weakness of, clinical implications of, 105
Rhomboid minor muscle
  actions of, 11*t*, 104
  anatomy of, 104, 104*f*
  innervation of, 11*f*, 11*t*, 104
  strength testing of, 104–105, 104*f*–105*f*
  weakness of, clinical implications of, 105
Rib pain, 2, 3*f*
Rib stress fractures, sports-related, 5*t*
Rod Laver arm, 63, 63*f*
Rotation. *See also specific tests*
  active motion of, 42
    with arm at 90 degrees, 44–45, 45*f*–46*f*
    with arm at side, 42–43, 43*f*–44*f*
  Codman's paradox in, 77, 77*f*
  dynamometer values in, 96, 96*t*
  end points in, 37
  external, 16–17, 16*t*
    with arm at 90 degrees, 16*t*, 44–45, 45*f*–46*f*
    with arm at side, 42–43, 43*f*–44*f*
    functional positions for, 50, 51*f*
    normal range of, 16*t*
    180 degree rule for, 36
    in overhead athletes, 29–37, 41–42
    scapular, 55*t*, 56–58, 57*f*
  glenohumeral motion in, 37–42
    clinical studies of, 38–42, 38*t*–41*t*
    versus combined motions, 38–42, 38*t*–40*t*
    distribution of
      by age, 41, 41*t*
      by diagnosis, 41, 41*t*
    in dominant *versus* non-dominant shoulder, 39, 39*t*–40*t*
    reliability of measurements of, 39–40
    versus scapulothoracic motion, 22–25, 23*t*, 37–39, 37*t*
    in standing *versus* supine position, 39–40, 40*t*
    visual observation of, 40–41
  internal, 16, 16*t*, 17–18
    with arm at 90 degrees, 16*t*, 43–44, 44*f*–45*f*
    functional positions for, 50, 50*f*
    glenohumeral deficit of, 29–37, 47, 47*f*, 61
    with hand up the back, 48, 48*f*
    in lateral decubitus position, 47, 47*f*
    normal range of, 16*t*
    180 degree rule for, 36
    in overhead athletes, 29–37, 41–42
    in posterior instability, 199, 199*f*
  lateral, 17
  measurement of, 29–48
    end feel in, 43*f*, 48–49, 49*t*
    functional, 49–50, 50*f*–51*f*
    in lateral decubitus examination, 47, 47*f*
    Maitland scheme of, 48–49, 49*t*
    in standing examination, 42–45, 43*f*–46*f*
    in supine examination, 46–47, 46*f*–47*f*
    techniques for, 42–48

  medial, 17
  in overhead athletes, 29–37, 30*t*–33*t*, 41–42
  passive motion of, 42
    with arm at 90 degrees, 43–45, 44*f*–45*f*
    with arm at side, 42–43, 43*f*–44*f*
  scapular, 46–47, 46*f*, 55*t*
    along vertical axis, 56–57, 57*f*
    downward, 55, 56*f*
    external, 55*t*, 56–58, 57*f*
    internal, 55*t*, 56–58, 57*f*
    upward, 53–55, 54*f*–55*f*, 55*t*
Rotator cuff disease, 126–158
  abrasion sign in, 140, 140*f*
  versus acromioclavicular disorders, 245
  age and, 126–127, 127*t*, 157–158, 157*t*
  in athletes, 128, 128*f*, 134–136, 138, 163–164
  versus axillary nerve palsy, 110
  biceps pathology and, 220–221, 221*f*
  biomechanics of, 127–128
  coracoid impingement sign in, 147–148, 147*f*
  crepitus in, 140, 140*f*
  Dawbarn's sign in, 141
  diagnostic injection in, 148–151, 150*f*
  etiology of, 2
    theories of, 126–129
  examination for, 138–151
    accuracy of tests in, 142–144, 142*t*–144*t*
    combined tests for, 157–158
    diagnostic values of tests in, 143, 143*t*
    sensitivity and specificity of tests in, 142*t*–144*t*
  glenohumeral motion in, 41*t*
  historical perspective on, 126
  Hornblower's sign in, 156–157, 156*f*
  instability and, 163–164
  Jobe sign in, 152–153, 152*f*
  Kennedy-Hawkins sign in, 144–145, 144*f*
  lag signs in, 116, 154–157
  lift-off sign in, 153, 153*f*
  likelihood ratios in, 157*t*
  local tenderness in, 138–140, 139*f*–140*f*
  mechanisms of, 6*t*
  muscle defects in, 8*t*, 115, 115*f*
    palpation of, 139–140, 139*f*–140*f*
  Neer impingement sign in, 141–144, 142*f*
  Neer impingement test for, 148–151, 150*f*
  painful arc syndrome in, 146–147, 146*f*
  pain in, 2, 128–129, 137–138
    activities aggravating, 4, 5*t*
    distribution of, 2, 3*f*, 138, 138*f*–139*f*
    patterns of, 5*t*
    versus posterior instability, 201, 201*f*
  post-test probability for, 157–158, 157*t*
  regression analysis in, 157*t*, 158
  relocation sign in, 193
  rent sign in, 140–141, 141*f*
  and scapular motion, 70–71, 135
  shrug sign test in, 80*t*
  Speed's test for, 148, 148*f*
  sports-related, 5*t*, 29

strength testing for, 151–158
tendon defects in, palpation of, 140–141, 141*f*
weakness with, 2
Whipple test for, 148, 148*f*
Yocum sign in, 145, 145*f*
Rotator cuff impingement, 129–158
in athletes, 134–136, 138
biceps pathology and, 220–221, 221*f*
contact in flexion and, 136–138, 136*f*
coracoid, 131–133, 131*f*
biceps tendon in, 221, 221*f*
functional, 133
iatrogenic, 131–133
idiopathic, 132
pain in, 131–132
posterior glenoid osteotomies and, 132–133
posttraumatic, 132–133
testing for, 147–148, 147*f*
Trillat procedure and, 131–132
coracoid sign of, 147–148, 147*f*
examination for, 138–151
accuracy of tests in, 142–143, 142*t*–144*t*
diagnostic values of tests in, 143, 143*t*
sensitivity and specificity of tests in, 142*t*–144*t*
internal, 29, 133–136, 134*f*, 164, 165*f*
anterior, 136, 196–197, 196*f*
arthroscopic findings of, 133–135, 133*f*, 135
cadaveric studies of, 135, 135*f*–136*f*
versus internal contact, 135
in occult instability, 196–197, 196*f*
osteophytes and, 135, 135*f*
physical therapy for, 136
physiologic contact in, 135
radiographic studies of, 134–135, 134*f*
scapular dyskinesia and, 135
SLAP lesions with, 136, 223
stage I, 136
stage II, 136
stage III, 136
Neer sign of, 141–144, 142*f*
scapular motion in, 70–71, 135
secondary, 193
subacromial, 129–131
acromial shape and, 130–131, 130*f*
biceps tendon in, 221, 221*f*
diagnostic injection in, 148–151, 150*f*
radiographic studies of, 129–130, 129*f*–130*f*
secondary, posterior shoulder tightness
test in, 75
types of, 129–138
Rotator cuff muscles, 90, 169
Rotator cuff tears, 126–127.
See also Rotator cuff disease
age and, 126–127, 127*t*, 157–158, 157*t*
biomechanics of, 127–128
combined tests for, 157–158
compressive forces in, 127–128
imaging studies of, 126–127, 127*t*
partial, Ellman classification of, 133, 133*t*
post-test probability for, 157–158, 157*t*

regression analysis of, 157*t*, 158
rent sign of, 140–141, 141*f*
Rowe test(s)
for inferior instability, 204, 204*f*
for posterior instability, 201, 201*f*, 203
prone, for anterior instability, 196
standing, for anterior instability, 195, 196*f*
Rowing injuries, 5*t*

S
Saha's zero position, 78, 79*f*
Sarcoma, soft tissue, of biceps tendon, 226, 226*f*
Savoie test, for SLAP lesions, 240, 240*f*
Scalloped shoulder, 8, 9*f*, 110, 110*f*
Scaphoid sign, 8, 9*f*, 110, 110*f*
Scaption, 17, 17*f*
Scapula
asymmetry of
observation of, 10, 10*f*
in scoliosis, 81, 81*f*
functions of, 51
malpositioning of. *See* Scapular dyskinesia(s)
motions of, 22–26, 51–61
abnormal or asynchronous, 58. *See also* Scapular
dyskinesia(s)
clinical evaluation of, 58–61
crepitus with, 81
difficulty in assessing, 51
in elevation
in abduction, 57
biomechanics of, 53–58
in flexion, 57
versus glenohumeral motion, 51–52
kinetic chain of, 67–71
mean, 55*t*
nomenclature for, 51
in overhead athlete, 51
posture and, 69–70, 69*f*
rotator cuff problems and, 70–71, 135
in supine position, 46–47, 46*f*
visual inspection for, 47
pain in, localization of, 81–82, 82*f*
palpation of, 81–82
positioning of
with inclinometers, 60–61
Kibler's positions for testing, 59–60, 59*f*
lateral slide test of, 58–60, 59*f*
protraction of, 53–55, 54*f*–55*f*, 82, 82*f*
resting position of, 52–53
and Lennie test, 52–53, 53*f*
retraction of, 54–55, 54*f*
rotation of, 46–47, 46*f*, 55*t*
along vertical axis, 56–57, 57*f*
downward, 55, 56*f*
external, 55*t*, 56–58, 57*f*
internal, 56–58, 57*f*
upward, 53–55, 54*f*–55*f*, 55*t*
setting phase of, 52
snapping, syndrome of, 81–82
tilt of, 55–57, 55*t*, 56*f*

Scapular assistance test (SAT), 64, 64*f*
Scapular distance, 58, 59*f*
Scapular dyskinesia(s), 26, 51, 61–67
  definition of, 61
  demonstrable or voluntary, 67, 67*f*
  etiology of, 61
  evaluation of, 64–65
  identification and diagnosis of, 65–66
  and internal impingement, 135
  as normal adaption to pain, 66–67
  scapular assistance test in, 64, 64*f*
  scapular flip sign in, 64–65, 65*f*
  SICK scapula, 63–64, 63*f*–64*f*
  tennis shoulder, 63, 63*f*
  type I, 62, 62*f*
  type II, 62, 62*f*
  type III, 62, 62*f*
  type IV (symmetric), 62
  types of, 61–62
  weighted scapular flexion test in, 65
Scapular flip sign, 64–65, 65*f*
Scapular plane, 52
  elevation in, 17, 17*f*, 27*f*, 52
Scapular rotator muscles, 90
Scapular size, 58
Scapular stabilization, 46, 46*f*
Scapular winging, 58
  demonstrable or voluntary, 67, 67*f*
  grading of, 103
  mild, 103
  moderate, 103
  nerve palsies in, 58, 58*f*, 65–66, 82, 99–100,
      99*f*–100*f*
  observation of, 10, 10*f*, 58, 58*f*
  serratus anterior weakness and, 102–103, 103*f*
  severe, 103
  testing for, 99–100, 100*f*, 102–103, 103*f*
  trapezius weakness and, 65–66, 99–100, 100*f*
Scapular Y radiograph, 13–14, 13*f*
Scapulohumeral muscles, strength testing of, 107–120
Scapulohumeral pivotors (muscles), 90
Scapulothoracic joint, motion of
  versus glenohumeral motion, 22–26, 25*t*, 37–38, 37*t*
  with glenohumeral motion. *See* Glenohumeral-
      scapulothoracic rotation, combined
Scapulothoracic rhythm
  altered, 26
  reverse, 81
Scoliosis, scapular asymmetry in, 81, 81*f*
Seizure disorders, posterior instability in, 198–199
Sensitivity, definition of, 258–259
Sensory testing, 10
Serratus anterior muscle
  actions of, 11*t*, 102
  anatomy of, 102, 103*f*
  divisions of, 102
  fatigue in, 104
  innervation of, 11*t*, 102
  strength testing of, 102–104, 103*f*
    optimal position for, 104, 104*f*

weakness, in scapular winging, 58, 58*f*, 99–100,
      102–103, 103*f*
Setting phase of scapula, 52
Shearing force, in rotator cuff disease, 127–128
Shelf, putting items on, range of motion for, 50*t*
Shoulder. *See specific entries*
Shoulder blades, medial, pain in, 2
Shoulder examination. *See also specific tests and disorders*
  general principles of, 1–14
  neurovascular examination in, 10–13
  patient confidence/comfort in, 14
  patient history in, 1, 1*t*, 7
  physical examination in, 6–14, 6*t*
  radiography in, 13–14, 13*f*
  strength testing in, 88–122
Shrug, resisted, in trapezius testing, 100, 100*f*
Shrug sign, 80, 80*f*, 80*t*
SICK scapula, 63–64, 63*f*–64*f*
Side-to-side comparisons, 8–10, 9*f*–10*f*, 244, 244*f*, 245
  in overhead athletes, 35–36
Significance, measures of, 260, 260*t*
Sitting position, and range of motion, 21–22
SLAP. *See* Superior labrum injury, anterior to
      posterior (SLAP)
"SLAPrehension" test, 238, 238*f*
Sleep, pain during, 4, 5*t*
Snapping scapula syndrome, 81–82
Snyder's classification, of SLAP lesions, 216, 217*f*
Soft tissue sarcoma, of biceps tendon, 226, 226*f*
Spasm, as end feel, 49
Specificity, definition of, 259
Speed's test
  for acromioclavicular disorders, diagnostic
      values of, 251*t*
  for biceps pathology, 228–229, 228*f*
    diagnostic values of, 228–229, 228*t*–229*t*
  for rotator cuff disease, 148, 148*f*
    accuracy of, 142*t*–144*t*, 148
    diagnostic values of, 143*t*, 148
    sensitivity and specificity of, 142*t*–144*t*, 148
  for SLAP lesions, 224*t*
    sensitivity and specificity of, 224*t*, 234*t*
Spinal accessory nerve
  muscle innervated by, 11*t*, 99
  palsy, and scapular winging, 65–66, 99–100, 100*f*
Splinter hemorrhages, 13
Sports injuries, 1*t*, 5–6, 5*t*–6*t*. *See also specific sports
      and injuries*
Sprengel' syndrome, observation of, 7, 7*f*
Spring scale dynamometer, 95–96, 95*f*, 95*t*
Springy block, 49
Spur, anterior acromial, 130, 130*f*
Stability
  biceps tendon in, 217–218
  biomechanics of, 167–170
  circle concept of, 169–170, 170*f*
  clinical tests for, validity of, 186*t*
  disorders of. *See* Instability
  ligaments in, 169–170, 169*t*
  normal anatomy of, 162, 162*f*–163*f*

Standing position
glenohumeral motion in, 39–40, 40*t*
and range of motion, 21–22
rotation measurements in, 42–45, 43*f*–46*f*
Standing Rowe test, for anterior instability, 195, 196*f*
Statistical terms and analysis, 258–261
Sternoclavicular (SC) joint, 244, 255–256
arthritis of, 256
dislocation of, 255–256
disorders/injuries of, 255–256
examination in, 255–256
history of, 255–256
low incidence of, 255
fracture of, 255–256
physeal, 255–256, 256*f*
hyperostosis of, 256
pain in, 2
subluxation of, 255–256
demonstrable or voluntary, 256
swelling of, evaluation of, 256
Stiffness, 71. *See also* Mobility
Strain gauge dynamometer, 95, 95*f*
Strength testing, 10, 88–122
age and, 91
applications of, 88
arm dominance and, 91
basic principles of, 89
of biceps brachii muscle, 120–121
of deltoid muscle, 107–110, 109*f*
diurnal variation in, 91–92
dynamometers for, 94–97
electromyographic, 89–90
environmental factors in, 91–92
evaluator variables in, 91
extremity positioning in, effects of, 92–93
factors affecting, 90–93
patient or individual, 90
technical or methodologic, 90
force-length relationship (Blix's curve) in, 89, 89*f*
gender and, 91
of humeroscapular muscles, 120–122
of infraspinatus muscle, 114–116, 116*f*, 153
isokinetic, 95, 95*f*, 97–98
lag signs in, 89, 154–157
of latissimus dorsi muscle, 101–102
manual, 93–94, 98
muscle isolation in, 89, 92–93
optimal position for, 92, 93*t*
pain in, 92
patient motivation in, 92
of pectoralis major muscle, 105–106, 106*f*
of pectoralis minor muscle, 106–107, 107*f*
purpose of, 90
of rhomboid muscles, 104–105, 104*f*–105*f*
for rotator cuff disease, 151–158
of scapulohumeral muscles, 107–120
of serratus anterior muscle, 102–103, 103*f*–104*f*
strength-to-function relationship in, 98
of subscapularis muscle, 116–119, 117*f*–119*f*,
153, 153*f*

of supraspinatus muscle, 111–114, 112*f*–113*f*, 151–153,
151*f*–153*f*
systems for, validity and reliability of, 93–98
of teres major muscle, 110–111
of teres minor muscle, 119–120, 120*f*
of thorax muscles, 98–107
of trapezius muscle, 98–101, 100*f*–101*f*
of triceps muscle, 121–122, 121*f*
Strength-to-function relationship, 98
Subacromial impingement, 129–131
acromial shape and, 130–131, 130*f*
biceps tendon in, 221, 221*f*
diagnostic injection in, 148–151, 150*f*
radiographic studies of, 129–130, 129*f*–130*f*
secondary, posterior shoulder tightness test in, 75
Subacromial injection
in acromioclavicular pathology, 249–250, 254
anterior, 150, 150*f*
in biceps pathology, 232
diagnostic, 148–151, 232, 249–250
lateral, 150–151, 150*f*
posterior, 150, 150*f*
procedure for, 149–151, 150*f*
side effects of, 151
therapeutic, 149–150
volume of anesthetic for, 150
Subcoracoid impingement, 131. *See also* Coracoid
impingement
Sublabral hole, 215, 215*f*, 219
Subluxation, 162. *See also* Instability
anatomical restraints to, 169–170
anterior
demonstrable or voluntary, 206, 206*f*
test for, 80–81, 81*f*
biceps tendon, 221
demonstrable or voluntary, 198, 198*f*, 205–207, 256
evaluation of, 205
inferior, 203–204
demonstrable or voluntary, 206–207, 206*f*
posterior
demonstrable or voluntary, 205–206, 206*f*
test for, 80–81, 81*f*, 202, 202*f*
sternoclavicular, 255–256
superior, test for, 80–81, 81*f*
Subscapular bursitis, 82, 82*f*
Subscapularis lag sign, 156, 156*f*
Subscapularis muscle
actions of, 11*t*, 117
anatomy of, 116, 116*f*
atrophy of, impossibility of visualizing, 116
belly press test of, 118–119, 118*f*
innervation of, 11*t*, 116
lift-off test of, 117–119, 117*f*, 153, 153*f*
resisted belly press test of, 119, 119*f*
resisted lift-off test of, 118, 118*f*
in rotator cuff disease, 153, 153*f*
strength testing of, 116–119, 117*f*–119*f*, 153, 153*f*
Subscapularis muscle tightness test, 76
Subscapularis nerve, 116
Subscapularis tendon, in pulley system, 213–214

Subscapularis tendon injury, 4, 117
Subscapular nerve, muscles innervated by, 11*f*, 11*t*, 111
Sulcus sign, in laxity testing, 179–180, 185*t*–186*t*,
    187–189, 188*f*, 203–204
Superior glenohumeral ligament, 162*f*
  in pulley system, 213–214
  stability functions of, 169–170, 169*t*
Superior glenoid
  biceps tendon attachment to, 214–215, 214*f*
  labrum attachment to, 214–215, 215*f*
Superior instability, 218–219
Superior labrum, 163*f*
  biceps tendon attachment to, 214–215, 214*f*
  instability of, 164–165, 218–220
  peeling off/peeling back of, 34–35, 219, 219*f*
  "trapped," 222
Superior labrum injury, anterior to posterior (SLAP),
    216–217
  versus acromioclavicular disorders, 245
  active compression sign (O'Brien's sign) in, 235–236,
    235*f*–236*f*
  age and, 224
  anterior glide test (Kibler test) for, 233–234, 233*f*
  arthroscopy of, 240–241
  biceps load test I for, 236–237, 236*f*
  biceps load test II for, 237, 237*f*
  classification of, 216–217, 217*f*
  clunk test for, 233, 233*f*
  coexisting pathologies with, 223–224, 223*t*
  compression rotation sign in, 232–233, 232*f*
  crank test for, 234–235, 234*f*
  diagnosis of, challenge of, 222–226
  distribution by type, 224
  glenohumeral motion in, 41*t*
  incidence by type, 222*t*
  instability in, 164–165, 218–220
  internal impingement with, 136, 223
  magnetic resonance imaging of, 225
  Mayo shear test for, 239–240, 239*f*
  mechanisms of, 4, 6*t*, 222–223, 223*t*
  pain in
    activities aggravating, 4, 5*t*
    patterns of, 5*t*, 224
  pain provocation test for, 237–238, 238*f*
  physical examination findings in, 222
  preoperative examination in, 225, 225*t*
  pseudolaxity in, 34, 219
  relocation test for, 238–239, 239*f*
  rotator cuff disease with, 128, 136
  Savoie test for, 240, 240*f*
  shrug sign test in, 80*t*
  "SLAPrehension" test for, 238, 238*f*
  sports-related, 5*t*, 29–35
  supination sign of Yergason in, 228
  tests for, 232–240
    combined, 240, 240*t*
    diagnostic accuracy of, 225–226, 225*t*, 233*t*
    specificity and sensitivity of, 224–225, 224*t*, 234*t*
  type I, 216
  type II, 216–217, 217*f*
  type III, 216–217
  type IV, 217
  type V, 216
  type VI, 216
Supination sign of Yergason, 142*t*, 144*t*, 224*t*,
    227–228, 228*f*
Supinator muscle, innervation of, 11*f*
Supine position
  glenohumeral motion in, 39–40, 40*t*
  laxity and translations in, 183
  and range of motion, 21–22
  rotation measurements in, 46–47, 46*f*–47*f*
  scapular motion in, 46–47, 46*f*
Suprascapular nerve
  injection studies of, 113
  muscles innervated by, 11*f*, 11*t*, 114
  palsy of, 115*f*
Supraspinatus lag signs, 154–155, 154*f*–155*f*
Supraspinatus muscle
  actions of, 11*t*
  anatomy of, 111, 112*f*
  atrophy of
    conditions associated with, 8*t*
    observation of, 8, 8*f*
  innervation of, 11*f*, 11*t*, 111
  in rotator cuff disease, 139, 139*f*, 151–153,
    151*f*–153*f*
  strength testing of, 111–114, 112*f*–113*f*, 151–153,
    151*f*–153*f*
    Blackburn position for, 112, 112*f*
    drop arm sign in, 151–152
    "empty can" position for, 112–113, 112*f*–113*f*,
      152–153, 152*f*
    "full can" position for, 113, 113*f*,
      152–153, 152*f*
    Jobe position for, 112–113, 112*f*–113*f*,
      152–153, 152*f*
    optimal position for, 93*t*
    optimal positions for, 112, 112*f*
  tenderness of, palpation for, 139, 139*f*
Supraspinatus tendon
  footprint of, 111–112, 112*f*
  in pulley system, 213–214
  in rotator cuff impingement, 129, 129*f*
  stability function of, 170
Surface electromyography, 89–90
Surprise test
  for anterior instability, 198
  diagnostic values of, 192*t*, 198
Swimmers
  rotational injuries in, 35
  rotational range of motion in, 32*t*
  serratus anterior fatigue in, 104
  total arc of motion in, 36
Symptoms
  severity at onset, 1–2
  standardized checklist for, 1, 2*f*
Synovial cysts
  of acromioclavicular joint, 246, 246*f*
  of biceps tendon, 226

T

Tennis players
  rotational injuries in, 29–37, 30*t*–33*t*
  rotational range of motion in, 30*t*, 32*t*
  total arc of motion in, 35–37
Tennis shoulder, 63, 63*f*
Tensile forces, in rotator cuff disease, 127–128
Tension overload
  in instability, 219
  in rotator cuff disease, 128
Teres major muscle
  actions of, 11*t*, 111
  anatomy of, 110–111, 111*f*
  innervation of, 11*f*, 11*t*, 111
  strength testing of, 110–111
Teres minor muscle
  actions of, 11*t*, 120
  anatomy of, 119–120, 119*f*
  drop sign test of, 120
  innervation of, 11*f*, 11*t*, 120
  Patte test of, 120, 145–146, 145*f*
  strength testing of, 119–120, 120*f*
Thermal capsular shrinkage, 164
Thoracic outlet syndrome, pain in, 2, 3*f*
Thoracodorsal nerve, muscle innervated by, 11*t*, 101
Thorax
  pain in, 2, 3*f*
  relationship of bones to, motion studies of, 22–25, 23*f*–25*f*
Thorax muscles, strength testing of, 98–107
Thrower's test, 207, 207*f*
Thumb, hyperlaxity of, 207, 207*f*
Tightness test(s)
  pectoralis minor muscle, 76–77, 76*f*–77*f*
  posterior shoulder, 74–76, 74*f*–75*f*
  subscapularis muscle, 76
Tilt, scapular, 55–57, 55*t*, 56*f*
Tissue approximation, as end feel, 49
Torque, dynamometer measurement of, 94–97, 96*t*
Total motion concept, 36
Traction injury
  to infraspinatus muscle, 114
  mechanism of, 5*t*
  superior labrum, 222–223, 223*t*
Transdeltoid palpation, 140–141
Translation of humeral head, 171–182
  anatomical restraints to, 169–170
  anteroposterior
    drawer tests of, 182–184, 182*f*–183*f*
    load and shift test of, 185–186, 185*f*–186*f*
    measurement of, 182–187
    Protzman test of, 187, 187*f*
    push-pull test of, 186–187, 187*f*
    total, 178, 178*t*
  cadaveric studies *versus* physical findings of, 178, 178*t*
  clinical feel of, 181–182, 181*f*
  force for, 171, 178–179
  Hawkins classifications of, 179–182, 180*f*–181*f*
  inferior
    hyperabduction test in, 189–190, 189*f*
    measurement of, 187–190

    sulcus sign in, 187–189, 188*f*, 203–204
    true (luxatio erecta), 188–189, 188*f*, 203
  labrum as chock block to, 167, 167*f*
  literature review of, 172*t*–177*t*
  in millimeters, 179–180, 179*f*
  in percent head diameters, 180
  quantitative measures of, 179–182
  sulcus sign in, 179–180, 187–189, 188*f*, 203–204
Trapezius muscle
  actions of, 11*t*, 99
  anatomy of, 98–99, 99*f*
  atrophy of
    observation of, 8, 8*f*, 99–100, 99*f*
    and scapular winging, 65–66, 99–100, 100*f*
  innervation of, 11*t*, 99
  lower, 99
    testing of, 101, 101*f*
  middle, 99
    testing of, 100–101, 100*f*
  pain in, acromioclavicular joint problems and, 2, 3*f*, 249, 250*f*
  shrug sign test of, 80, 80*f*, 80*t*
  strength testing of, 98–101
  upper, 99
    testing of, 100, 100*f*
Trapshooting injuries, 5*t*
Trendelenburg test, 68
Triceps muscle
  actions of, 11*t*, 121
  anatomy of, 121, 121*f*
  innervation of, 11*t*
  lateral head of, 121
  long head of, 121
  medial head of, 121
  strength testing of, 121–122, 121*f*
Triceps tendinitis, sports-related, 121
Trillat procedure, and coracoid impingement, 131–132
t-test, 260*t*
Tucking in shirt, range of motion for, 50*t*

U

Ulnar nerve, muscles innervated by, 11*t*, 12*f*
Ultrasound, of rotator cuff tears, 126–127, 127*t*
Undressing of patient, 6–7, 6*f*–7*f*
Upper Body Exercise Table (UBXT), 97
Upward rotation, scapular, 53–55, 54*f*–55*f*, 55*t*
Utility (statistical), 260–261

V

Validity
  of clinical tests for stability, 186*t*
  construct, 258
  content, 258
  definition of, 258
  determination of, 258
  face, 258
  of range of motion measurements, 18–19
  of strength testing systems, 93–98
Venting of joint, in laxity testing, 171
Vertical axis, scapular rotation along, 56–57, 57*f*

Visceral pain, referred to shoulder, 2, 4*f*
Visual estimation, of range of motion, 19
Volleyball players, infraspinatus atrophy in, 114
Voluntary scapular dyskinesia, 67, 67*f*
Voluntary scapular winging, 67, 67*f*
Voluntary subluxation, 198, 198*f*, 205–207
    anterior, 206, 206*f*
    evaluation of, 205
    inferior, 206–207, 206*f*
    posterior, 205–206, 206*f*
    sternoclavicular, 256

W
Wall push-up, for muscle testing, of serratus anterior
        muscle, 102–103, 103*f*
Warm-up, for strength testing, 91–92
Washing opposite shoulder, range of motion for, 50*t*
Weakness, 2
    testing for, 88–122. *See also* Strength testing
Web neck syndrome, observation of, 7, 7*f*

Weighted scapular flexion test, 65
Weightlifting injuries, 5, 5*t*–6*t*, 105–106, 244
Whipple, Terry L., 148
Whipple test, 148, 148*f*
Wilcoxon rank, 260*t*
Winging, scapular. *See* Scapular winging
Women
    physical examination of, 6–7, 6*f*–7*f*
    range of motion in, 21, 21*t*
    strength testing in, 91

Y
Yergason sign, 142*t*, 144*t*, 224*t*, 227–228, 228*f*
Yocum sign, 142*t*, 145, 145*f*

Z
Zero position(s), 15, 16*f*
    laxity in, 170–171, 171*f*
    of Nobuhara, 79–80, 79*f*
    of Saha, 78, 79*f*